PRENATAL ASSESSMENT OF MULTIPLE PREGNANCY

PRENATAL ASSESSMENT OF MULTIPLE PREGNANCY

Edited by

Isaac Blickstein MD
Department of Obstetrics and Gynecology
Kaplan Medical Center
Rehovot
and
The Hadassah-Hebrew University School of Medicine
Jerusalem
Israel

and

Louis G Keith MD PhD
Department of Obstetrics and Gynecology
The Feinberg School of Medicine
Northwestern University
and
The Center for Study of Multiple Birth
Chicago
Illinois
USA

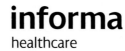

informa
healthcare

First published in the United Kingdom in 2007 by Informa Healthcare, Telephone House, 69–77 Paul Street, London EC2A 4LQ. Informa Healthcare is a trading division of Informa UK Ltd. Registered Office: 37/41 Mortimer Street, London W1T 3JH. Registered in England and Wales Number 1072954.

Tel.: +44 (0)20 7017 5000
Fax.: +44 (0)20 7017 6699
Website: www.informahealthcare.com

A CIP record for this book is available from the British Library.

Library of Congress Cataloging-in-Publication Data

Data available on application

ISBN-10: 0 415 38424 9
ISBN-13: 978 0 415 38 424 7

Distributed in North and South America by
Taylor & Francis
6000 Broken Sound Parkway, NW, (Suite 300)
Boca Raton, FL 33487, USA

Within Continental USA
Tel: 1(800)272 7737; Fax: 1(800)374 3401
Outside Continental USA
Tel: (561)994 0555; Fax: (561)361 6018
E-mail: orders@crcpress.com

Distributed in the rest of the world by
Thomson Publishing Services
Cheriton House
North Way
Andover, Hampshire SP10 5BE, UK
Tel.: +44 (0)1264 332424
E-mail: tps.tandfsalesorder@thomson.com

Composition by C&M Digitals (P) Ltd, Chennai, India
Printed and bound by Replika Press Pvt Ltd

Dedication

I dedicate this book to my parents and to the three women in my life: my wife and my two daughters.

Isaac

This book is dedicated to the memory of my late parents, Jennette and Myron Keith, who instilled within me the knowledge and appreciation of what it meant to be a twin, to the members of my mother's birth family whose legacies generously supported the efforts of the Center for Study of Multiple Birth, and to my identical twin brother, Donald, whose presence is ever with me although he is unable to stand beside me.

Louis

Contents

Contributors

Chapters contributed to are in square brackets.

C V Ananth PhD MPH [8]
Department of Obstetrics, Gynecology
  and Reproductive Sciences
University of Medicine and Dentistry of
  New Jersey
Robert Wood Johnson Medical School
New Brunswick, NJ
USA

Z Appelman MD [6,9]
Institution of Genetics
Kaplan Medical Center
Rehovot
Israel

B Arabin MD PhD [15,19]
Department of Perinatal Medicine
Isala Clinics Sophia
Dr Van Heesweg 2
AB Zwolle
The Netherlands

A Barash MD [18]
The IVF Unit
Kaplan Medical Center
Rehovot
Israel

J J de Sousa Barros MD PhD [3]
Faculty of Medicine
University of Coimbra
Coimbra
Portugal

A Ben-Arie MD [17]
Department of Obstetrics and Gynecology
Kaplan Medical Center
Rehovot
Israel

C M Bilardo MD [15]
Department of Prenatal Diagnosis
Academic Medical Centre
Amsterdam
The Netherlands

I Blickstein MD [1,10,14,15]
Department of Obstetrics and Gynecology
Kaplan Medical Center
Rehovot
and
The Hadassah-Hebrew University
  School of Medicine
Jerusalem
Israel

G H Bręborowicz MD PhD [11,14]
Department of Perinatology and Gynecology
University of Medical Sciences
Poznan
Poland

T Chyczewski RN RDMS [10]
9759 Forestview Drive
Mokena, IL
USA

G Clerici MD PhD [20]
Centre of Perinatal and
  Reproductive Medicine
University Hospital Monteluce
Perugia
Italy

C Derom PhD [1,2]
CME UZ-Leuven
Gasthuisberg O&N
Leuven
Belgium

R Derom MD PhD FRCOG [1,2]
Association for Scientific Research in
    Multiple Births
Destelbergen
Belgium

G C Di Renzo MD PhD [20]
Centre of Perinatal and Reproductive
    Medicine
University Hospital Monteluce
Perugia
Italy

N M Fisk PhD FRCOG [13]
Centre for Fetal Care
Queen Charlotte's Hospital
London
UK

R Hackmon MD [16]
Ultrasound Unit
Department of Obstetrics and Gynecology
Rabin Medical Center
Beilinson Campus
Petah Tiqva
Israel

A Herman MD [8]
Department of Obstetrics and Gynecology
Assaf Harofeh Medical Center
Zerifin
Israel

M Karoshi MD [21]
North Middlesex University Hospital
Edmonton
London
UK

L G Keith MD PhD [21]
Department of Obstetrics and Gynecology
The Feinberg School of Medicine
Northwestern University
Chicago, IL
and
The Center for Study of Multiple Birth
Chicago, IL
USA

A Kurjak MD [5]
Department of Obstetrics and Gynecology
Medical School University of Zagreb
Hospital 'Sveti Duh'
Zagreb
Croatia

R Luzietti MD PhD [20]
Centre of Perinatal and Reproductive
    Medicine
University Hospital Monteluce
Perugia
Italy

G A Machin MD PhD [2,3,4,14]
3931 Cherrilee Crescent
Victoria
British Columbia
Canada

A Matias MD PhD [13]
Department of Obstetrics and Gynecology
University Hospital of S. João
Porto
Portugal

R Maymon MD [8]
Department of Obstetrics and
    Gynecology
Assaf Harofeh Medical Center
Zerifin
Israel

I Meizner MD [16]
Ultrasound Unit
Department of Obstetrics and
    Gynecology
Rabin Medical Center
Beilinson Campus
Petah Tiqva
Israel

M M Mignosa MD [20]
Centre of Perinatal and Reproductive
    Medicine
University Hospital Monteluce
Perugia
Italy

A Monteagudo MD [5]
Department of Obstetrics and
  Gynecology
New York University School
  of Medicine
New York, NY
USA

N Montenegro MD [13]
Department of Obstetrics and
  Gynecology
University Hospital of S. João
Porto
Portugal

D A Netta MD PhD [19]
Division of Maternal–Fetal Medicine
Department of Obstetrics, Gynecology and
  Reproductive Sciences
University of Medicine and Dentistry of
  New Jersey
Robert Wood Johnson Medical School
New Brunswick, NJ
USA

J Nizard MD [19]
Department of Perinatal Medicine
Isala Clinics Sophia
Zwolle
The Netherlands

A K Oleszczuk MD [16]
Department of Ophthalmology
Medical Institute of the Department
  of Defense
Warsaw
Poland

J J Oleszczuk MD PhD [16]
McKinsey and Company, Chicago
Chicago, IL
USA

Y Or MD [18]
The IVF Unit
Kaplan Medical Center
Rehovot
Israel

E Pergament MD PhD FACMG [9]
Obstetrics and Gynecology
Northwestern University Medical School
Chicago, IL
USA

M Respondek-Liberska MD [12,13,14]
Research Institute Polish Mother's
  Memorial Hospital
Medical University of Lodz
Rzowska
Lodz
Poland

M Ropacka MD PhD [11,14]
Department of Perinatology and
  Gynecology
University of Medical Sciences
Poznan
Poland

A Rosati MD [20]
Centre of Perinatal and Reproductive
  Medicine
University Hospital Monteluce
Perugia
Italy

E R Sabbagha MD [10]
Department of Obstetrics and
  Gynecology
Northwestern University Medical School
Chicago, IL
USA

R E Sabbagha MD [10]
Department of Obstetrics and
  Gynecology
Northwestern University Medical School
Chicago, IL
USA

K Spencer MSc DSc CBiol CCem CSci
  EurClinChem MIBiol FRSC FRCPath [6,7]
Department of Clinical Biochemistry
Harold Wood Hospital
Romford
UK

M J O Taylor BA MRCGP MRCOG PhD [13]
Peninsula Medical School
Exeter Fetal Care Centre
Royal Devon and Exeter Hospital (Heavitree)
Exeter
UK

I E Timor-Tritsch MD [5]
Department of Obstetrics and Gynecology
New York University School of Medicine
New York, NY
USA

E Vaisbuch MD [17]
Department of Obstetrics and Gynecology
Kaplan Medical Center
Rehovot
Israel

J van Eyck MD PhD [19]
Department of Perinatal Medicine
Isala Clinics Sophia
Zwolle
The Netherlands

N Veček MD [5]
Department of Obstetrics and Gynecology
Medical School University of Zagreb
Hospital 'Sveti Duh'
Zagreb
Croatia

A Wtoch MD [12,13,14]
Fetal Cardiology Center
Silesian Medical Academy
Katowice
Poland

Preface

When we began the collaboration that resulted in the publication of our monograph, Iatrogenic Multiple Pregnancy: Clinical Implications in 2001, little could we imagine that the last sentence of the preface that suggested our imaginations had not been exhausted would, in reality, be prophetic. But it was. In the ensuing years, we edited Triplet Pregnancies and their Consequences and the second edition of Multiple Pregnancy: Epidemiology, Gestation and Perinatal Outcome. This latter volume, with its 110 chapters would have seemed, at face value, to have been the definitive work on the topic. It not only comprised a total and complete revision of the first edition published 10 years previously, but it covered every possible niche on the topic and proved to be the most comprehensive document on multiples ever brought forward by obstetricians. It was impressive to readers and to critics as well, so much so that it won the first prize in the British Medical associations Book of the Year Award list for 2005 in the category of Obstetrics and Gynecology against some very stiff competition.

Even while appreciating the numerous qualities of this effort, especially in terms of its up-to-date content, we began to wonder if a shorter version might not have an appeal of its own. Part of our concern was our impression, gained from numerous conversations at congresses around the world, that clinicians often were confronted with specific aspects of the prenatal care of multiples for which there was controversy or multiple approaches. Simple examples suffice to illustrate this point: the issues of proper understanding of placentation and non-invasive screening. The same may be said for assessing aberrations of the normal growth patters of twins and then standards for their assessment. The list goes on and on.

Soon it became apparent that these needs could be addressed in a "spin off" book which would ultilize the textual material of the second edition but format it in a slightly different manner. Once an agreement with our publisher had been signed, we sought permission from each of the authors who had contributed to the second edition to reformat their words, sometimes in a single chapter and other times combined with the words of another author from another chapter. All contributors agreed and this became the proforma for the present book. Isaac Blickstein performed the reformatting and both Isaac and Louis Keith edited this material once again for clarity and uniformity of style.

This volume therefore contains a total of 21 chapters, all of which address a single topic. Together these chapters illuminate "Prenatal Diagnosis of Multiples". Subjects that are not germane to this topic are not included and can be found in the Second Edition of Multiple Pregnancy. The result is shorter, more compact, and more "user friendly" for the busy practitioner, the resident, or the student who is faced with clinical dilemmas on a daily basis and wants something to read "between seeing patients", as it were.

Isaac Blickstein and Louis Keith

Acknowledgments

Cover

Farewell. Monoamniotic set including an anencephalic twin (right), 3D image taken a few hours before birth, courtsey B. Caspi, Kaplan Medical Center, Israel.

How is multiple pregnancy defined?

INTRODUCTION

According to Cicero, a renowned Roman orator and statesman, Hippocrates (a preeminent physician of ancient Greece) suspected that a pair of brothers were twins.[1] Hippocrates reached this conclusion because they both became ill at the same time, and their disease progressed to a crisis and subsided in the same length of time for each of them. Hippocrates' conclusion was not accepted by the astrologer Posidonius the Stoic who challenged this diagnosis and explained this coincidence by the fact that the two brothers were conceived and born under the same constellation.

Centuries later, in the first edition of his book *Inquiries into Human Faculty and its Development*, Francis Galton (1883) commented:[2]

The reader will easily understand that the word 'twins' is a vague expression, which covers two very dissimilar events – the one corresponding to the progeny of animals that usually bear more than one at a birth, each of the progeny being derived from a separate ovum, while the other event is due to the development of two germinal spots in the same ovum. In the latter case they are enveloped in the same membrane, and all such twins are found invariably to be of the same sex.

This definition represents a considerable part of the foundation of modern medical thinking, and remained in use, albeit in a refined nature, until the end of the 20th century.

THE EFFECT OF INFERTILITY TREATMENT

An important observation about the twinning process was made during the late 19th century, when Hellin described the mathematic relationship between the rates of twins and higher-order multiples. This relationship, the so-called Hellin's law, suggests that if the twinning rate is X, then the triplet rate is X^2, the quadruplet rate is X^3, and so forth. Hellin's law is an approximation, however, for naturally occurring multiples when tested in a population at large. As such, it disregards secular trends in twinning rates as well the effect of maternal age and race.

The first recorded deviation from Hellin's law, that is, the difference between the expected and observed numbers of multiples in a given population, did not occur until the last two decades of the 20th century – the era of iatrogenic multiple pregnancies. Figure 1.1 shows the comparison between the expected (based on Hellin's law, from the twin birth rate) and the observed triplet birth rates in the United States during three distinct periods: (a) before the availability of ovulation induction agents; (b) at the beginning of the 1980s – the start of the epidemic of multiple gestations; and (c) at the late 1990s – the peak of the epidemic. The difference between the expected and observed rate of triplets was negligible in the era of natural twinning before the use of ovulation induction and obeyed quite neatly Hellin's law. However, with the increasing number of iatrogenic multiples, either from ovulation induction or from assisted reproduction technologies (ART), the deviation from

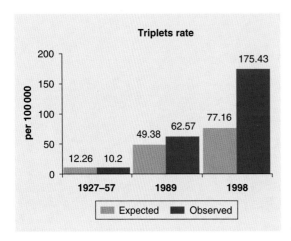

Figure 1.1 Expected (by Hellin's Law) vs observed triplets rate, before, in the middle and at the peak of the 'epidemic' of multiple pregnancies

natural twinning is increasingly evident. A similar conclusion was reached by Fellman and Eriksson, who studied secular data from Finland for 1881–1990 and from Sweden since 1751.[3]

The frequency of twins and higher-order multiples is not the only change that occurred following the widespread implementation of infertility treatment over the past two decades. Another major change is the ratio between dizygotic (DZ) and monozygotic (MZ) twins. In spontaneous conceptions, MZ twins comprise about one-third and DZ two-thirds. In contrast, MZ comprise about 5% of all twin births following iatrogenic pregnancies and DZ the remainder. Table 1.1 is derived from the East Flanders Prospective Twin Survey (EFPTS), in which zygosity is known for all twins, and shows the frequency of MZ twins by mode of conception. As was shown in East Flanders and in other studies, MZ twinning is increased following ovulation induction as well as following *in vitro* (IVF) procedures. An evaluation of a population-based dataset of single embryo transfers following IVF found an incidence of 2.3% monozygotic twins, a figure 6 times higher than after spontaneous pregnancies as quoted in the literature.[4] The largest series with complete zygosity assessment derives from

the EFPTS and confirms that the overall frequency of MZ twinning following all assisted conceptions – 4.5% – is 10 times the spontaneous rate (0.45%). Interestingly, the frequency of MZ twinning following ART procedures (2.6%) was 6-fold the spontaneous rate, in full accord with estimates derived from single embryo transfer pregnancies.[5]

The advent of infertility treatment radically changed the definition of twinning, as conceptualized based on spontaneous conceptions. To appreciate this change, one may imagine how Cicero and Galton (cited above) would consider the so-called 'Angela' case.[6] This Italian woman was at the same time and in one pregnancy a surrogate mother for two unrelated couples, and when she delivered unlike-sexed twins, postnatal blood typing (confirmed by DNA fingerprinting) allowed identification of each baby's genetic parents. This is presumably the first time in which the twins were not genetically related to each other, nor was there any genetic relationship to the mother. Thus, at the present time, simple definitions of twinning are unsuitable to encompass the whole spectrum of multiple gestation as seen by modern, technologically capable clinicians.

SUPERFETATION AND SUPERFECUNDATION

Superfecundation, defined as the fertilization of two or more ova released during the same menstrual cycle by sperm from separate acts of coitus, is frequently and erroneously confused with superfetation. In superfetation, which is an entirely different phenomenon, the fertilization and creation of another conceptus is assumed to take place when the female is already pregnant. In humans, superfetation has been discarded by scientific arguments, namely the arrest of subsequent ovulation after the initial ovulation and the inability of sperm to reach the fertilization site in the Fallopian tube. However, modern infertility treatment can theoretically circumvent these obstacles in one of two manners. The first is

Table 1.1 Zygosity of spontaneous and iatrogenic twin and triplet maternities (1964–2000)

Zygosity	Twins			Triplets		
	Spontaneous	AIO only	ART	Spontaneous	AIO only	ART
Trizygotic	—	—	—	9 (24%)	71 (87%)	38 (84%)
Dizygotic	2360 (54%)	637 (92%)	602 (96%)	22 (60%)	11 (13%)	3 (7%)
Monozygotic	1924 (44%)	49 (7%)	14 (2%)	6 (16%)	0 (0%)	1 (2%)
Unknown	106 (2%)	3 (1%)	8 (1%)	0 (0%)	0 (0%)	3 (7%)
Total	4390 (100%)	689 (100%)	624 (100%)	37 (100%)	82 (100%)	45 (100%)

Difference between spontaneous and iatrogenic: $p < 0.001$ for twins and triplets; difference between artificial induction of ovulation (AIO) only and assisted reproductive technologies (ART): $p < 0.001$ for twins, not significant for triplets transfer of sperm directly to the Fallopian tube by a procedure characterized as gamete intrafallopian transfer (GIFT). If this procedure is performed when the patient is already pregnant, and follicles are pushed to ovulate under the influence of hCG, a 'retrograde' fertilization may occur. Obviously, such a gestation is likely to develop in the Fallopian tube because the preceding gestational sac blocks the uterine cavity.[7]

A second possibility arises from the fertilization of oocytes *in vitro*, a routine procedure in ART. Once created *in vitro*, zygote transfer directly to the Fallopian tube by a procedure known as zygote intrafallopian transfer (ZIFT) and performed inadvertently during an early gestation may create a heterotopic superfetation.[8]

It is questionable if the ovulatory-inhibitory effect of an intrauterine pregnancy is the same in the presence of an extrauterine pregnancy. Indeed, it is speculated that the latter produces a lesser quantity of progesterone because of a smaller quantity of trophoblastic tissue and a diminished effect on the corpus luteum. In such circumstances, it is therefore possible that an ovarian follicle might escape the progesterone-induced ovarian suppression. This may be the reason why heterotopic superfetations are repeatedly mentioned in the older[9] as well as in the more recent literature.[10,11]

The diagnosis of superfetation is often conjectured and speculative. In contrast, the diagnosis of superfecundation, especially the heteropaternal pregnancy – when the twins are of different color or racial phenotype – is usually unquestionable. In the human, the best examples are those in which the twins born to the same woman are of different colors. Gould and Pyle cited a long list of prominent medical authorities that described such cases, the earliest of which was from 1714.[9] Interestingly, most cases in the past, but certainly not all of them, described black women (many of whom were servants) who acknowledged that shortly after being with their respective husbands, they had intercourse with a white man.[9] In recent years, the effect of modern infertility technologies also resulted in

some form of superfecundation. A mix-up at a Leeds *in vitro* fertilization (IVF) clinic in 2002 resulted in the delivery of twins of different colors to an infertile white patient. The blunder could have been at either the fertilization stage (using sperm of a different father, i.e. *heteropaternal* pregnancy) or the embryo transfer stage (using an embryo from a different couple, i.e. heterologous pregnancy).[12] DNA fingerprinting confirmed the former possibility. However, in its 'pure' sense, these heteropaternal twins were not a result of superfecundation because they were produced by inseminating retrieved eggs of the same ovulation cohort. Heteropaternal superfecundation seems to be an anecdotal and rare occurrence; however, Wenk and colleagues[13] identified three cases in a parentage-test database of 39 000 records and quoted a frequency of 2.4% heteropaternal superfecundations among DZ twins whose parents were involved in paternity suits. James[14] has suggested that about one pair in 400 is heteropaternal in the population of DZ twins born to married white women in the USA.

Superfecundation is by no means equivalent to heteropaternity, however. Estimates from the Galton Institute in London[14] suggest at least one dizygotic twin maternity in 12 is preceded by superfecundation, with varying frequencies depending on the population's coital rates and rates of double ovulation. Monopaternal superfecundation may also occur in assisted reproduction. Amsalem and colleagues[15] reported the transfer of two embryos on day 3 and the development of five separate embryonic sacs. Genetic analysis of the twin pregnancy and of the three embryos that were reduced confirmed monopaternal superfecundation.

THE DEFINITION

In order to formulate the most appropriate definition of twinning, it is necessary to consider the following:[16]

(1) The definition should include *multiple gestations that do not end with more than one fetus/neonate*. Thus, cases of singletons following embryonic or fetal demise, or

following spontaneous or iatrogenic reduction, should be considered as a multiple gestation. The registration of singletons that had a missed ('vanished') twin or are delivered along with a fetus papyraceous is also important. For example, Pharoah and Cooke[17] pointed out that registration of such cases as singletons does not permit a true evaluation of single fetal demise on the prevalence of cerebral palsy in twins. This definition should also include combinations of a fetus and a complete hydatidiform mole, a circumstance that is clearly a twin pregnancy.

(2) A pregnancy should be defined as *intracorporeal* rather than intrauterine to include multiple gestations of the heterotopic type. These are encountered much more frequently following assisted reproduction. The definition should exclude twins produced by cloning, but may include monozygotic (MZ) twins in whom zygotic splitting occurred *in vitro*.

(3) The *number of zygotes* at the beginning of gestation should be considered in the definition in order to include cases of conjoined twins, and inclusion of a set of MZ twins among a higher-order multiple pregnancy. This, however, is not always possible.

(4) The *production time* of the zygote(s) should be incorporated in the definition to include cases of superfecundation, which may occur during ovulation induction and assisted reproductive technologies (ART). The definition should enable consideration of two embryos produced in the same ovulatory cycle but transferred on different occasions as *biologic twins* that develop as singletons in different pregnancies. As an exception to the definition, and due to the advent of cryopreservation, it may also include thawed embryos produced in different cycles but transferred simultaneously in one cycle.

(5) The definition disregards the source of zygote(s) in order to include multiple pregnancies resulting from transferred fertilized donor eggs, or multiples developing in a surrogate womb.

Bearing in mind these points, the following definition of multiple pregnancy is proposed.

Irrespective of the final number of fetuses/neonates, a multiple pregnancy is the result of intracorporeal development of more than one zygote and/or the intracorporeal development of a split zygote, which was produced in the same or in a different ovulatory cycle.

Only the future will reveal whether the definition is sufficiently comprehensive for all types of spontaneous and iatrogenic multiple pregnancies.

REFERENCES

1. Schaff P. NP NF1-02. St. Augustin's City of God and Christian Doctrine. Available from http://www.ccel. org/s/schaff/npnf102/htm/iv.V.2.htm. (accessed 10 March 2007)

2. Galton F. History of twins. In: Inquiries into Human Faculty and its Development, 1st edn. London: Macmillan, 1883.

3. Fellman JO, Eriksson AW. Biometric analysis of the multiple maternities in Finland, 1881–1990, and in Sweden since 1751. Hum Biol 1993; 65: 463–79.

4. Blickstein I, Jones C, Keith LG. Zygotic splitting rates following single embryo transfers in in-vitro fertilization: a population-based study. N Engl J Med 2003; 348: 2366–7.

5. Derom C, Derom R. The East Flanders Prospective Twin Survey. In: Blickstein I, Keith LG, eds. Multiple Pregnancy, 2nd edn. London: Taylor & Francis, 2005: 39–47.

6. Simini B. Italian surrogate 'twins'. Lancet 1997; 350: 307.

7. Steck T, Bussen S. Conception during pregnancy. Hum Reprod 1997; 12: 1835–6.

8. Krenn V, Marx A, Wiedemann R et al. Superfetation occurring in connection with gamete intrafallopian

transfer: a case report. Virchow's Arch 1995; 426: 647–9.

9. Gould GM, Pyle WL. Prolificity. In: Anomalies and Curiosities of Medicine (Popular Edition). Philadelphia: WB Saunders, 1896.

10. Litschgi M, Dietrich H. A case of superfetation. Geburtshilfe Frauenheilkd 1979; 39: 248–52.

11. Kobayashi F, Sagawa N, Konishi I et al. Spontaneous conception and intrauterine pregnancy in a symptomatic missed abortion of ectopic pregnancy in the previous cycle. Hum Reprod 1996; 11: 1347–9.

12. Dyer C. Human error and systems failure caused IVF mix up. BMJ 2004; 328: 1518.

13. Wenk RE, Houtz T, Brooks M, Chiafari FA. How frequent is heteropaternal superfecundation? Acta Genet Med Gemellol 1992; 41: 43–7.

14. James WH. The incidence of superfecundation and of double paternity in the general population. Acta Genet Med Gemellol 1993; 42: 257–62.

15. Amsalem H, Tsvieli R, Zentner BS et al. Monopaternal superfecundation of quintuplets after transfer of two embryos in an in vitro fertilization cycle. Fertil Steril 2001; 76: 621–3.

16. Blickstein I, Keith LG. The spectrum of iatrogenic multiple pregnancy. In: Blickstein I, Keith LG, eds. Iatrogenic Multiple Pregnancy: Clinical Implications. Carnforth, UK: Parthenon Publishing, 2001: 1–7.

17. Pharoah PO, Cooke RW. Registering a fetus papyraceus. Registration is important for research into cerebral palsy. BMJ 1997; 314: 441–2.

Placentation in twins and triplets

2

Placentation in multiple pregnancies is influenced by the number of zygotes as well as by the number of blastocysts and, before or after implantation, the division of the inner cell mass. If, in the past, the relationship between the number of the zygotes, their divisions, and the gross morphology of the placenta was not always clear, this need be the case no longer. With a minimum of instruction, anyone looking at the placenta of a multiple pregnancy should be able to grasp the link between this structure and the origin of the pregnancy.

Single placentas are generally characteristic of monozygotic (MZ) pregnancies and are monochorionic. When they are dichorionic, the single placental mass is a result from fusion of two separate placental disks. When two placentas are present, they are almost always dichorionic. Most, but not all, instances of two placentas arise from the dizygotic (DZ) twinning process; some are also present in MZ twinning in which division occurs before implantation (Figure 2.1).

It is not generally appreciated that twin placentation differs widely by race. Table 2.1 documents marked differences in the rates of monochorionic and dichorionic placentation in distinct geographic regions inhabited by different ethnic groups. Considering the extent of these differences, any assessment of zygosity based solely on the number of placental disks is of little value. Rather, it is necessary and crucial to consider the number and structure of the membranes as well as the number of placental disks in order to determine zygosity accurately.

The principles addressed in the preceding paragraph also pertain to triplet and higher-order placentation. With regard to triplets, a fused placental mass is more common, regardless of zygosity, simply because of crowding within the uterus. Figure 2.2 shows the mechanisms of MZ, DZ, and trizygotic (TZ) triplets with different types of membranes. It is readily apparent that examination of the membranes alone cannot establish zygosity if the placental

Table 2.1 Geographic distribution of the relative frequencies of placental structures of twins

		Dichorionic		
	Monochorionic	Single and fused	Double or separate	Unknown
Ibadan, Nigeria	5.0	51.1	41.2	2.7
Aberdeen, UK	18.7	34.5	41.0	5.6
Oxford, UK	22.5	33.0	42.5	2.0
Birmingham, UK	19.6	80.4		—
East Flanders, Belgium	26.3	37.2	35.3	0.1
Japan	61.8	19.7	18.5	—

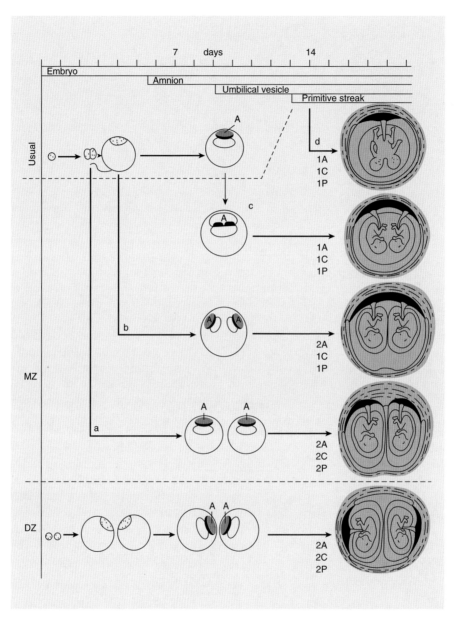

Figure 2.1 The arrangement of the adnexa (fetal membranes) in twinning. MZ, monozygotic; DZ, dizygotic; A, amnion; C, chorion; P, placenta. Image courtesy of O'Rahilly R, Müller F. *Human Embryology and Teratology.* New York: Wiley-Liss, 1992

mass is trichorionic. Similarly, if the placental mass is dichorionic, the zygosity may be MZ or DZ. Finally, only when the (single) placenta is monochorionic can one truly establish monozygosity, regardless of the number of fetuses. Thus, the principle stated in the preceding paragraph, i.e. that placental examination by itself is insufficient to establish zygosity in all cases, can be extended to the membranes as well. The general rule in triplets is to have a

Table 2.2 Placental structures of triplets

Number of chorionic membranes	Number of amniotic membranes	Denomination
3	3	trichorionic–triamniotic
2	3	dichorionic–triamniotic
	2	dichorionic–diamniotic
1	3	monochorionic–triamniotic
	2	monochorionic–diamniotic
	1	monochorionic–monoamniotic

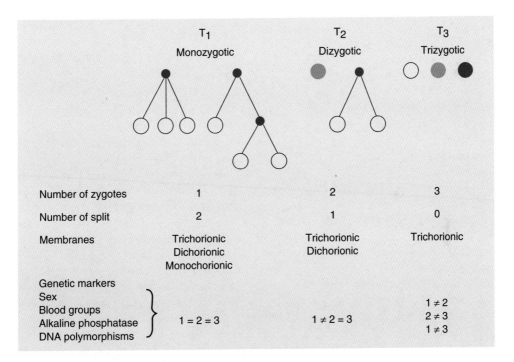

Figure 2.2 Stylized presentation of zygosity and placentation in triplets (T)

single placental mass, and a single placental mass can result from MZ, DZ, or TZ origins. Table 2.2 outlines placental structure in triplets and complements data presented in Figure 2.2.

The relationship between zygosity and placental structure in twins leads to three clinical aphorisms, the last one of which is of paramount importance. As stressed in the preceding commentary, one can conclude from proper examination of the placental membranes (as opposed to the number of placentas) that a twin pair is monozygotic. The clinical aphorisms are as follows (see Figure 2.1 for visual confirmation):

(1) Dizygotic twins are dichorionic;
(2) Monozygotic twins are either monochorionic or dichorionic;
(3) A monochorionic placenta is proof of monozygosity.

Only three well-documented exceptions to this third rule have been published,[1-3] so that the diagnosis of monozygosity is very close to certainty in monochorionic twins. In a consecutive series of 1438 monochorionic twin pairs from the East Flanders Prospective Twin Survey, all were of the same sex. Follow-up data are available in a random sample of 491 pairs in which the diagnosis of monozygosity was confirmed phenotypically and/or according to a similarity questionnaire. In addition, DNA analysis of fetal tissue samples collected on the maternal side of the cotyledons of each member of the pair in 166 random placentas failed to show any discordance of the markers studied.

The aphorisms for triplets (see Figure 2.2 for visual confirmation) are as follows:

(1) Trizygotic triplets are trichorionic;
(2) Dizygotic triplets are either di- or trichorionic;
(3) Monozygotic triplets are tri-, di-, or monochorionic;
(4) Dichorionic triplets are either mono- or dizygotic;
(5) Monochorionic triplets are monozygotic.

A unique feature of placentation in multiple pregnancies is the high prevalence of marginal and velamentous insertion of one or more umbilical cords. Among singletons, these variations are found in less than 10%, and 2% of cases, respectively, although slightly different rates have been published in various reports.[4] A more complete analysis of velamentous insertion in twins is founding data from the East Flanders Prospective Twin Survey. In many, but not all instances, marginal insertions are symmetric, i.e. present in both twins, all three triplets, or all four quadruplets if the placenta is monochorionic.[4,5] Marginal or velamentous insertion of the cord is associated with preterm birth and low birth weight, and, if present, should always be noted in the delivery record, the operation report, or the formal report of the pathologic examination of the placenta.

Table 2.3 Anastomoses in 39 monochorionic placentas. From reference 6

Artery-to-artery only	4
Artery-to-artery + artery-to-vein	11****†
Artery-to-artery + vein-to-vein	2†
Vein-to-vein only	0
Artery-to-vein only	2*
Artery-to-vein + vein-to-artery	3**†
Artery-to-vein + vein-to-vein	2
Artery-to-vein + vein-to-vein + artery-to-artery	4**†
Artery-to-vein + vein-to-artery + artery-to-artery	4*
Artery-to-vein + vein-to-artery + artery-to-artery + vein-to-vein	3**
No anastomoses seen	4

*Case of transfusion syndrome; †probable case of transfusion syndrome

Most monochorionic placentas show anastomoses between the arteries (A) and the veins (V) at the fetal surface (see Chapter 4). These may be A–A, A–V, or V–V. If large enough, A–A and V–V anastomoses are visible to the naked eye. However, injection techniques are usually required to demonstrate small A–A and V–V anastomoses. Arteriovenous anastomoses can only be demonstrated by special techniques. The complexity and variety of the anastomotic connections in monochorionic twin placentas are shown in Table 2.3[6] and described more fully in Chapter 4. A systematic study of placental vascular anastomoses in fused dichorionic twin placentas was performed by Cameron,[7] who found two arterio-arterial anastomoses in a series of 534 dichorionic placental masses. In these instances, the twins were probably monozygotic.

In the East Flanders Prospective Twin Survey, no vascular communications were demonstrated in a series of 200 dichorionic twins. Undoubtedly, an A–A or V–V anastomosis is a rare event in dichorionic placentation.

The impact of the different types of placental vascular communications is presently not entirely understood. Clearly, hemodynamic imbalance must result from a one-way fetus-to-fetus passage of blood. Numerous authorities are of the opinion that the superficial A–A and/or V–V anastomoses compensate for exchanges in the deep A–V channels, and that the feto-fetal transfusion syndrome is likely to originate when superficial anastomoses are absent, small, or few in number.

The placentation of monochorionic triplets is entirely comparable to that of monochorionic twins, particularly with regard to vascular anastomoses and the presence or absence of a diamniotic dividing membrane. Monochorionic triplets can have one, two, or three amniotic membranes. Published injection studies have yet to demonstrate the presence of vascular anastomoses in monochorionic triplets.

However, it can be assumed that they are present, just as they are present in the placentas of monochorionic twins, and in two cases of monochorionic quintuplets.[8,9]

Placentation in pregnancies numbering four or more fetuses follows the same pattern described for triplets. Theoretically, the placentation of quadruplets can be of 12 types. Tetra-, tri-, di-, and monochorionic cases have been described.

HETEROKARYOTYPIC MONOCHORIONIC TWINS

Phenotypic as well as genotypic discordances are common among monozygotic twins despite the similarity in appearance. Considerable evidence supports the contention that most monozygotic twins are, in fact, not 'identical' at all.[10] There are several possible causes for genotypic differences in monochorionic twins, including post-zygotic non-disjunction events or variations in gene expression, asymmetric

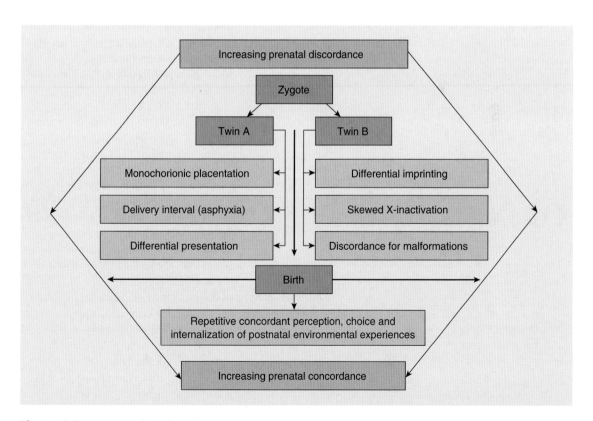

Figure 2.3 Acquisition of discordance in twins from conception to mature extrauterine existence. Adapted from reference 12

X-chromosome inactivation, and parental imprinting effects[11] (see Figure 2.3). Discordant structural anomalies and discordant growth as a result of placental factors (twin–twin transfusion, unequal placental sharing, and velamentous cord insertion) also may lead to significant phenotypic discordances.[13,14]

Prior to invasive genetic diagnosis, all heterokaryotypic monochorionic twins came to attention post-partum, albeit rarely. For example, Rohrer et al[15] reported on less than two dozen monochorionic twins discordant for the Turner syndrome published until 2004, with only a few cases published for discordant autosomal aneuploidy.[14] However, the exact frequency of heterokaryotypic monochorionic twins remains largely unknown and is probably underestimated for three main reasons. First, because 1 in 7 dichorionic same-sex twins are monozygotic, they may be wrongly assumed to be dizygotic, especially when associated with different gender or with a discordant karyotype. Second, karyotypic analysis is unpracticed for early embryonic/fetal death (including 'vanished' twins), which might be monochorionic, but discordant for a non-viable chromosomal abnormality.[14] Third, as long as single sac sampling is performed during amniocentesis, the possibility of heterokaryotypic monochorionic twins will continue to be overlooked.[14]

Post-zygotic mitotic errors such as non-disjunction and anaphase lagging involving the X-chromosome, and autosomes are believed to cause heterokaryotypic twinning.[11] In anaphase lag, the fertilized oocyte (single cell zygote) is trisomic (47, XY+21) and undergoes post-zygotic division ('trisomic rescue') to form 47, XY+21 and 46, XY cell lines. An alternative explanation hypothesizes fusion of two distinct, but impinging cell masses to form dizygotic monochorionic twins.[3,16–19]

In a recent study, Lewi et al[14] documented the difficult diagnosis of heterokaryotypic twins. In these authors' experience, chorionic villus sampling could miss the diagnosis and, therefore, dual amniocentesis of both amniotic sacs should always be performed, irrespective of chorionicity.

REFERENCES

1. Bieber FR, Nance WE, Morton CE et al. Genetic studies of an acardiac monster: evidence of polar body twinning in man. Science 1981; 213: 775–7.
2. Redline RW. Nonidentical twins with a single placenta – disproving dogma in perinatal pathology. N Engl J Med 2003; 349: 111–14.
3. Souter VL, Kapur RP, Nyholt DR et al. A report of dizygous monochorionic twins. N Engl J Med 2003; 349: 154–8.
4. Benirschke K, Kaufmann P. Pathology of the Human Placenta, 3rd edn. New York: Springer-Verlag, 1995.
5. Matayoshi K, Yoshida K. Observation of 11 cases of triplets and their outcome. Presented at the Sixth International Congress on Twin Studies, Rome, 1989: 92.
6. Strong SJ, Corney G. The Placenta in Twin Pregnancy. Oxford: Pergamon Press, 1967.
7. Cameron AH. The Birmingham twin survey. Proc Soc Med 1968; 61: 229–34.
8. Gibbs CE, Boldt JW, Daly JW, Morgan HC. A quintuplet gestation. Obstet Gynecol 1984; 16: 464–8.
9. Neubecker RD, Blumberg JM, Townsend FM. A human monozygotic quintuplet placenta: report of a specimen. J Obstet Gynaecol Br Commonw 1962; 69: 137–9.
10. Machin GA. The phenomenon of monozygosity. In: Blickstein I, Keith LG, eds. Multiple Pregnancy. Epidemiology, Gestation and Perinatal Outcome. Abingdon, UK, Taylor and Francis: 2005; 201–13.
11. Hall JG. Twinning. Lancet 2003; 362: 735–43.
12. Keith L, Machin G. Zygosity testing. Current status and evolving issues. J Reprod Med 1997; 42: 699–707.
13. Lewi L, Van Schoubroeck D, Gratacos E et al. Monochorionic diamniotic twins: complications and management options. Curr Opin Obstet Gynecol 2003; 15: 177–94.
14. Lewi L, Blickstein I, Van Schoubroeck D et al. Diagnosis and management of heterokaryotypic monochorionic twins. Am J Med Genet 2006; 140: 272–5.

15. Rohrer TR, Gassmann KF, Rauch A, Pfeiffer RA, Doerr HG. Growth of heterokaryotic monozygotic twins discordant for Ullrich–Turner syndrome during the first years of life. Am J Med Genet A 2004; 126: 78–83.

16. Miura K, Niikawa N. Do monochorionic dizygotic twins increase after pregnancy by assisted reproductive technology? J Hum Genet 2005; 50: 1–6.

17. Ginsberg NA, Ginsberg S, Rechitsky S, Verlinsky Y. Fusion as the etiology of chimerism in monochorionic dizygotic twins. Fetal Diagn Ther 2005; 20: 20–2.

18. Redline RW. Nonidentical twins with a single placenta – disproving dogma in perinatal pathology. N Engl J Med 2003; 349: 111–14.

19. Yoon G, Beischel LS, Johnson JP, Jones MC. Dizygotic twin pregnancy conceived with assisted reproductive technology associated with chromosomal anomaly, imprinting disorder, and monochorionic placentation. Pediatr 2005; 146: 565–7.

3

Postpartum placental examination

INTRODUCTION

The importance of the pre- and postnatal determination of chorionicity, amnionicity, and zygosity is outlined in numerous studies in the literature and described in detail in Chapter 2 of this book. According to the 'Declaration of rights and statement of needs of twins and higher order multiples', 'every twin and their parents have the right to expect accurate recording of placentation and the diagnosis of zygosity of the same-sex multiple at birth'.[1] In the past, before the advent of ultrasound and DNA-based zygosity studies, the classification of so-called 'fraternal' or 'identical' twins was mainly a postpartum event.

For some decades prior to the 1970s, macro- and microscopic postpartum placental examination and study of phenotypic characteristics remained the primary methods of determining zygosity. More recently, however, widespread use of modern ultrasonographic technology, mainly with high-resolution transvaginal probes in the first trimester, has improved the antepartum prediction of chorionicity and amnionicity to such an extent that this diagnosis is not only possible but of crucial importance for the management of multiple gestations.[2] Ultrasound is currently the best diagnostic technique for antenatal identification of placentation type, with almost 100% accuracy.[3,4] However, when performed in the second and third trimesters, suboptimal sensitivity and specificity are reported.[5,6] This circumstance reflects that ultrasound is not a 100% perfect tool with unlimited capacity for all kinds of prenatal diagnosis. A number of problems hinder it, including advanced gestational age, poor resolution capacity, overlying fetuses, a single placental site, rupture of the dividing membrane by fetal or iatrogenic trauma, and the sonographer's experience or lack thereof.[7–9]

Ultrasound scanning has become an integral part of prenatal care in industrialized countries, whereas this is not the case in parts of the world where few women have access to antenatal care. In these instances, histologic examination of the placentas and fetal membranes is also not practical.

The determination of zygosity is important for medical reasons, for scientific research, and because parents and their children want to satisfy their curiosity or remove any doubts. As the determination of zygosity in later life is time-consuming and expensive, it is particularly important to point out that the most favorable conditions for determining zygosity are present at birth.[10]

Adequate and methodic examination of the placenta at birth by the delivery-room physician can provide the necessary information for zygosity diagnosis and reduce the numbers of sets of twins that require additional research for zygosity determination. Over recent decades, there has been a sharp increase in the incidence of multiple gestations in association with older maternal age of child-bearing and access to modern reproductive technologies. Monochorionic placentation is more common after infertility treatment using assisted reproductive medicine than in naturally conceived twins and higher-order multiple gestations.[11] In this context it is especially important that contemporary obstetricians are aware of the potential advantages of using the placenta for the clinical recognition of zygosity, as it is now clear that monozygous twins are neither phenotypically nor genotypically perfectly identical.[12–14]

The remarkable success of using placentation is that it is a paradigm in which, for all practical purposes, monochorionic placentation is equivalent to a monozygotic multiple gestation. Although descriptions of dizygotic–monochorionic twins have been reported,[15,16] they must be exceptional, and monochorionic placentation remains an excellent predictor of monozygosity. The placenta should be carefully observed by the obstetrician or the midwife immediately after its delivery in all cases of twins and higher-order multiple pregnancies. When needed, pathologic confirmation of the chorion state can be requested, using histologic observation of the interamniotic membrane[17–19] (see Chapter 4). In most instances, placental/membranous examination, along with knowledge of the fetal gender, allows the accurate establishment of zygosity in a sizeable number of cases.[20] Confusion arises only in situations when concordant-sex pairs have dichorionic placentation, or in those rare instances when chorionicity cannot be accurately determined through examination of the membranes. In such circumstances, the most accurate method for determining zygosity is through DNA analysis using a skin biopsy specimen, umbilical cord tissue, or buccal smear.[21]

This chapter provides a framework for health-care providers to examine placentas from multiple gestations. Those who deliver multiple pregnancies will find guidelines for handling the placenta in the delivery room, so that they can gather as much information as possible regarding the diagnosis of chorionicity and zygosity assessment. A number of distinct steps must be clearly and sequentially followed for the best possible results.

DELIVERY OF THE PLACENTA

General

In order to obtain the best specimens, delivery of the placenta must be performed carefully, to preserve the anatomic connections between amnions and chorions and the placental masses. To do this, the physiology and clinical management of the third stage of labor must be rigorously respected. The goal is spontaneous delivery of the placenta, that is, one in which little or no external help is necessary.

To begin with, accurate identification of the umbilical cords is important, to ensure that each is properly assigned to the appropriate twin or multiple. The best way to do this is by placing one or more clamps on the terminal part of the umbilical cord of each newborn during delivery. Two clamps are used to label the umbilical cord of the second baby, three clamps for the third, and so on.

Vaginal delivery

In vaginal delivery, the third stage of labor begins as the baby is born, and ends with extrusion of the placenta and fetal membranes. It involves separation of the placenta, its vaginal descent, and its extrusion. After the birth of each fetus there is a time lag during which the uterine contractions slow down or even disappear. When there is more than one placental disk, premature separation of one of them may take place after delivery of the corresponding fetus and before delivery of the other fetus(es). As a rule, the placentas remain inside the uterine cavity, and it is only after the birth of the last child that delivery of the placenta begins to follow the same mechanisms as those of a placenta from a singleton pregnancy. Separation of the placentas begins normally within a few minutes post-delivery, but may take as long as an hour.

Do not try to remove the placentas manually. Because of the lesser contractile force of the myometrium, the overdistended uterus and the larger volume of the placental mass, complications are more frequent. When these require some sort of intervention, such as manual placental extraction, manipulations change the anatomy of the organ, making it more difficult afterwards to identify placentation type adequately.

Immediately after the birth of the babies, the consistency and height of the uterine fundus must be assessed. Attempts to accelerate placental expulsion through expression and vigorous massaging may turn out to be dangerous, and are frequently useless. A hand is often placed upon the abdominal wall at the level of the uterine fundus to check whether the uterus is well contracted rather than atonic and filled with blood behind a separated placenta. If the uterus remains well contracted and the amount of vaginal bleeding is normal, placental separation should be allowed to evolve spontaneously.

The initial signs and symptoms of placental separation are clear: the uterus contracts and the fundus becomes hard and globular. This is followed by a gush of blood from the vagina and lengthening of the umbilical cords. Clamps placed on the umbilical cords fall away, indicating that the placenta has started to descend. The safest way of knowing that the placenta is in the vagina is by touching it in its inferior portion with a finger introduced into the introitus. Once the placenta is in the vagina, spontaneous delivery is anticipated. At this point the woman usually feels the urge to bear down once again and expels the placenta in the process. Should this not take place, however, the mother should be encouraged to push to increase her intra-abdominal pressure, which might be sufficient to ensure expulsion. If these efforts should fail or spontaneous expulsion is impossible because of epidural anesthesia, after ensuring the uterus is well contracted and the placenta is in the vagina, it is then safe to place a hand on the abdomen, pushing and lifting the uterine body in the cephalad direction to propel the separated placenta from the vagina.

When the placenta reaches the introitus, the umbilical cords can be grasped with one hand and elevated under gentle tension, which, in turn, lifts the placenta out of the vagina. However, this maneuver may at times cause rupture of blood vessels near the insertion site of the umbilical cords on the chorionic plate. Moreover, if there are insertional abnormalities, these may tear, causing disruption and damage of the pathologic architecture.

The umbilical cord should never be pulled to draw the placenta out of the uterus. Instead, when the placentas reach the introitus, it is preferable to put an instrument tray near the perineum underneath the placental masses to support them. The woman is then advised to push, and the placenta easily bulges through the vulva and leaves the perineum, sliding towards the instrument tray or the palms of the hands. Next, in a slow and gentle downward movement as the hands move down, the traction exerted by the intrinsic weight of the placentas as the movement is being carried out helps to complete expulsion of the placenta, as well as of the membranes. If the membranes have not loosened completely or are too long, an assistant with a hand placed upon the woman's abdomen should push the uterine body in the cephalad direction simultaneously with the downward movement of the operator's hands. This maneuver frees the adherent membranes from any thin attachments. When the membranes begin to tear, they must be grasped with a clamp and peeled off with soft traction movements.

Cesarean delivery

In cesarean sections, the placenta may be removed manually immediately after delivery of the babies by placing a whole hand inside the uterus and gently freeing the placenta(s) from their beds.[22] This may cause hemorrhage, however, if the uterus is not well contracted. Because of this, to preserve the placenta's anatomy and hasten its delivery, I prefer to place my hand inside the abdomen behind the uterine fundus and, with gentle massage, stimulate contraction as soon as the fetuses have been delivered, thus promoting a spontaneous non-traumatic separation of the placenta, which bulges through the uterine incision as the uterus contracts. After placental expulsion, by carrying on massaging the uterus, one also reduces bleeding and the risk of postpartum hemorrhage.

EXAMINATION OF THE DELIVERED TWIN PLACENTA

The specific techniques and value of placental membrane examination for the determination of zygosity are described by several authors.[23,24] Twins are currently classified according to the structure of their membranes as dichorionic or monochorionic.[25] Ideally, delivery-room examination of the placenta should include identification of the number of placental masses and amniotic cavities, inspection of the membranes, umbilical cords, fetal and maternal surfaces of each placental disk, and cord length measurements, as well as palpation of the villous tissues. This examination also aims at observing the presence and components of each intertwin septum. These procedures enable immediate identification of placental abnormalities, such as discordant variations in the pattern of placentation for each twin, and the presence of vascular anastomoses that may explain clinical features such as discordant twin development or growth. However, the main goal of delivery-room placental examination in a multiple pregnancy is to check whether the placenta is monochorionic or dichorionic, which, along with the gender of the newborns, makes it possible to determine zygosity in more than half of twins.

The best way to proceed is to place the placenta on a table and take a few moments to manipulate it gently under proper illumination, so that the disks, membranes, and cords are oriented and the separate amniotic cavities reconstructed as closely as possible to their intrauterine positions in order to define the overall arrangement of the specimen and make the examination easier. Afterwards, it is necessary to separate and dissect the dividing membranes. Anatomically speaking, placentas from twin gestations may consist of two well-separated disks or one disk with several membrane patterns.

In the first instance, there are either two well-separated disks with one amniotic sac for each, or two distinct disks with sac membranes creating a distinct shared septum, sometimes with overlapping or shared amniochorionic membranes, so-called 'irregular chorionic fusion'. All of these are dichorionic–diamniotic placentations.

In the second instance, the placenta may consist of two fused placental disks with two distinct amniotic sacs (dichorionic–diamniotic fused placenta) or a true single disk with either one (monochorionic–monoamniotic placentation) or two distinct amniotic sacs (monochorionic–diamniotic placentation). Although placentation types are limited to three in twin gestations, in higher-order multifetal pregnancies a combination of monozygotic and dizygotic fetuses is expected, and placentation may be of one or several varieties. In the examination of twin placentas and, most of all, those from higher-order multifetal pregnancies, numerous membranes need to be identified, oriented, elevated, and held. You may choose to do this by yourself, or ask for help from an assistant.

The dichorionic placenta

The dichorionic–diamniotic twin placenta may consist of two entirely separate disks, each with its own cord and chorioamnionic sac (Figure 3.1). In such cases, the fertilized ova were implanted in very distinct zones of the uterine mucosa, each with its decidua capsularis, which in turn made contact with each other, but are now readily separated. Each placental disk may be examined as if the placenta in question were one of a singleton pregnancy. The fetal surface of the placenta and the free membranes form a continuous layer covered by amnion, with the underlying chorion which had enclosed the umbilical cord and the fetus. With the fetal surface lying up, first identify the opening of the membranes for the exit of the

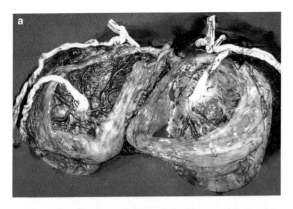

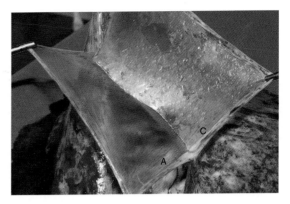

Figure 3.3 General appearance of the fetal membranes. From the border of the opening of the sac it is easy to strip the amniotic layer from the chorion. The amnion (A) is a thin translucent layer of tissue loosely attached to the chorion (C)

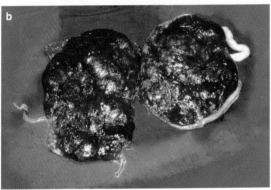

Figure 3.1 Dichorionic–diamniotic twin placenta. (a) Fetal surfaces of two well-separated placental masses each with its umbilical cord and amniotic cavity. (b) Maternal surfaces. When two distinctly separated placental disks are found, the diagnosis is evident: we are dealing with a dichorionic twin placenta

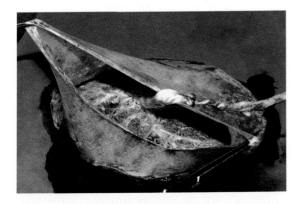

Figure 3.2 Reconstruction of the chorioamniotic cavity. Note the opening for the exit of the fetus

fetus. By grasping them at the border and lifting, the amniotic cavity may be reconstructed (Figure 3.2). Using one's fingers or atraumatic forceps, it is possible to dissect the membranes from the top to the bottom of the amniotic sac and identify the amnion and the chorion of each placenta (Figure 3.3). Normally, the free membranes meet the placental surface at the margin of the vascular or chorionic plate, as in any normal singleton placenta.

When the placental masses are separated but have partially fused or overlapping membranes, the membrane borders can be grasped and elevated to rebuild the amniotic sacs and identify a shared septum, forming the dividing membrane between two amniotic cavities (Figure 3.4). The septum may be attached to the chorionic surfaces across a greater or lesser extension of one or the two placental masses. On overall examination, the meeting plane of the membranous sacs is seen as irregularly positioned, the membranes of one twin overlapping the placental disk of the other, at times significantly. This is not abnormal. Rather, what happened was that during the process of development the chorion of the surface of one or more placentas was stripped off, and the surface was then covered by the membranes of another fetus.[26]

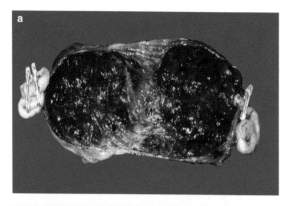

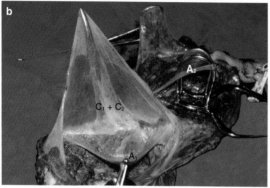

Figure 3.4 Dichorionic–diamniotic twin placenta. (a) Maternal surfaces of two distinct placental portions with partially overlapped membranes (M). (b) The dividing membrane has four layers (amnion–chorion–chorion–amnion). Notice that the two chorionic layers ($C_1 + C_2$) are adherent and the two amnions (A_1 and A_2) have been dissected from the chorionic layer

Grasp the edges of the dividing membrane with fingers or hemostatic forceps and gently lift it and stretch it. On inspection, this septum is thick and opaque, and four layers are identified by dissection: the amnion and chorion from each twin. Using an atraumatic forceps or other suitable device, carefully identify at the edge of the dividing membrane the amniotic membranes on both sides of the septum and a layer of chorionic tissue that remains in the middle. One of the thin, avascular amnions of one placental side is easily peeled off, followed by the other. Directly in the middle is the chorionic membrane, composed mainly of two chorions, one from each twin (Figure 3.4). The two chorions that are an extension of the underlying placentas' chorionic tissue may separate to allow the four membranes to be completely isolated. By proceeding with separation of the two layers of chorion one reaches the chorionic plate. Further dissection, however, would disrupt the fetal surface of the placenta, as the villous tissue frees itself from the underside of the chorionic membrane.

When two distinct and separated placental disks are found, the diagnosis is obvious: dichorionic twin placentation. However, in a dichorionic–diamniotic twin placenta the two placental portions (chorion frondosum) may be intimately fused (dichorionic–diamniotic fused). This presents as a single-disk twin placenta with an identifiable thick and opaque septum attached across the chorionic surface, clearly

Figure 3.5 Dichorionic–diamniotic fused single-disk placenta. (a) Maternal surface. Notice the collision zone of the villous tissue (arrows). There are two more or less symmetric placental portions as can be seen from the differential appearances of the maternal surface of the placenta. (b) The septum (S) attached across the chorionic plate between the two umbilical cords and the circulation territories of each fetus. (c) Identification of the fetal membranes. They were stretched slightly to reconstruct the amniotic cavities (T_1 and T_2). There is a thick and opaque dividing membrane (S) characteristic of the dichorionic variety. (d) Dissection of the dividing membrane. Identify the layers at the top of the septum and grasp them with artery forceps or with your fingers. There are two layers of amnion on either side (A_1 and A_2), beneath which there are two layers of chorion (C_1 and C_2). (e) General appearance of the intertwin septal membranes. The amnion (A_1) of the first twin is being peeled off the chorion layer (C_1) and the chorionic surface (Cs_1). Notice the transparency characteristic of the amniotic layer. (f) General appearance of the intertwin septal membranes. Note the amnion layer (A_2), chorion layer (C_2), and the chorionic surface (Cs_2) of the second twin. (g) The two central chorions are being separated; this attempt will be met with success only up to the point of attachment of the membranes on the surface of the placental disk (arrow). (h) Notice the disruption of the placental surface across the line of attachment (arrows) by the attempt to strip further the chorionic membranes from the surface of the placenta. The amniotic membranes (A_1 and A_2) are rolled to make their location more visible

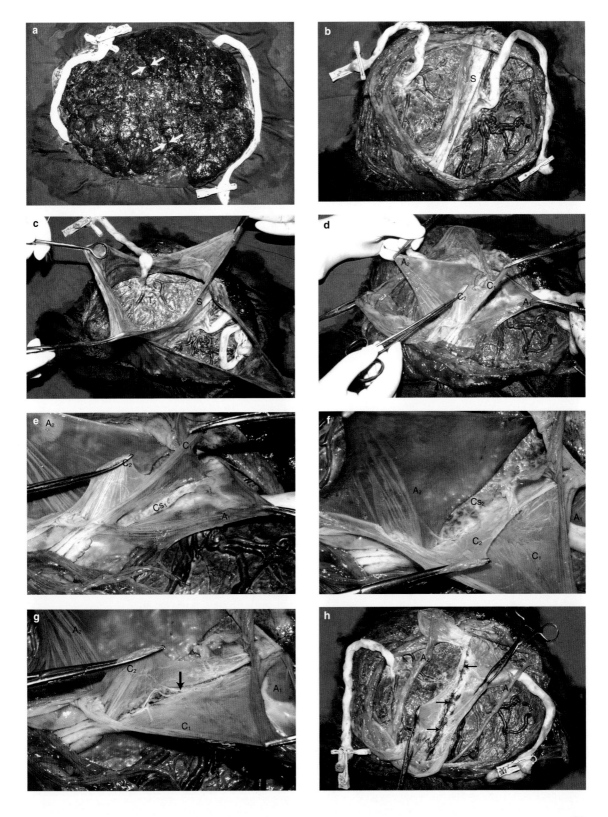

demarcating the two sides of the placental disk and the circulatory areas of each twin (Figure 3.5). It represents two distinct ova implanted side by side, which, because of their great proximity, collided physically during embryonic growth. Accordingly, the insertion line of the dividing membrane also coincides with the border of the fetal surfaces of the two placental masses (Figure 3.5a, b, and c). When carefully dissected, three distinct layers of the dividing membrane are clearly observable, corresponding to the two amnions, between which is a third layer corresponding to the two fused chorions. Often these can also be separated with careful dissection, although this may prove difficult if the chorionic layers are thin or fused (Figure 3.5d, e, and f).

The chorionic layer of the dividing membrane is an extension of the chorionic tissue of the underlying placental components. When one arrives at the chorionic plate by separating the two leaves of the chorionic layer, further dissection is impossible because the septum is firmly anchored to the fetal surface of the placental disk. Indeed, the chorionic membranes cannot be completely stripped off the placental mass without disrupting it because of the extensive ramifications of the chorionic villi from their undersurfaces. If one attempts to cleave them further, the surface of the placenta is disrupted, ultimately proving the existence of the two chorionic membranes (Figure 3.5g and h). In conclusion, same-sex twins with a separate or fused dichorionic placenta may be monozygotic or dizygotic, but opposite-sex twins are dizygotic.

The monochorionic placenta

In practical terms, the examination of monochorionic–diamniotic placentation is similar to that of a dichorionic fused placenta, as a monochorionic placenta presents as a single disk, and must be examined for the presence or absence of a dividing membrane. The nature of the dividing membrane located between twins is an important piece of information based upon the thickness and the insertion place of the membrane. With the fetal surface of the placental disk lying up, lifting the chorioamniotic membrane by its borders restores the two amniotic sacs and identifies the dividing membrane. In such circumstances, a single chorionic sac encloses two juxtaposed amniotic cavities (Figure 3.6a and b). The septum may be whole, contain a gap that allowed for the exit of the second fetus, or exist in a completely torn state. It is simple and easy to check in the most general way whether the membrane represents a fused dichorionic single disk or a true monochorionic placentation. In the latter, no interposed chorionic tissue lies between the two amnions, whereby the diamniotic septum is seen to be much more delicate, translucent, and thinner than the septum of a dichorionic–diamniotic placenta. Moreover, the septum can easily be elevated from the fetal surface of the placenta because two amnions are not anchored to the chorionic plate, and their attachment point is extremely variable and independent of the vascular

Figure 3.6 Monochorionic–diamniotic twin placenta. (a) Maternal surface of a true single-disk twin placenta. As can be seen, there is no differential appearance through the maternal surface, and it is not possible to identify a distinct junctional zone. (b) Note the placental septum (S), dividing two amniotic sacs. Since there is one placental portion, the main question is whether the placenta is mono- or dichorionic. An overall examination of the membranes of the septum is necessary as they connect to the placental surface. (c) Note the line of 'attachment' of a delicate diamniotic septum (S). The membranes are held up to show their transparency. (d and e) The dividing membranes are being separated in a slow downward movement. There are only two sheets of very thin translucent amniotic tissue (A_1 and A_2) loosely attached to each other. (f) The two layers of amnion (A_1 and A_2) may be readily separated, and at their base it is easy to peel them off the underlying chorionic surface leaving a single continuous chorionic plate (Cp). (g) Umbilical cord of the acardiac twin embedded in the intertwin membrane in a case of monochorionic twins with twin-reversed arterial perfusion sequence. (Image courtesy of I. Blickstein)

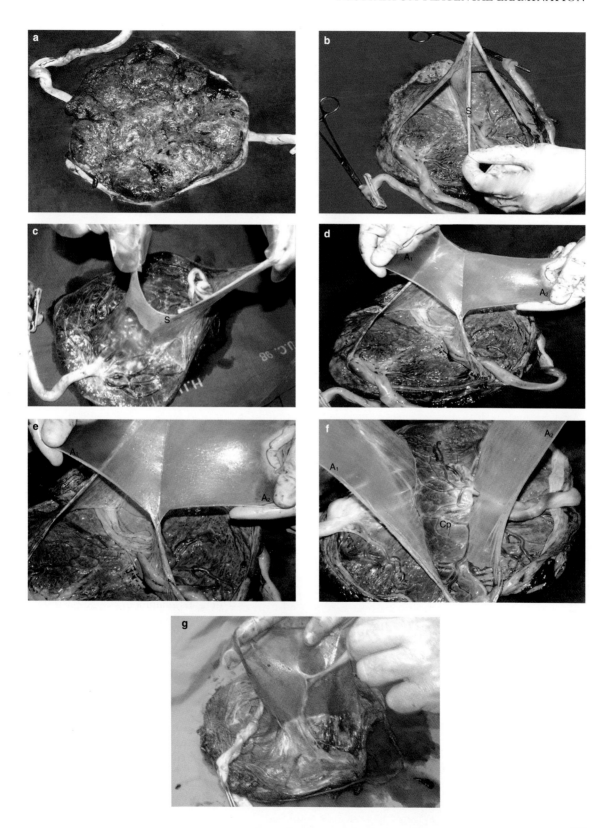

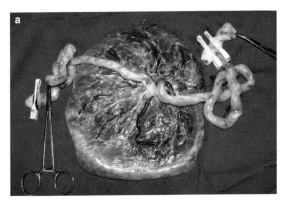
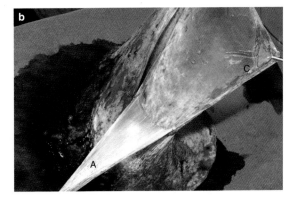

Figure 3.7 Monochorionic–monoamniotic twin placenta. (a) No septum or any amniotic folds between the umbilical cords inserted closely next to each other. (b) Examination of this pattern of placentation is similar to that of a singleton placenta. A, amnion; C, chorion

pattern of the chorionic plate (Figure 3.6c). It is easy to peel apart the two leaves of amnion from each other (Figure 3.6d and e). When the amniotic membranes arrive at their insertion area on the placental surface, continuing to strip the amnions away clearly leaves a single continuous chorionic plate underneath (Figure 3.6f), demonstrating that the dividing membrane includes only the amniotic layers reflected from the fetal surface of the placenta. Such a maneuver would not be possible unless the placenta was monochorionic and the twins monozygotic.

Monochorionic placentation is linked to the majority of complications in twin pregnancies. Abnormal cord insertions are significantly more common in twin pregnancies, mainly in monochorionic placentations, being almost invariably present among higher-order multiple gestations. Abnormal insertions may take a velamentous form in which the umbilical cord inserts into the fetal membranes. The insertion may be into the intertwin membrane, as is visible in Figure 3.6g, in which the umbilical cord of an acardiac twin is attached to the septum, with vessels passing through the septum to the chorionic plate. In acardiacs the placentas are always monochorionic and may be diamniotic (Figure 3.6g) or monoamniotic.

The examination of a monochorionic–monoamniotic placenta is similar to that of a

placenta from a singleton pregnancy, in that, after proper orientation of the placental disk, a single-disk placenta is identified with no dividing membrane and both umbilical cords inside the same cavity. The outer free reflected membranes form a sac, with the wall composed of the amnion juxtaposed with the chorion, that may be examined in the usual fashion (Figure 3.7). The chorioamniotic membrane can be lifted to rebuild the amniotic cavity. Particular attention should be paid to looking for a rupture site, in case a dividing membrane has been torn earlier in the gestation or by an iatrogenic traumatic disturbance, even though this is extremely rare. The umbilical cords may be inserted within a few centimeters of each other or widely separated, and occasionally a single, branched umbilical cord can be observed. If no septal tissue is found along the fetal surface of the placenta and between the umbilical cord insertion sites, and if it is certain that the amnion layer is complete and intact with no signs of a membrane fold, the pattern of placentation is monochorionic–monoamniotic, with both fetuses in the same chorioamniotic cavity, and monozygotic.

Higher-order multifetal placentas

Placentas of higher-order multifetal pregnancies may be multichorionic and multiamniotic,

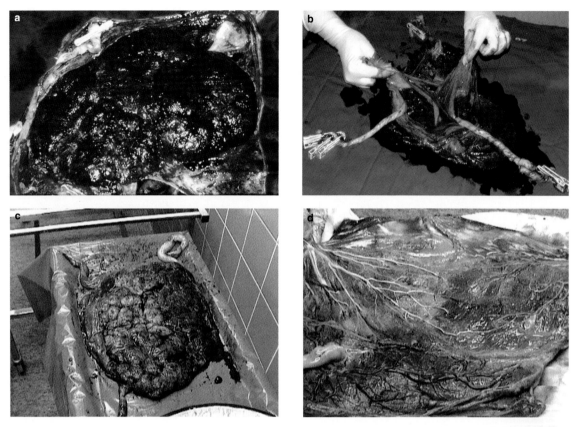

Figure 3.8 Trichorionic–triamniotic triplet placenta. (a) As can be seen, it is possible to identify three placental portions on the maternal surface. (b) Fetal surfaces. All the dividing membranes have four layers (amnion–chorion–chorion–amnion). (c) Maternal surface of dichorionic triplet placenta. (Image courtesy of M. Ropacka.) (d) Fetal surface of dichorionic triplet placenta. (Image courtesy of M. Ropacka)

and are often a mixture of different chorionic types.[17] Placentas from higher-order multiple gestations are potentially more complex, but here also a number of simple steps can help to identify their particularities. The easiest way is to identify the number of placental disks and sacs for each disk by reconstructing them in a manner that approximates the interior of the uterine cavity, using the hands of an assistant (Figure 3.8a and b). It is easier to handle each separate disk as a singleton placenta and examine the components of each dividing membrane separately, as summarized in the general description of a twin placenta. It may be possible to identify placental portions from the differential appearances of the placental maternal surfaces and the junctional zone of the placental parenchymas (Figure 3.8c and d). As is the case with twins, the nature of the membrane wall separating two cavities that belong to the same placental portion is an essential diagnostic finding for zygosity determination. A thick and opaque dividing membrane that cannot be easily torn apart represents dichorionic placentation, whereas a monochorionic–diamniotic membrane appears more translucent, and its two amnions are juxtaposed with only a sparsely cellular matrix separating them, without the additional presence of chorion. Dissect the first dividing membrane and, if after the removal of the amniotic membrane of each side a layer of tissue remains in the middle, the sac is then separated by a chorion, and placentation is dichorionic. Repeat the same procedure for each of the remaining dividing membranes until all the sacs have been stripped of amnion. When a membrane that separates two cavities is composed solely of amnions, the two cavities will have been transformed into a single one after dissection of the membrane. If at the end, after all the dividing membranes have been stripped of amnion, the two leaves of the adjoining sacs' chorionic membranes do not separate, it is because they are fused and are not easily separable by blunt dissection, the number of cavities being equal to the number of chorionic membranes.

In conclusion, it is possible, important and necessary to identify the pattern of placentation through careful examination of the placenta and fetal membranes after their delivery. In a considerable number of situations, this task provides undeniably good results as far as diagnosis of zygosity is concerned. It is easy to perform a general examination of the placenta immediately after birth in the delivery room. The only thing that is indispensable is proper knowledge of the nature of the two patterns of dividing membranes and the way they present themselves.

The need for sufficient practice in carrying out this task cannot be stressed sufficiently, as only properly trained physicians or midwives have the skills required to ensure reliable results. Until this degree of expertise and practice has been attained, chorionicity should be confirmed histologically. A fragment of the septum and the zone where the septum joins the chorial surface of the placenta, called the T-zone, may be collected for histologic examination, as explained in reference 19 and shown in Chapter 4.

REFERENCES

1. Council of Multiple Birth Organization (COMBO). Declaration of rights and statement of needs of twins and higher order multiples. Twin Res 1998; 1: 52.
2. Bajoria R, Kingdom J. The case for routine determination of chorionicity and zygosity in multiple pregnancy. Prenat Diagn 1997; 17: 1207–25.
3. Carroll SG, Soothill PW, Abdel-Fattah SA et al. Prediction of chorionicity in twin pregnancies at 10–14 weeks of gestation. Br J Obstet Gynaecol 2002; 109: 182–6.
4. Malinowski W. Reliability of sonographic diagnosis of chorionicity and amnionicity in twin pregnancy. Ginekol Pol 2002; 73: 763–70.
5. Stenhouse E, Hardwick C, Maharaj S et al. Chorionicity determination in twin pregnancies: how accurate are we? Ultrasound Obstet Gynecol 2002; 19: 350–2.
6. Bracero LA, Byrne DW. Ultrasound determination of chorionicity and perinatal outcome in twin pregnancies using dividing membrane thickness. Gynecol Obstet Invest 2003; 55: 50–7.
7. Scardo JA, Ellings JM, Newman RB. Prospective determination of chorionicity, amnionicity, and zygosity in twin gestations. Am J Obstet Gynecol 1995; 173: 1376–80.
8. Strohbehn K, Dattel BJ. Pitfalls in the diagnosis of nonconjoined monoamniotic twins. J Perinatol 1995; 15: 484–93.
9. Devlieger RG, Demeyere T, Deprest JA et al. Ultrasound determination of chorionicity in twin pregnancy: accuracy and operator experience. Twin Res 2001; 4: 223–6.
10. Derom R, Vlietinck RF, Derom C et al. Zygosity determination at birth: a plea to the obstetrician. J Perinat Med 1991; 19(Suppl 1): 234–40.
11. Wenstrom KD, Syrop CH, Hammitt DG, Van Voorhis BJ. Increased risk of monochorionic twinning associated with assisted reproduction. Fertil Steril 1993; 60: 510–14.
12. Machin GA. Some causes of genotypic and phenotypic discordance in monozygotic twin pairs. Am J Med Genet 1996; 61: 216–28.
13. Gringras P, Chen W. Mechanisms for differences in monozygous twins. Early Hum Dev 2001; 64: 105–17.
14. Gringras P. Identical differences. Lancet 1999; 353: 562.
15. Souter VL, Kapur RP, Nyholt DR et al. A report of dizygous monochorionic twins. N Engl J Med 2003; 349: 154–8.
16. Redline RW. Nonidentical twins with a single placenta – disproving dogma in perinatal pathology. N Engl J Med 2003; 349: 111–14.
17. Machin GA, Keith LG. An Atlas of Multiple Pregnancy: Biology and Pathology. Carnforth, UK: Parthenon Publishing, 1999.

18. Keith L, Machin G. Zygosity testing. Current status and evolving issues. J Reprod Med 1997; 42: 699–707.

19. Riethmuller D, Liegeon B, Deliencourt C et al. Value of histologic examination of the interamniotic membrane in the twin placenta for confirmation of chorionicity diagnosis. J Gynecol Obstet Biol Reprod (Paris) 1999; 28: 817–19.

20. Derom R, Bryan E, Derom C et al. Twins, chorionicity and zygosity. Twin Res 2001; 4: 134–6.

21. Hall JG. Twinning. Lancet 2003; 362: 735–43.

22. Holmgren G, Sjoholm L, Stark M. The Misgav Ladach method for cesarean section: method description. Acta Obstet Gynecol Scand 1999; 78: 615–21.

23. Benirschke K. Accurate recording of twin placentation: a plea to the obstetrician. Obstet Gynaecol 1961; 18: 334–47.

24. Nylander PP. The value of the placenta in the determination of zygosity – a study of 1052 Nigerian twin maternities. J Obstet Gynaecol Br Commonw 1969; 76: 699–704.

25. Benirschke K, Kim CK. Multiple pregnancy 1. N Engl J Med 1973; 288: 1276–84.

26. Benirschke K, Kaufman P. Multiple pregnancy. In: Benirschke K, Kaufman P, eds. Pathology of the Human Placenta, 2nd edn. New York: Springer-Verlag, 1990; 679.

Advanced placental examination

4

INTRODUCTION

Twin and higher-order multiple pregnancy (HOMP) placentas should be examined routinely because:

(1) Chorionicity is not always determined correctly by prenatal ultrasound, and is relevant to any adverse pregnancy outcomes;

(2) If placentation is proved to be monochorionic (MC) by pathology, twins are monozygotic (MZ) (with very rare exceptions);

(3) Explanations of growth discordance, fetal demise, neurologic injury, extent of chorioamnionitis/fetal inflammation depend on chorionicity;

(4) The usual 'rules' about twin pathology are regularly broken, so that only familiarity with norms allows sophisticated exceptions to be recognized, e.g. 'hybrid' MC/dichorionic (DC) twin placentas, succenturiate lobes in MC placentas masquerading as 'DC' by ultrasound.

The minimal clinical data required for meaningful pathology reporting of twin and HOMP placentas include gestational age, sexes, birth weights, and significant clinical complications. It is preferable to know whether conception was spontaneous or assisted, and whether there has been multifetal reduction. The cords should be clearly identified, preferably with one and two clamps for twins A and B, respectively.

DICHORIONIC TWIN PLACENTATION

DC twin placentas may be separate or fused, as seen by ultrasound or in the pathology laboratory. Viewed from the maternal side, fused DC placentas are completely seamless, with what appears to be a continuous parenchymal mass. On the fetal side, however, the membranous septum is palpably thick, sometimes with a ridge of viable residual placental tissue in its base, corresponding with the 'twin peak sign' seen on ultrasound. The septum is translucent but not transparent. Sclerosed chorionic vessels form a fine reticulum (Figure 4.1). There are rarely any interfetal vascular connections, and chorionic vessels running toward the base of the septum from each fetus are deviated

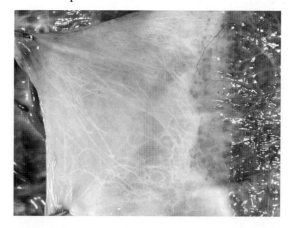

Figure 4.1 In these fused, dichorionic (DC) placentas, viable parenchymal tissue is seen in the base of the septum. The DC septum has a fine, reticular pattern of sclerosed chorionic vessels

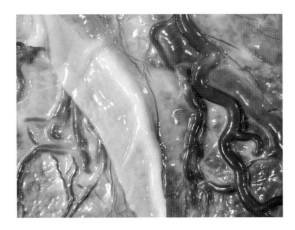

Figure 4.2 At the dichorionic (DC) septum, chorionic plate vessels turn parallel to the septum, but rarely transgress it

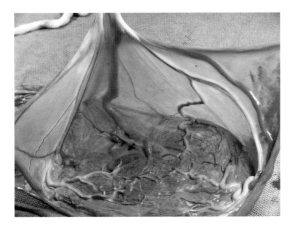

Figure 4.3 When the cord of the second-born dichorionic (DC) twin inserts into the septal membranes it creates a special kind of vasa previa

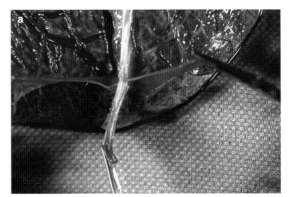

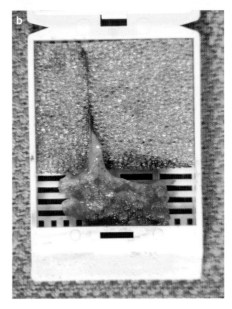

Figure 4.4 (a) The two amniotic layers of a dichorionic (DC) septum can be peeled apart, leaving the chorionic component, which is firmly attached to the placental disk. (b) Elsewhere in the septum, a block is made of the DC septal T-junction

from their path to run parallel with the septal base (Figure 4.2). Although instances of interfetal vascular connections have been described in DC twins,[1,2] these are exceptionally rare. Velamentous cord insertion is common in DC twins. Sometimes this velamentous insertion is into the septum, creating a special type of vasa previa if it belongs to the 'upper', second-born twin (Figure 4.3).

DC placentation should be recorded permanently by making a 'T-junction' block (Figure 4.4). Separate DC placentas can be weighed

separately, allowing the calculation of fetal/placental (F/P) ratios for each twin, especially when there is significant growth discordance. It is also possible to cut fused DC placentas apart along the base of the septum if both F/P ratios are required. Marked growth discordance in DC twins has a different causation and natural history than in MC twins.[3] Growth discordance in DC twins can be caused by placental abnormality of the smaller twin, including: small placental mass, velamentous or marginal cord insertion, and parenchymal pathology such as increased perivillous fibrin deposition and/or maternal floor infarction.[4] Differential parenchymal pathology secondary to thrombophilia strongly suggests dizygosity, with differential genetic thrombophilia of one twin but not the other.

DC placentation does not designate zygosity in like-sexed twins, because one-third of MZ twins are DC. Paraffin-processed placental parenchymal blocks constitute a valuable resource for later DNA extraction and genetic testing, including zygosity studies.

Adverse outcomes in DC twins are caused by factors similar to those in singletons, having no connection with twinning *per se*. There are no special vascular considerations, such as apply to MC twin placentation.

MONOCHORIONIC TWIN PLACENTATION

The MC twin or HOMP placenta is a single placenta, not two placentas fused together. The difference in structure from DC placentas is highly significant, because the complete absence of chorion in the membranous septum of MC twin placentas allows fetal chorionic plate vessels from both twins to have unrestricted access to the whole placental surface, where they usually form connections of various kinds. In consequence, the cardiovascular systems of MC twins are interdependent, and any deterioration in one twin will inevitably affect the other. In addition, specific patterns of intertwin vascular connections are required for the development of twin–twin transfusion (TTT) and twin reversed arterial perfusion (TRAP). It is important to realize that MC twin gestations are completely surrounded by a seamless single hollow sphere of chorion, both placental and free-membranous. There is no single chorion component in the septum, as is sometimes supposed.

Examining the septum

A large proportion (95%) of MC twin placentas are diamniotic (DA). However, the MC–DA septum is sometimes difficult to find by ultrasound, so some placentas will arrive in the pathology laboratory with serious questions about monoamniotic (MA) versus DA status. If the amniotic membrane has been completely stripped from the placenta, it is not possible to arrive at a definite diagnosis. However, it is rare for the amnion to strip off in MC–MA placentas, largely because cord insertions are close together and anchor the amnion down close to the fetal surface. In contrast, the MC–DA amnion frequently strips. By unraveling the two membrane components from the cord insertions and laying them down again on the placental surface, it is easy to see if there is too much excess of membrane for placentation to have been MA.

Because the septum of MC–DA placentas consists of two layers of amnion only, laid back-to-back, there is no chorionic component. The septum is very thin and totally transparent. There are no sclerosed chorionic vessels. Cords cannot be velamentously inserted into the septum because there is no chorionic component. The septum meets the placental surface cleanly, without a 'twin peak' or wedge of placental tissue.

By sampling an undisturbed portion of the septum, a membrane roll can be made to confirm MC–DA placentation (Figure 4.5). (This septal membrane roll is also a permanent record of monozygosity.) A T-junction block is not necessary if the placenta is fresh and injection studies are planned.

Documenting the cord insertions and placental diameters

Cord insertions are documented as central, eccentric, marginal, or velamentous. Two placental diameters are measured, the major one lying through both cord insertion points and the other at right angles to those insertions, at a point roughly halfway between the cord insertions – this corresponds with the vascular equator. The major diameter is usually longer than the vascular equator. The vascular equator does not correlate with the base of the membranous septum, and that septum probably moves during gestation,

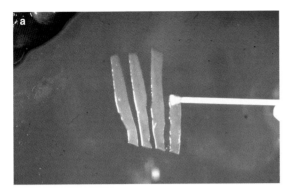

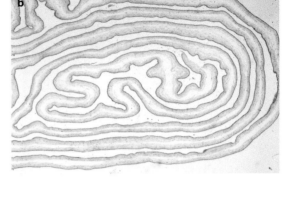

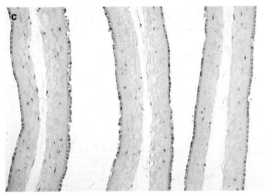

Figure 4.5 For monochorionic (MC) twins, a membrane roll of the septum leaves the chorionic vessels intact for perfusion studies. With rare exceptions, the MC septal membrane roll is a permanent record that the twins are monozygotic (MZ). (a) Making the membrane roll. (b) Low-power microscopy of the tissue roll. (c) High-power view shows two layers of amnion arranged back-to-back without interposed chorion

particularly if there are discrepancies in amniotic fluid volumes (see Chapter 13). It is not known whether the ratio of the major diameter to the vascular equator affects the number of equatorial vascular anastomoses.

Growth discordance in MC twins is almost entirely caused by asymmetric cord insertions, such that the larger twin has a central insertion, whereas the smaller twin has a marginal/velamentous insertion. In this circumstance, the smaller twin perfuses a smaller proportion of the parenchyma and is metabolically challenged (Figure 4.6). A single umbilical artery of the smaller twin can exacerbate the effect of discordant cord insertion. Velamentous cord insertions increase the risks in MC twins.[5]

The MC twin placenta should be weighed, although there are no studies of F/P weight ratios in MC twinning.

Preparing the chorionic plate vessels

It is unusual in clinical practice for pathologists to carry out perfusion studies in MC

twin placentas, despite the fact that it is these very vascular structures that are almost

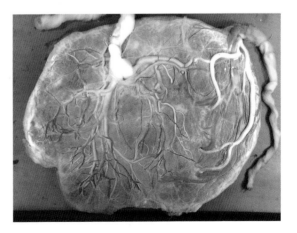

Figure 4.6 Asymmetric cord insertions in monochorionic (MC) twins cause unequal sharing of the parenchyma, leading to growth discordance. The twin on the right has a thin, marginally inserted cord. Venous return (red dye) constitutes only about 25% of the total parenchyma, the remainder draining to the larger twin on the left

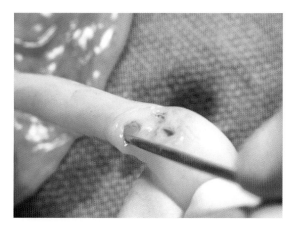

Figure 4.7 A cautious cut-down into the cord, 3–5 cm from its insertion, allows the venous catheter to be threaded into the chorionic plate veins for perfusion

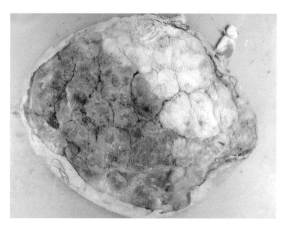

Figure 4.8 A view of the maternal surface of a monochorionic (MC) twin placenta with fetal demise of one twin. The vascular equator appears as a serrated or 'patchwork quilt' effect, because some cotyledons at the equator have been infarcted by the lack of arterial perfusion from the dead twin. Other cotyledons remain viable because they are perfused by the survivor. Thus the vascular equator is not a smooth line. The pale placental zone on the right corresponds with the dead fetus

entirely responsible for the dire consequences of MC placentation. Perfusion studies are simple and quick to perform on fresh MC placentas, and pathology assistants can be trained to do the work. The presence of the anastomosis of Hyrtl between the umbilical arteries in the cord within 1–2 cm of its insertion makes it necessary to catheterize only one artery in each cord. Size 5 French gauge umbilical vascular-access catheters are used for arteries and veins (Figure 4.7). They are primed with normal saline. A cut-down is made about 3–4 cm away from the cord insertion, and the vessel lumen is dilated with a probe. Several wash-outs may be required, particularly in the vein, for the removal of postpartum clots. The catheter tips may be threaded out into several vascular branches to dislodge clots and clean their distal ends. Blood and clots can be massaged back up the cord and out through the cut-down sites. When the vessels have been thoroughly cleaned out, arterial and venous catheters are tightly tied in with thread or string to prevent back-leakage. It is best to mimic the *in vivo* status by using blue dye for the artery and red for the vein. In the unusual event that there is no arterioarterial (a→←a) connection, a green dye can be used for the arterial

tree of the other twin. Venovenous (v↔v) connections are uncommon, so there may be an opportunity to use yellow dye for the second venous dye. The use of several dye colors makes it very clear as to which vessels are present at the vascular equator. In cases where one fetus has died or there has been multifetal or selective termination, the two zones of placental parenchyma are remarkably distinct, and form a mosaic or patchwork serrated effect at the vascular equator (Figure 4.8). This indicates that the equatorial zone of the two twin perfusion zones consists of a series of interdigitating cotyledons of varying sizes, some connected to one twin, some to the other, and some to both.

Types of vascular connections

Both a→←a and v↔v connections cross the equator on the surface above the chorionic plate and are direct, end-to-end anastomoses. There is usually one a→←a connection per

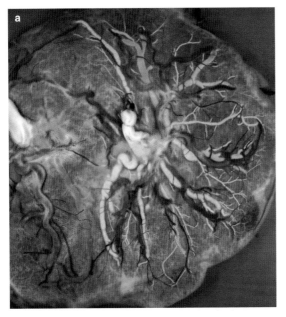

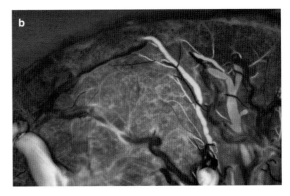

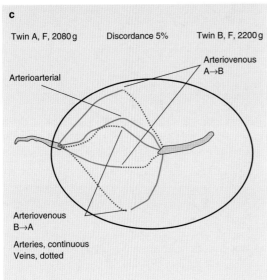

Twin A, F, 2080 g   Discordance 5%   Twin B, F, 2200 g

Arteriovenous
A→B

Arterioarterial

Arteriovenous
B→A

Arteries, continuous
Veins, dotted

Figure 4.9 (a) Perfusion study shows an arterioarterial connection and several, bidirectional arteriovenous connections. Arteries in blue, veins of left twin in red, veins of right twin in yellow. (b) Close-up view of upper half of placenta. Near the upper margin of the placenta there is an arteriovenous connection from left to right. The artery (blue) from the left twin perfuses an equatorial cotyledon from which the draining vein (yellow dye) runs to the twin on the right. In the mid-zone there is an arterioarterial connection. Immediately below, there is an arteriovenous connection from right to left; an artery from the twin on the right supplies an equatorial cotyledon from which venous blood (red) drains to the left twin. (c) Line diagram of vascular connections and clinical outcome

placenta. In contrast v↔v connections are found in about 20% of MC placentas, and there may be more than one per placenta. Artery-to-vein (a→v) connections are also common, and there are frequently several, sometimes operating in opposite directions (Figure 4.9). The structure of a→v connections is frequently misunderstood. These connections represent a 'hybrid' cotyledon at the equator which is perfused by an artery of one twin, but drains to the other twin via the venous end of the connection. The artery of the 'donor' twin perforates the chorionic plate via a foramen to leave the fetal surface and reach the underlying placental parenchyma. The corresponding vein emerges back onto the fetal surface via the same foramen, but proceeds to the cord insertion of the other twin (Figure 4.10).

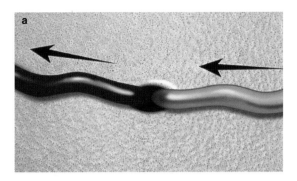

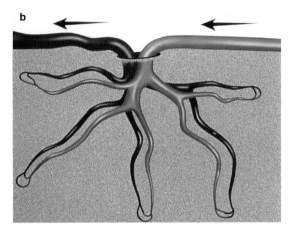

Figure 4.10 Diagrammatic representation of an arteriovenous connection. (a) Surface view. The feeder artery (from the right) and draining vein (running to the left) meet at the foramen through the chorionic plate, but there is no direct vascular connection on the surface. (b) Side view. The artery and vein penetrate the chorionic plate foramen together. Circulation through the parenchymal capillaries is normal, and net transfusion from donor artery to recipient vein takes place down a pressure gradient. If this were the causative arteriovenous connection in a case of twin-to-twin transfusion, it is only necessary to coagulate the surface vessels, even though the transfusion actually takes place in the underlying parenchyma

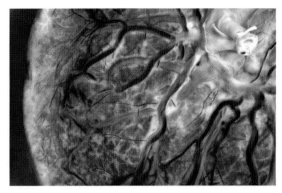

Figure 4.11 Detail of perfusion of a normal singleton placenta. Note that arterial and venous branches run in pairs in the cotyledonary foramens. This arrangement is exactly replicated in a monochorionic (MC) arteriovenous connection, except that the feeder artery and draining vein are connected to different twins

This characteristic surface appearance identifies a→v connections. The diameters of the surface vessels presumably reflect the size of the supplied cotyledons. The structure of a→v connections exactly mimics the feeder vessels of a normal cotyledon (twin or singleton) in that the artery and vein traverse a common foramen (Figure 4.11). In the case of an MC a→v connection, the artery is supplied by the donor twin, whereas the vein is connected to the recipient. There is no transfusion directly on the surface. It is not necessary to perfuse dye on the arterial side until it is seen emerging up the corresponding vein; the very presence of a feeder artery and draining vein at the mouth of their common foramen is sufficient for the diagnosis of a functional a→v connection. Because of the arteriovenous pressure gradient, there is always a net flow from donor to recipient. The numbers and diameters of all three types of connections should be recorded. There are usually several connections in uncomplicated MC gestations.

Defining the vascular equator and assessing parenchymal sharing

In cases of discordant growth and cord insertion, injection studies allow a good estimate of unequal sharing. The vascular equator is a somewhat wavy line defined by the several points where an a→v anastomotic feeder and draining vessels abut (head-to-head) on the chorionic plate.

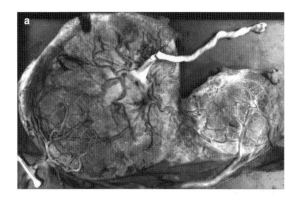

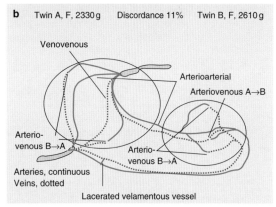

b   Twin A, F, 2330 g   Discordance 11%   Twin B, F, 2610 g

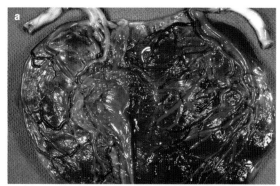

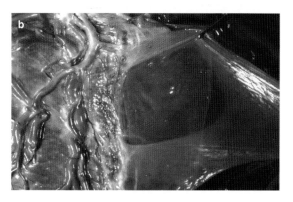

Figure 4.12 (a) This monochorionic (MC) placenta has a large succenturiate lobe, with vessels running in the free membranes. Because there were 'two distinct placental masses', this placenta was diagnosed by ultrasound as being dichorionic (DC), despite the absence of a twin peak sign. In fact, the septum was very thin and typically MC in appearance. (b) Line drawing

Uncommon anatomic variants of MC twin placentation

Bilobed MC placentas

As in singleton placentas, about 1–2% of MC twin placentas are bilobed or have large succenturiate lobes (Figure 4.12). If chorionicity at ultrasound has been designated by the number of 'placental masses' rather than by septal membrane thickness and 'twin peak sign', bilobed MC placentas may have been misdiagnosed as 'DC'. Bilobed MC placentas

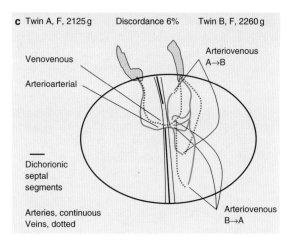

c   Twin A, F, 2125 g   Discordance 6%   Twin B, F, 2260 g

Figure 4.13 (a) This is a 'hybrid' dichorionic/monochorionic (DC/MC) placenta. It may have arisen just at the moment when the trophoblast was separating from the inner cell mass. This placenta was diagnosed by ultrasound as DC, but most of it was MC, with connecting fetal vessels. (b) Close-up. The transparent window in the septum is the MC component. (c) Line drawing

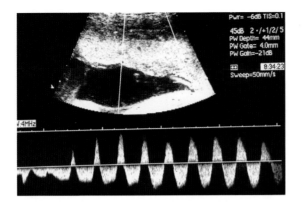

Figure 4.14 Arterioarterial anastomoses can be diagnosed *in utero* by the typical bidirectional pulsatile flow seen by Doppler study

contain average numbers and patterns of vascular connections, so the development of TTT is possible, a matter for dismay if 'dichorionicity' has been diagnosed on the basis of 'placental masses'.

Hybrid DC/MC placentas

These are very rare. One portion of the membranous septum is DC, whereas the remainder is MC, with usual interfetal vascular connections (Figure 4.13). These cases are likely to have been diagnosed as DC by ultrasound. They probably result from a twinning process at the cusp between 2 and 3 days postconception, i.e. there is a partial attempt at DC twinning.

Uncommon vascular connections at the equator

These connections include a→←a connections that dip below the chorionic plate for very short distances (Figure 4.14). These are difficult to diagnose at fetoscopy. Equatorial cotyledons are occasionally perfused by an artery from each twin but drained by veins to both twins. Alternatively, a cotyledon may be supplied by arteries from both twins, but drain venously to one twin only (Figure 4.15). These variants should not affect fetoscopic assessment and management.

Concentric placental vascular and parenchymal allocation

This is very rare and would be difficult to delineate at fetoscopy (Figure 4.16).

SPECIAL FEATURES OF MONOCHORIONIC–MONOAMNIOTIC PLACENTAS

Cords are usually entwined and/or knotted (Figure 4.17). This can cause fetal brain damage or demise of one or both fetuses. There may be extensive chorionic plate and umbilical vascular thrombosis. Most MC–MA placentas have closely adjacent cord insertions, i.e. less than 4 cm distance, with the result that large a→←a and v↔v connections are usually present between the roots of the cords, preventing the development of TTT. MA twins with TTT usually have cords inserted far apart.

EXAMINATION OF MONOCHORIONIC TWIN PLACENTAS AFTER FETOSCOPIC LASER COAGULATION

Appearances of the laser sites vary according to the time interval since coagulation. Veins are usually more effectively coagulated than arteries, and may show segments of thrombosis extending toward the recipient cord insertion (Figure 4.18). The purpose of perfusion studies is to determine

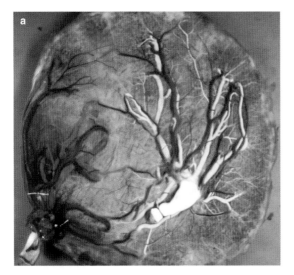

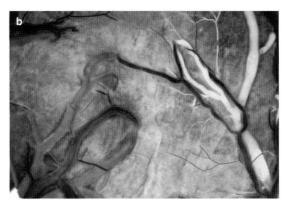

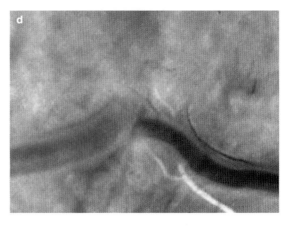

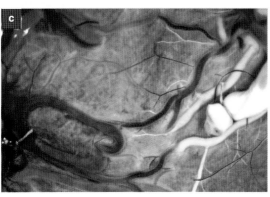

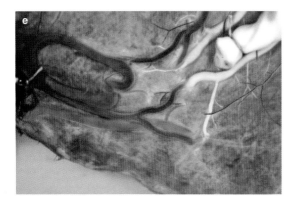

Figure 4.15 Complex equatorial cotyledons. (a) General view of a placenta with an arterioarterial connection and numerous, bidirectional arteriovenous connections. Veins of left and right twins in red and yellow, respectively. (b) There is a standard arteriovenous connection from right to left (red vein). (c) Close-up view of mid-zone. There is an arterioarterial connection towards the lower edge. At the top edge there is a complex arteriovenous connection primarily draining to the left twin (red vein), but with some drainage back also to the right twin (yellow). (d) Detail of (c), showing the complex cotyledon. (e) Toward the lower edge there is a complex cotyledon supplied by an artery from the left twin, but draining into red and yellow veins. (f) Line diagram of the placenta overall. (g) Overall view of another case with a complex equatorial cotyledon at the mid-zone. (h) This shows an arterioarterial connection within which left (red) and right (yellow) veins drain from a common cotyledon. (i) Line drawing of this case

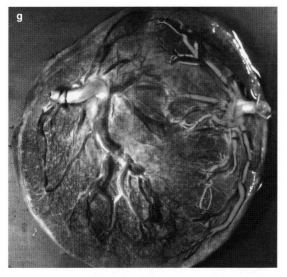

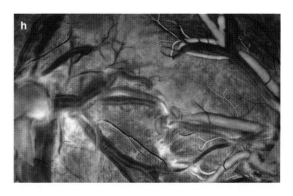

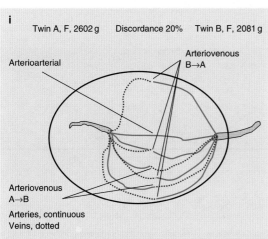

i

Twin A, F, 2602 g   Discordance 20%   Twin B, F, 2081 g

Arterioarterial

Arteriovenous
B→A

Arteriovenous
A→B

Arteries, continuous
Veins, dotted

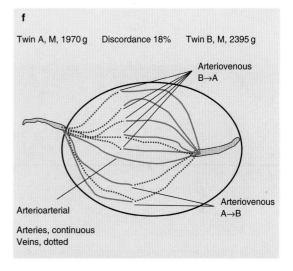

f

Twin A, M, 1970 g   Discordance 18%   Twin B, M, 2395 g

Arteriovenous
B→A

Arterioarterial

Arteriovenous
A→B

Arteries, continuous
Veins, dotted

whether there are any persisting interfetal connections. Microscopy of the corresponding cotyledon shows bland villous infarction.

PATTERNS OF PLACENTAL SHAPE, CORD INSERTIONS, AND VASCULAR CONNECTIONS IN SOME SPECIFIC COMPLICATIONS OF MONOCHORIONIC PLACENTATION

Severe growth discordance

Central and peripheral cord insertions are usually present.

Twin-to-twin transfusion

In severe cases, there is a dominant, causative a→v connection, which may be the only connection (Figure 4.19). In less severe cases there are other connections that have been unable to compensate effectively for the causative a→v connection. In addition, a→v connections in the opposite direction are common, and a→←a connections may also be seen (Figure 4.20).

Twin reversed arterial perfusion

Cord insertions are closely adjacent, such that the circulation of the acardiac fetus

39

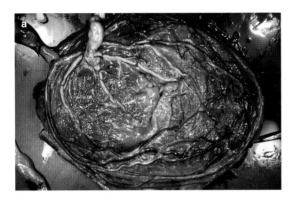

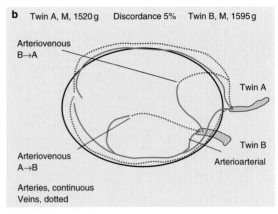

Figure 4.16 In this case, the parenchymal zone of the smaller twin is enclosed within the zone of the larger twin, creating a concentric arrangement. The vascular anatomy would be very difficult to map by ultrasound or at fetoscopy. (a) Perfusion study. (b) Line drawing

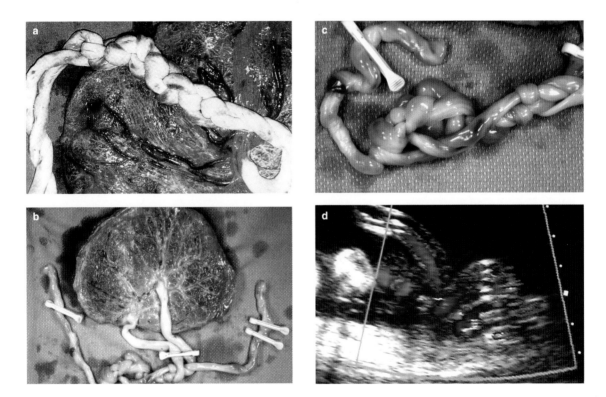

Figure 4.17 Almost all monochorionic–monoamniotic (MC–MA) twins have entwined, braided, and/or knotted cords. (a) These twins survived intact. (b) Both twin fetuses in this case died from cord entwining. (c) Close-up view of complex knotting and braiding. (d) Because braiding occurs in almost all MC–MA pregnancies, it should be looked for in the ultrasound examination, especially in cases where the membranous septum is thin and it is not clear whether the twins are diamniotic (DA) or MA

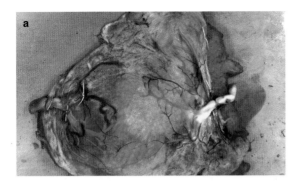

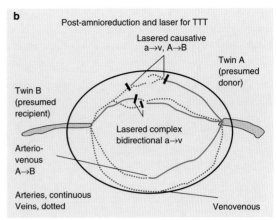

Figure 4.18 This case had fetoscopic laser coagulation for severe twin-to-twin transfusion (TTT). (a) Perfusion study. A thrombus is seen extending along the vein towards the cord of the recipient from the laser site at the vascular equator. (b) Line drawing

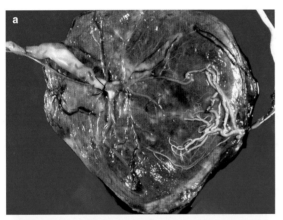

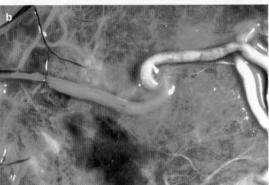

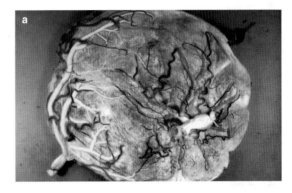

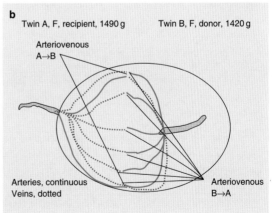

Figure 4.19 (a) This postpartum perfusion study shows the single, causative arteriovenous connection, upper right. Note that the donor cord is velamentously inserted, with markedly unequal sharing. (b) Detail of the causative anastomosis

Figure 4.20 (a) In this case of mild twin-to-twin transfusion, there are several bidirectional arteriovenous connections. These were not quite able to equilibrate, so mild disease developed. (b) Line drawing

41

is virtually a side-branch of the pump twin umbilical vessels (Figure 4.21). There may be thrombosis in the v→v connection (Figure 4.22).

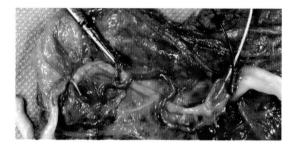

Figure 4.21 Twin reversed arterial perfusion. The cords are inserted very close together, with large arterioarterial and venovenous connections between their bases. The acardiac cord is to the left

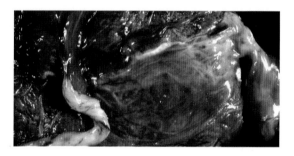

Figure 4.22 Thrombosis in the venovenous return from the acardiac to the pump twin is caused by sluggish flow. Emboli from the venovenous thrombosis would run immediately to the brain of the pump twin

Fetal demise

This may be caused by severe growth discordance, TTT, TRAP, and discordant lethal malformation (e.g. cystic hygroma with hydrops). In addition, selective termination for fetal anomaly and multifetal reduction will produce similar placental findings. With the exception of TRAP, the presence of the vascular connections places the surviving co-twin at risk for hemorrhagic hypotension into the placental portion and body of the demised twin. Depending on

the interval between fetal demise and delivery, it may be possible to determine the number and type of vascular connections between the dead and surviving fetuses (Figure 4.23).

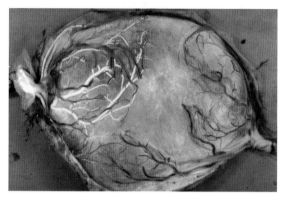

Figure 4.23 Looking for residual vascular connections after fetal demise of one twin. Success depends on the time interval between death and delivery, but may explain any cerebral pathology in the survivor

HIGH-ORDER MULTIPLE PREGNANCY PLACENTAS, INCLUDING THOSE WITH MULTIFETAL REDUCTION

As mentioned in Chapter 2, most naturally conceived triplet placentas either contain MC twins or are entirely MC (Figure 4.24). In the case of

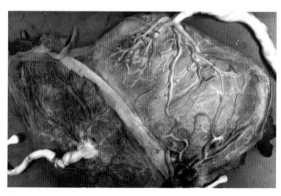

Figure 4.24 Higher-order multiple gestations usually contain monochorionic (MC) twins or consist of MC triplets. Here there is a dichorionic (DC) triplet with an MC twin pair. There are vascular connections between the MC twins, but none to the DC triplet

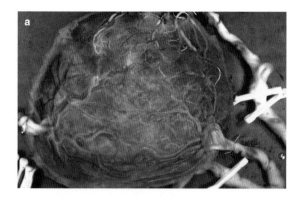

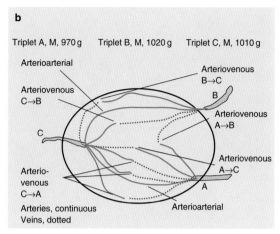

Triplet A, M, 970 g   Triplet B, M, 1020 g   Triplet C, M, 1010 g

Arterioarterial

Arteriovenous
B→C

Arteriovenous
C→B

B

Arteriovenous
A→B

C

Arteriovenous
A→C

Arterio-
venous
C→A

A

Arteries, continuous
Veins, dotted

Arterioarterial

Figure 4.25   (a) A ring of vessels connects all three fetuses in this monochorionic (MC) triplet placenta. (b) Line drawing

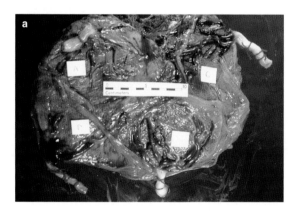

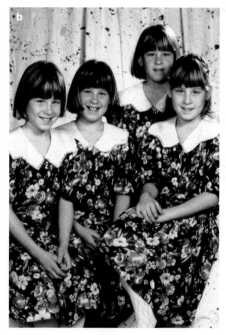

Figure 4.26 This is a spontaneously conceived monochorionic (MC) quadruplet pregnancy. (a) The placenta was MC, tetra-amniotic. (b) The quadruplets are clearly monozygotic (MZ)

DC triplets, and relying on cord identifications by the attending obstetrician, triplet placentas can be thoroughly examined for chorion status, which, in the case of MC twins or triplets, also designates zygosity. Appropriate septal membrane histology is prepared. TTT may occur in DC and MC triplets. In MC triplets with TTT, there is usually one recipient, one primary donor, and an accessory donor boosting the primary donor via an a→a connection. MC triplets usually show ring-like connections between all three fetal circulations (Figure 4.25). Quadruplet placentas may contain combinations of DC and MC placentation (Figure 4.26). Careful sampling of septal membranes is necessary.

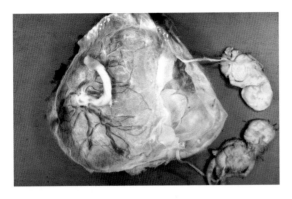

Figure 4.27 Following multifetal pregnancy reduction, the corresponding papyraceous fetuses are identified. In this case, trichorionic triplets were reduced to a singleton

Following multifetal reduction, papyraceous fetuses are found, usually at the periphery of the surviving placental parenchyma(s) (Figure 4.27). It is rarely possible to delineate chorionic relationships, and this is not necessary, because attempted fetal reduction of one MC fetus usually results in severe injury to the other twin.

ROUTINE PATHOLOGY

In addition to the special considerations listed above, DC and MC twin placentas should be examined and sampled for pathologic disorders that are also common in singleton placentas: chorioamnionitis and fetal inflammation, cord lesions (e.g. single umbilical artery, hematomas, thromboses, knots, etc.), abruption and marginal hemorrhage, and the full array of standard parenchymal lesions (e.g. fetal and maternal infarcts, intervillous thrombosis, maternal-floor infarction/increased perivillous fibrin deposition, villitis, choriangiomas, thromboses in chorionic plate and stem villous vessels).

REFERENCES

1. Foschini MP, Gabrielli L, Dorji T et al. Vascular anastomoses in dichorionic diamniotic-fused placentas. Int J Gynecol Pathol 2003; 22: 359–61.
2. Lage JM, Vanmarter LJ, Mikhail E. Vascular anastomoses in fused, dichorionic twin placentas resulting in twin transfusion syndrome. Placenta 1989; 10: 55–9.
3. Chauhan SP, Shields D, Parker D et al. Detecting fetal growth restriction or discordant growth in twin gestations stratified by placental chorionicity. J Reprod Med 2004; 49: 279–84.
4. Redline RW, Jiang JC, Shah D. Discordancy for maternal floor infarction in dizygotic twin placentas. Hum Pathol 2003; 34: 822–4.
5. Machin GA. Velamentous cord insertion in monochorionic twin gestation. An added risk factor. J Reprod Med 1997; 42: 785–9.

5

Diagnosing chorionicity and amnionicity by ultrasound

INTRODUCTION

The early diagnosis of chorionicity and amnionicity forms the basis of the modern perinatal approach in multiple pregnancy. Without knowing these basic parameters, it is virtually impossible to manage multifetal pregnancy adequately. At the outset it must be emphasized that the determination of chorionicity and amnionicity, as well as dating the gestation, are not only most accurate but also easiest to perform in the first trimester. An additional advantage of scanning the pregnancy at these early stages is that, owing to the amount of amniotic fluid, numerous anomalies, such as those of the body contours, brain, limbs, etc., which are visible at this stage of the pregnancy can be detected. Likewise, natural spontaneous reductions, which occur commonly in multifetal gestations, can easily be documented. Of equal importance, early diagnosis of multifetal pregnancies allows the perinatologist or the obstetrician to counsel the patient properly for fetal as well as maternal risks.

It follows that an early approach to sonographic evaluation is absolutely essential in multifetal pregnancies. Whereas a short 2–3-min ultrasound examination performed by an experienced sonographist with a modern machine can reliably assess chorionicity and amnionicity during the first trimester, the same task performed during or beyond the second trimester may be an extremely labor-intensive and tedious process. More important, at the end of such examination even experienced sonographers occasionally incorrectly assign chorionicity and amnionicity.

DETERMINING CHORIONICITY AND AMNIONICITY IN THE FIRST TRIMESTER

In the first trimester, the optimal value of ultrasound is best attained using transvaginal sonography (TVS). TVS is superior in providing information at early gestational ages. In contrast, transabdominal sonography (TAS) generates images with lower resolution, which diagnostically are less explanatory than the comparable image provided by the vaginal ultrasound probe.

It is axiomatic that resolution quality is highly dependent upon the machine and the transducer used. Top-of-the-line equipment, with transducer frequencies of 5–8 MHz, should also be able to provide excellent resolution. Some less expensive machines with high-frequency probes should be able to provide at least a diagnostic quality image.

First-trimester multifetal pregnancy is best evaluated as a function of its gestational age. Assessments should be based upon counting the chorionic sacs, counting the embryos or fetuses and the number of beating hearts, and finally on assessing the nature of the amniotic and chorionic sacs.

Determination of chorionicity

The chorionic sacs are implanted and detectable by sonography on one side of the central cavity line (created by the arising endometrial linings of the anterior and the posterior wall) within the appropriately thick decidua. The sacs appear as round sonolucent structures, flanked by a bright echogenic ring

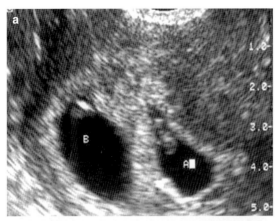

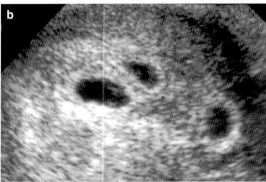

Figure 5.1 Determination of the number of chorionic sacs. (a) At 5 postmenstrual weeks the number of chorions in this twin pregnancy is clear. Note the hyperechoic chorionic rings. (b) The same can be said about this trichorionic triplet pregnancy at the same age

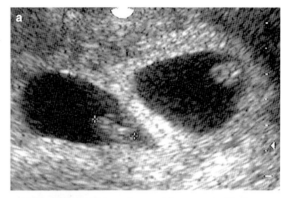

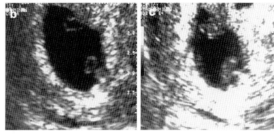

Figure 5.2 Determining the number of fetuses in a multifetal pregnancy. (a) Two embryos and two heartbeats are seen at 6 postmenstrual weeks and 2 days. (b) Two yolk sacs are seen within one chorionic sac. (c) In the same pregnancy two embryos are seen. Note that the amnions are not yet seen, as at this time they are snugly surrounding the embryos

representing the chorion (Figure 5.1). Their sizes range between 2 and 5 mm in diameter, and they can be detected as early as 4–5 postmenstrual weeks,[1,2] depending upon the resolution of the transvaginal probe.[2–5] By simply counting the number of chorionic sacs, one can determine whether the pregnancy is dichorionic (Figure 5.1a), trichorionic (Figure 5.1b), or multichorionic. In spite of the experience of the sonographer, Doubilet and Benson[6] reported that TVS undercounted multiple gestations at the gestational age of 5–6 postmenstrual weeks. As far as the terminology of the 'sac' is concerned, 'chorionic sac' is the correct term based upon nomenclature commonly used in embryology texts. On the other hand, 'gestational sac' is a term used in ultrasound, and it does not correctly indicate the histologic nature of the 'sac' (i.e. chorionic or amnionic).

Determination of the number of embryos

At around 5 weeks or definitely by the sixth well-dated postmenstrual week, TVS can visualize the yolk sacs and embryos. However, to use the number of chorionic sacs and the number of yolk sacs alone to determine the number of embryos can be misleading. Therefore, it is wise to wait until the embryonic heartbeats are visible at or shortly after 6 postmenstrual weeks. At this stage, the yolk sacs are located in the extraembryonic space and the fetal pole is almost attached (Figure 5.2). The embryonic

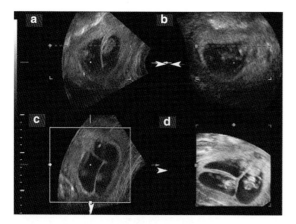

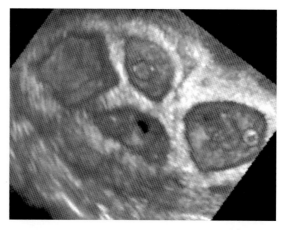

Figure 5.3 3D multiplanar view in determination of accurate number of gestational sacs. Transvaginal multiplanar view of a triplet pregnancy at 12 weeks. This example illustrates the possible pitfall regarding undercounting of gestational sacs. The advantages of the coronal section are presented (c). In the transverse section, only two gestational sacs are present (a), whereas on sagittal section (b) only a single gestational sac is seen. On the coronal section, three gestational sacs with the Y-sign are seen (c). The most informative mode of 3D sonography is its surface-rendering mode (d). Using this mode, in addition to the correct number of embryos, the separation phenomenon can be seen which was unobtainable with conventional sonography. Using conventional 2D sonography, sagittal (a) and transverse sections (b) of the uterus are seen. The first two images (a and b) represent the limits of 2D in which a twin pregnancy is diagnosed. However, on the third, coronal plane section (c) three gestational sacs are clearly seen. The diagnosis of triplets was finally confirmed by 3D reconstruction (d)

Figure 5.4 3D diagnosis of an accurate number of gestational sacs. In contrast to 2D manual slicing, an analysis of 3D volugrams with 3D surface-rendering mode reveals the accurate number of this quadruplet gestation

heart becomes sonographically evident by the end of the fifth or the early sixth postmenstrual week (35–42 postmenstrual days), initially with a rate of about 80–90 beats/min. Around the ninth postmenstrual week, the heart rate is around 150–160 beats/min. Because the number of embryos present in a multifetal pregnancy should rely on detection of the number of beating hearts, the final determination must wait until at least the sixth postmenstrual week. One should always be aware that natural cessation of embryonic

heartbeats (the so-called vanishing twin syndrome) is possible, and this probability should be considered when the follow-up scan is scheduled at around week 8–9 to determine amnionicity.

The number of yolk sacs is used to determine amnionicity in early first-trimester monochorionic twins.[7,8] In a sample of 20 monochorionic–diamniotic pregnancies and two monochorionic–monoamniotic pregnancies reviewed at less than 8 weeks' gestation, two yolk sacs were identified in all but one case, whereas the amniotic sac was not detected in any. At 8 weeks, the amniotic membrane was identified in only half of the monochorionic–diamniotic twin pregnancies. In the two monochorionic–monoamniotic twin sets, it was therefore concluded that sonographic identification of the number of yolk sacs in monochorionic twins enables the diagnosis of diamniotic twins early in the first trimester.

Three-dimensional volume acquisition (3D ultrasound) provides the possibility of simultaneous depiction of three orthogonal planes of examination. Moreover, it is possible to perform systematic examinations of acquired volumes with three different directions of scanning. For example, use of the frontal (coronal)

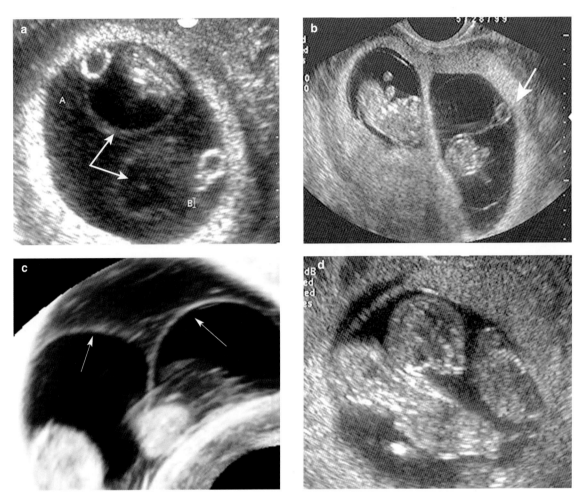

Figure 5.5 Determining the amnionicity. (a) At 7–7.5 postmenstrual weeks the amnions distance themselves from the embryonic body in this monochorionic–diamniotic twin gestation. The arrows point to the two distinctly seen amnions. (b) Shortly after the eighth postmenstrual week the amnions 'move' towards the shared chorion, 'pushing' the yolk sac/s (arrow) aside within the progressively narrowing extraembryonic celom. (c) Three-dimensional rendering of the amniotic membranes (arrows) in a monochorionic–diamniotic twin gestation. In this case, due to the early pregnancy (9 postmenstrual weeks), the membrane did not yet assume the typical T-shaped 'take-off'. (d) In the case of a monochorionic–monoamniotic gestation, at 9 postmenstrual weeks no membrane can be seen between the fetuses

plane enables examination of the uterine cavity in sections, a technical achievement which is unobtainable with conventional 2D sonography (Figure 5.3). Further, 3D sonography enables appropriate counting of gestational sacs without the risk of undercounting, even in the hands of less experienced sonographers. Therefore, interobserver variability in detecting the number of gestational sacs is significantly lower. Even quadruplets and quintuplets are recognizable without great difficulty (Figure 5.4). This advantage strongly suggests that where it is available, 3D ultrasound should become the new standard in the early management of high-order multiple pregnancies.

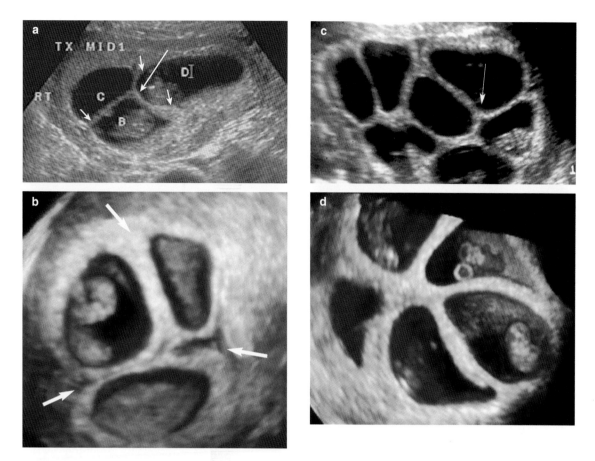

Figure 5.6 Determining chorionicity. (a) A trichorionic gestation at 8 postmenstrual weeks. Note the 'Y' sign at the meeting point of the three chorionic sacs (long arrow) and the delta ('twin peak') signs (short arrows) between two adjacent chorionic sacs. (b) A three-dimensional ultrasound rendering of an 8.5-week trichorionic–triamniotic triplet pregnancy. The arrows point to the triangular 'delta' or 'twin peak' signs. In one of the sacs the amnion is visible (small arrow). (c) This is a multichorionic and multiamniotic multifetal pregnancy. Each of the 12 live fetuses had its own chorion, amnion and tiny placenta. On the plane of this image, however, only eight could be included. The arrow points to one of the many 'Y' shared junctions created by three adjacent chorions. (d) A three-dimensional rendering of a quintuplet pregnancy with five chorions and five amnions (7 postmenstrual weeks)

Determination of amnionicity

At around 6.5–7 postmenstrual weeks, when the amnion starts to distance itself from the surrounding embryo, a high-resolution vaginal probe can visualize the tiny amniotic cavity and amniotic membrane for the first time. However, only at around 7 or 7.5 weeks can this process be reliably detected with most transvaginal probes (Figure 5.5a).

To reliably determine the number of amnions in a monochorionic pregnancy, it is wise to wait until at least the eighth postmenstrual week (Figure 5.5b). By this time the amnion and amniotic cavity are totally detached from the embryonic body. The yolk sacs are seen in the extraembryonic space 'pushed' towards the chorion, which becomes progressively restricted as a result of

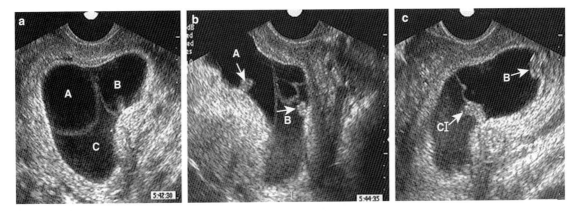

Figure 5.7 Unusual monochorionic–triamniotic gestation with three dead embryos. (a) The three amniotic sacs. (b) Embryos A and B. (c) Embryos C and B

the increasing amount of amniotic fluid.[2–4] Three-dimensional ultrasound is an additional and useful tool to assign amnionicity correctly at such early ages (Figure 5.5c and d).

THE MEMBRANES AS MARKERS OF CHORIONICITY AND AMNIONICITY

In some situations it is necessary to search for indirect clues of chorionicity. Of these clues, the first two are well known and clearly described in the literature. First, in a *dichorionic–diamniotic* twin pregnancy one can see a single fetus in each sac. The adjacent chorions create an easily recognized wedge-shaped structure that has been referred to in the literature for more than 20 years variably as the 'delta sign', 'lambda sign', or 'twin peak sign'.[9,10] Regardless of the number of chorions in a given multifetal pregnancy, this wedge-shaped 'twin peak sign' will always be seen between two adjacent chorionic sacs if examination is not delayed into the second trimester or beyond. In the case of a dichorionic twin pregnancy, two such wedge-shaped structures are seen (Figure 5.5b). However, in the case of a pregnancy with more than two chorionic sacs, one should be able to count more wedge-shaped structures than chorionic sacs (Figure 5.6a–d). Accordingly, the number of 'twin peak signs' is no indication of how many chorionic sacs exist within a given pregnancy.

The situation is entirely different for the *monochorionic–diamniotic* twin pregnancy. In these instances, the two adjacent amniotic sacs obliterate the extraembryonic space so that the amnions touch each other and form a relatively thin intertwin membrane. The junction of the two sacs with respect to the uterine wall at an approximately 90° angle creates a typical T-shaped junction or T-shaped 'take-off' (Figure 5.7). Because 3D ultrasound enables one to achieve a 'perfectly' oriented picture anytime, it may help in the orientation of the membranes (Figures 5.8 and 5.9).

The determination of the rare occurrence of *monochorionic–monoamniotic* multifetal pregnancies is relatively easy, even in the very early stages of gestation. At 8 postmenstrual weeks, it is clear that no amniotic membranes are present between the embryos and only one yolk sac is visualized (Figure 5.10a). Later, at or shortly after 9 postmenstrual weeks, this diagnosis is even easier to establish. It is important, however, to rule out the possibility of conjoined twins when the two embryos or fetuses assume a parallel, head-by-head position (Figure 5.10b). In this circumstance, one must determine whether the fetuses move away from each other and/or slide alongside each other to exclude conjoined twinning.

From the very outset, it is of paramount importance to look for cord entanglement between the fetuses in the monoamniotic

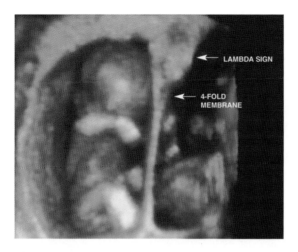

Figure 5.8 3D lambda ('twin peak') sign and intertwin membrane. Spatial reconstruction of the membrane's take-off site provides easier differentiation between dichorionic and monochorionic placentation. Furthermore, membrane thickness can be simultaneously evaluated

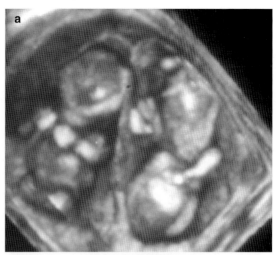

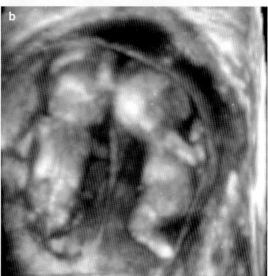

Figure 5.9 3D scan of dichorionic–diamniotic twins in the second trimester of gestation. With the 3D scan the same amount of detailed information is achieved in less time. Images (a) shows that both chorionicity and external frontal anatomy can be evaluated from a single image. Furthermore, orientation of one twin toward the other can be simultaneously assessed. (b) Twins seen from the back as well as the intertwin membrane

gestation, as this phenomenon is fraught with problems and has been visualized as early as 12 weeks. To detect cord entanglement so early in pregnancy, the sample-volume feature of the color Doppler mode is placed on the presumed bunch of cords seen between the two fetuses to detect consistently different pulse rates belonging to the two fetuses[11] (Figure 5.10c).

At times, a special and rare form of monochorionic twins together with one additional fetus in a dichorionic–diamniotic triplet pregnancy occurs (Figure 5.10d). Sometimes the monochorionic pair may have concordant anomalies or may even be conjoined (Figure 5.10e and f). Several studies highlight the efficacy of early and simple assessment of chorionicity and amnionicity in the first 14 weeks of multifetal pregnancy. Monteagudo et al[5] studied 212 pregnancies (64 twins, 87 triplets, 41 quadruplets, 18 quintuplets, one set of sextuplets, and one of septuplets). In all 15 'monochorionic' pregnancies, the number of yolk sacs matched the number of fetuses. No monochorionic–monoamniotic pregnancies were encountered in this study. Pathologic

examination of the available placentas confirmed all early sonographic diagnoses of chorionicity and amnioticity. Of equal importance, the time required to assess the pregnancy in trained hands was usually within

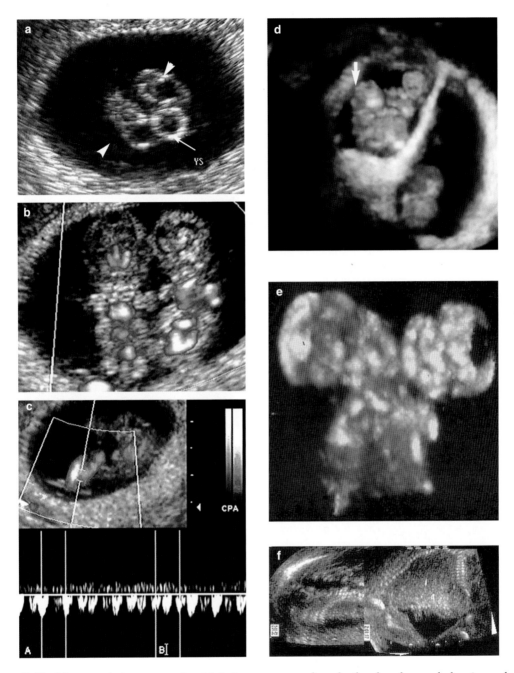

Figure 5.10 Monoamniotic pregnancies. (a) At 8 postmenstrual weeks the rhombencephalon (arrowheads) of the embryos is imaged together with the single yolk sac (YS, arrow). (b) At 9 postmenstrual weeks the fetuses are seen side by side. No membrane is seen between them and they were observed moving away from each other, ruling out conjoined organs. (c) The cords in these monoamniotic twins were consistently seen entangled. The sample-volume 'window' was placed on this area of cord between the fetuses. Different heart rates were elicited, proving the entangled nature of the cords. (d) Three-dimensional rendering of a dichorionic–diamniotic triplet pregnancy with a monochorionic twin pair (arrow). (e) Conjoined twins. Three-dimensional rendering of an omphalopagus pair at 18 postmenstrual weeks. (f) Conjoined twins. Cephalothoraco-omphalopagus

1–2 min.[3] Bromley and Benacerraf[7] concluded that the number of the visualized yolk sacs correlated with the number of amnions, and that the number of yolk sacs could be identified at least 2 weeks before the number of amnions. Copperman and colleagues[12] studied 47 twins conceived by *in vitro* fertilization and embryo transfer using TVS at 41 days after embryo transfer. The authors reported 100% accuracy in detecting 44 dichorionic–diamniotic and three monochorionic–diamniotic twins by sonography and concluded that this was because the TVS was performed at an early gestational age.

In summary, when scanning a twin pregnancy in the first trimester (Table 5.1):

(1) Chorionicity can be assessed by the fifth postmenstrual week.
(2) The number of embryos can be ascertained by the sixth postmenstrual week at the onset of cardiac activity.
(3) Amnionicity can be reliably assessed by the eighth postmenstrual week.
  • If each chorionic sac contains a single yolk sac and one embryo with cardiac activity then the amnionicity equals the chorionicity (dichorionic–diamniotic, trichorionic–triamniotic, etc.).
  • If a chorionic sac contains two yolk sacs and two embryos with cardiac activity, then either the number of amnions may be greater than the number of chorions (monochorionic–diamniotic), or the number of amnions and chorions may be equal (monochorionic–monoamniotic). In this latter case, one must wait until at least the eighth postmenstrual week when the amnions are clearly visible.
  • If a chorionic sac contains one yolk sac and two fetuses with cardiac activity, then the amnionicity and chorionicity are equal (monochorionic–monoamniotic).

Multifetal pregnancies of higher order

The higher the number of chorions and embryos/fetuses present in a multifetal pregnancy, the harder it is sonographically to assess their number, chorionicity, and amnionicity, as well as the combinations of chorionicity and amnionicity that may occur in multifetal pregnancies of higher order. The importance of this fact lies not only in the appropriate clinical management of these pregnancies, which present exceptionally high risks to mothers as well as their fetuses, but also in considering the possibility of multifetal pregnancy reduction and the issue of prenatal genetic diagnosis.

THE SECOND AND THIRD TRIMESTERS

Adequate first-trimester evaluation of a multifetal pregnancy makes subsequent second- and third-trimester ultrasound examinations much more meaningful, as well as simpler and shorter. Assessing amnionicity and chorionicity during the second and third trimesters may present serious challenges, even to the most expert practitioners of ultrasonography. The three basic determinants of chorionicity and amnionicity in the second and third trimesters are fetal gender, placental location, and interfetal membranes.

Determination of fetal gender

Most early studies of sonographic sex determination (sometimes called fetal 'sexing') used transabdominal ultrasound. These articles reporting TAS to determine fetal sex relied on examinations between 10 weeks and term. With the introduction of TVS, however, emphasis was placed on using this method for gender determination.[5,14] This latter approach relies on high-resolution, high-frequency probes; however, owing to their relatively shallow depth of penetration, such probes are difficult to use after 16–17 weeks, even though the fetus can sometimes conveniently move into the desired position. If, on the other hand, the fetus is in a breech presentation, transvaginal ultrasound can be used even later in pregnancy. The overall accuracy of sexing in various published articles is around 90% in males and about 97–98% in females. It is important to

Table 5.1 Sequential, gestational age-dependent sonographic appearance of embryonic structures in twin pregnancies. From reference 13

Timing of transvaginal scan (weeks)	Number of gestational sacs	Number of yolk sacs	Number of fetuses	Number of amniotic sacs	Chorionicity and amnionicity
4–5	two				dichorionic
	one				monochorionic
5–6	two	two			dichorionic
	one	two/one*			monochorionic
6–7	two	two	two		dichorionic
	one	two/one*	two/one[†]		monochorionic
7–8	two	two	two	two	dichorionic–diamniotic
	one	two/one*	two	two	monochorionic–dichorionic
	one	two/one*	two/one[†]	one	monochorionic–monoamniotic

*A single, double or partially divided yolk sac may be seen; [†]conjoined twins may be seen at this time mention, however, that visualizing the external genitalia in all fetuses presents a much greater degree of difficulty in a multifetal pregnancy of higher order.

In the common scenario, twins with different genders are always dizygotic (except for the exceedingly rare heterokaryotypic MC twins) and, hence, always dichorionic. If, however, in a set of twins the fetal sex is correctly determined by ultrasound in the second and third trimesters and it is found to be discordant, the pregnancy has to be considered dichorionic (Figure 5.11a).

In the second and third trimesters, the best imaging planes for the external genitalia are as follows: a median section showing the scrotum and the phallus pointing cephalad (Figure 5.11b) and on the axial plane, parallel to and below the flexed thighs (Figure 5.11c). For the female fetus, coronal planes through the labia (Figure 5.11d) or a median section through the downward pointing clitoris (Figure 5.11e) are most useful.

Lately, three-dimensional rendering of the genitalia has become available. If the technical parameters permit, clear pictures of the male and female genitalia are possible in the second and third trimesters (Figure 5.11f and g).

More accurate determinations of fetal gender began with the introduction of TVS. Two articles mentioned the accuracy of sex determination of twin pregnancies. One is relatively old and used TAS;[15] in spite of this, the authors correctly determined the gender in all 24 fetuses of 12 twin pregnancies. The other is a more recent[16] analysis of 100 twins at a gestational age of almost 30 weeks. Fetal gender was determined for both twins in 94% of the fetuses. All genders were correctly assessed, but it became increasingly difficult to determine with increasing gestational age. In this study, the finding of opposite gender in predicting dichorionicity had a sensitivity of 51.3% with a specificity of 100% and a positive predictive value of 100%. The negative predictive value, however, was only 39.3%. The same gender as a predictor of monochorionicity carried a sensitivity of 100% and a positive predictive value of 39.3%; however, the negative

predictive value was 100%. Additional articles[17,18] claim that chorionicity can be correctly assessed based on fetal gender in about 35% of cases discordant for gender.

Monteagudo and Timor-Tritsch[17] developed a simple algorithm to determine chorionicity and amnionicity in second- and third-trimester ultrasound. If male and female fetuses are seen in a twin pregnancy this must be dichorionic–diamniotic (DC–DA). However, like-sex twins are present in approximately 50% of DC–DA pregnancies. When like-sex twins are seen, the placenta or placentas must be evaluated in order to make the diagnosis of chorionicity (Figure 5.12).

Placental location

Assessing and determining the site as well as the number of placentas in a multifetal pregnancy is indicative of chorionicity and amnionicity, but does not yield an overly high sensitivity in the detection of dichorionicity or high specificity in determining monochorionicity. Simply stated, it is very difficult to distinguish a single from a fused placenta in twins (Figure 5.13a and b). This is true for all stages of the multifetal pregnancy. However, if the two placentas in the case of twins are detected on opposite sides of the uterine wall, and the placental cord insertions can be followed to those placentas which are situated at diagonally opposing uterine locations, this supports the diagnosis of two separate placentas, and hence dichorionicity (Figure 5.14a and b). This circumstance occurs in about one-third of twin gestations. Mahoney and colleagues[19] found a sensitivity of 32% when assessing two placental sites, and their predictive value was 100%. When only one placenta was detected, the accuracy of prediction for monochorionic pregnancy was only 49%. In the study of Scardo and co-workers,[16] the sonographic finding of a single placenta predicted monochorionicity with a sensitivity of 95.8%, specificity of 57.9%, positive predictive value of 51.8%, and a negative predictive value of 97.7%. If the authors had not mistakenly labeled one dichorionic placenta by ultrasound, which was

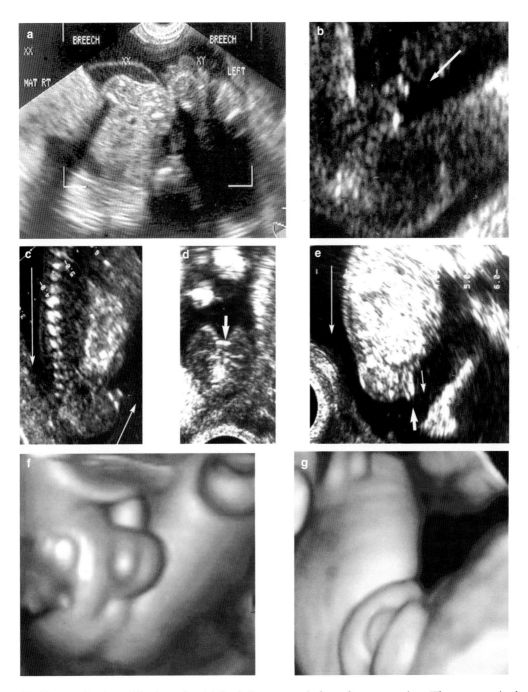

Figure 5.11 Evaluation of fetal gender. (a) Both fetuses are in breech presentation. The transvaginal scan revealed a female (XX) and a male (XY) fetus. A thick intertwin membrane is also seen. This is therefore a dichorionic–diamniotic twin pregnancy (reproduced with permission from reference 17). (b) At 16 postmenstrual weeks the male genitalia are clearly seen (arrow). (c) The phallus points cranially (upward arrow) in the opposite direction from that of the feet (downward arrow). (d) At the same age, the female genitalia are shown (arrow). (e) The clitoris points caudally (downward arrow) in the same direction as the feet (downward long arrow). (f) Three-dimensional ultrasound at times is able to show clearly the male genitalia. (g) Three-dimensional ultrasound image of the female genitalia

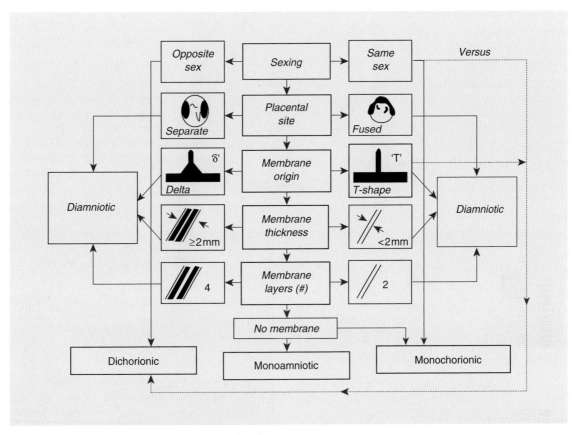

Figure 5.12 Several sonographic markers are available for assessment of chorionicity and amnionicity in the second and third trimesters. This algorithm can be used to make such an assessment

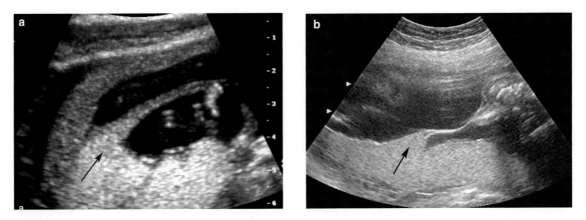

Figure 5.13 The 'lambda' ('delta', 'twin peak') sign in first-trimester dichorionic or multichorionic pregnancies. (a) The 'take-off' of the membrane (arrow) in the early first trimester is obvious. (b) The triangular 'take-off' of the intertwin membrane in the late first trimester (arrow)

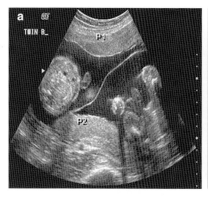
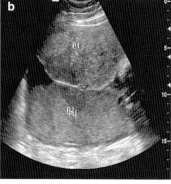

Figure 5.14 Detection of the placental sites. (a and b) The two placentas (P1 and P2) are on opposite sides of the uterus. These are clearly dichorionic twin gestations

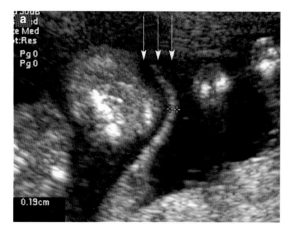
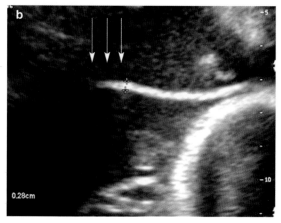

Figure 5.15 Technical aspects of intertwin membrane assessment. (a) If the membranes are parallel with the direction of the sound waves, measurement of the thickness yields a false value. The membrane measures 1.9 mm. (b) For better imaging of membrane thickness as well as detecting the layers, the membranes should be positioned at a 90° angle to the incandescent sound waves (arrows). The actual membrane thickness is 2.8 mm

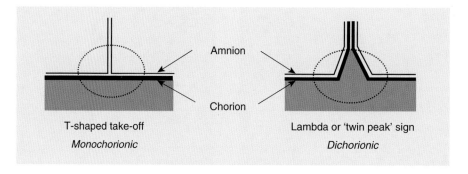

Figure 5.16 This line drawing depicts two kinds of intertwin membrane origins or 'take-offs'. At the left a T-shaped take-off represents a monochorionic placenta with two emerging amnions. There is only one chorion. On the right a dichorionic, fused placenta with wedge-shaped 'take-off' is seen creating the 'lambda' ('delta', 'twin peak') sign. The circles highlight the important feature of the two kinds of membrane origin

their only false detection in an extremely obese patient, their negative predictive value would have been 100%.[16]

A very effective way to determine placental location is to follow and trace the cord insertion, using color Doppler ultrasound. In twins the same method was used by Westover and associates[20] in 80 cases, at less than 24 weeks, 24–30 weeks, and more than 30 weeks. Successful visualization of both cords before 24 weeks was 100%, between 24 and 30 weeks six of eight cords were detected, and after 30 weeks only two of nine cords were successfully imaged. On the other hand, the correct prediction of insertion type, if the insertion was indeed seen, was 100% before 24 weeks, 85% between 24 and 30 weeks, and 90% past 30 weeks.

The interfetal membranes

The presence of an interfetal membrane must be assessed because the presence or absence of this structure can change the clinical management of a twin pregnancy. If no membrane is seen, a monochorionic–monoamniotic (MC–MA) twin pregnancy must be suspected. If two separate placental sites are identified, as described above, it is less important to scrutinize the membranes further. However, in cases in which a single placental site is identified, the following method can aid in classifying the pregnancy as DC or MC. Three important clues help to assess chorionicity and amnionicity:

(1) The origin of the membrane;
(2) The thickness of the intertwin membrane;
(3) The number of layers present in the intertwin membrane.

Identifying the origin of the membrane

Determining membrane thickness and counting the layers of the interfetal membrane with sonography is dependent upon the frequency of the ultrasound probe, the orientation of the membrane to the ultrasound transducer, and the experience of the sonographer. The higher the frequency of the ultrasound probe

the better is the resolution of the image. Having said this, as penetration of sound waves is limited, a lower frequency transducer may have to be used in very advanced gestations, potentially jeopardizing the actual imaging of these layers.

Membrane orientation in relation to the transducer probe is a key factor in trying to visualize the layers of the interfetal membranes (Figure 5.15). The membrane to be studied needs to be oriented at a right angle to the direction of the incoming sound waves to take advantage of the axial resolution of the machine, which is always superior to the lateral resolution of ultrasound equipment. A membrane placed parallel with the incoming sound waves will be poorly seen, and will appear thinner than it actually is owing to the less sharp lateral resolution of the equipment.

As discussed above, the 'lambda' ('delta' or 'twin peak') sign (Figure 5.16, right, and Figure 5.17) is a reliable indicator that the pregnancy is multichorionic, but its absence does not rule out the presence of dichorionicity.[10] In the MC placenta, the relationship of the two membranes to the uterine wall is at a 90° angle, and this 'T-shaped' take-off of the membrane (Figure 5.17, left) is a reliable sign of monochorionicity (Figure 5.18).

Determining membrane thickness

In DC twins, the opposing membranes are always thick because the interfetal membrane is composed of four layers, formed by a combination of each twin's chorion and amnion. Thick membranes measuring 2 mm or more (Figure 5.19a) have a predictive value between 89 and 95% for dichorionicity.[21,22] On the other hand, a thin membrane measuring less than 2 mm (Figure 5.20b) may have a predictive value of up to 82% for monochorionicity.[23] In addition, this thin membrane may be difficult to measure, and may be described as 'hair-like' or 'too thin to measure'.[12,21] Most authors agree that the assessment of membrane thickness is easiest in the first trimester, as progressive thinning of the membranes occurs as pregnancy progresses. Increasing fetal size,

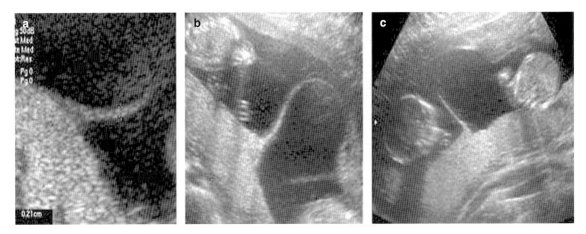

Figure 5.17 The 'lambda' ('delta', 'twin peak') sign in the second and third trimesters. The three images represent slight variations of the membrane 'take-off' in dichorionic gestations

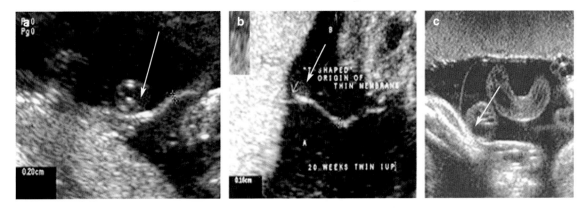

Figure 5.18 The T-shaped 'take-off' of intertwin membranes in monochorionic pregnancies (arrows) is easily detected in the first and second trimesters

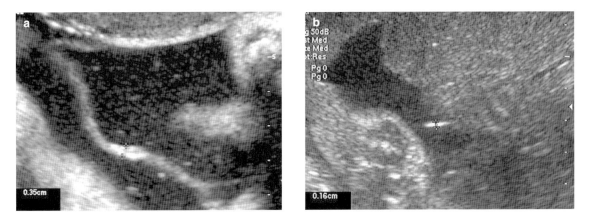

Figure 5.19 Assessing membrane thickness. (a) The correct position (at right angles to the sound waves) of the intertwin membrane in this dichorionic gestation measures 3.5 mm. (b) The intertwin membrane is thin (1.6 mm) in this monochorionic–diamniotic twin pregnancy

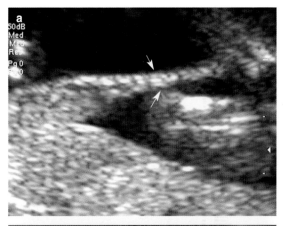

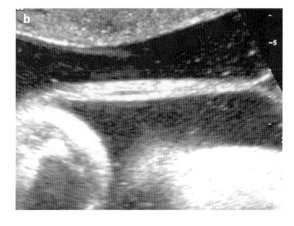

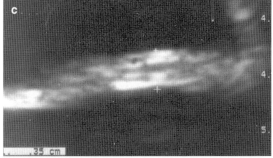

Figure 5.20 Assessing the layers in the membranes of dichorionic–diamniotic gestations. (a) In an early pregnancy the wedge-shaped 'take-off' and more than two membrane layers are seen. (b and c) Correctly positioned membranes examined with high-resolution transducers show clearly that there are four layers

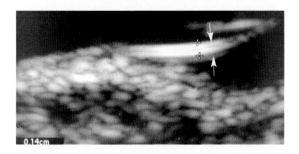

Figure 5.21 Assessing the layers in the membrane of a monochorionic–diamniotic gestation. Two layers are seen. Their combined thickness is 1.4 mm

crowding, and decreasing amount of amniotic fluid are all variables that make ultrasound difficult to use in assessing the membrane thickness, as well as counting membrane layers more difficult with advancing gestational age.

Counting the layers of the intertwin membrane

The membranes of a DC–DA placenta, when visualized through a microscope, have four layers (from one surface to the other: amnion–chorion–chorion–amnion), whereas those of an MC–DA placenta have two layers (amnion–amnion). The four layers of a DC–DA intertwin membrane (Figure 5.20) and the two layers of an MC–DA intertwin membrane (Figure 5.21) can be visualized by sonography, using a high-frequency transducer and obtaining a right-angled orientation of the probe in relation to the interfetal membrane (see above). The interfetal membranes of a DC–DA twin pregnancy appear relatively thick. When such a structure is identified, a DC pregnancy can be diagnosed in 89–90% of cases.[16,21] In contrast, if the membrane has a

61

thin 'hair like' appearance, it is more likely that only two opposing amnions are present. This circumstance is a reasonably good marker of monochorionicity.[22] It is important to note, however, that at times, the interfetal membranes of an MC–DA twin pregnancy can appear relatively thick. Therefore, to confirm the initial impression, interfetal membranes should be further scrutinized by 'zooming in' in an attempt to count the layers.

REFERENCES

1. Kurtz A, Wapner R, Mata J, Johnson A, Morgan P. Twin pregnancies: accuracy of first-trimester abdominal US in predicting chorionicity and amnionicity. Radiology 1992; 185: 759–62.

2. Goldstein SR. Early pregnancy scanning with endovaginal probe. Contemp Obstet Gynecol 1988; 27: 54–64.

3. Goldstein SR, Snyder J, Watson C, Danon M. Very early pregnancy detection with endovaginal ultrasound. Obstet Gynecol 1988; 72: 200–4.

4. Warren W, Timor-Tritsch IE, Peisner D, Raju S, Rosen M. Dating the pregnancy by sequential appearance of embryonic structures. Am J Obstet Gynecol 1989; 161: 747–53.

5. Monteagudo A, Timor-Tritsch IE, Sharma S. Early and simple determination of chorionic and amniotic type in multifetal gestations in the first fourteen weeks by high frequency transvaginal ultrasonography. Am J Obstet Gynecol 1994; 170: 824–9.

6. Doubilet PM, Benson CB. Appearing twin: undercounting of multiple gestations on early first trimester sonograms. J Ultrasound Med 1998; 17: 199–203.

7. Bromley B, Benacerraf B. Using the number of yolk sacs to determine amnionicity in early first trimester monochorionic twins. J Ultrasound Med 1995; 14: 415–19.

8. Hill LM, Chenevey P, Hecker J, Martin JG. Sonographic determination of first trimester twin chorionicity and amnionicity. J Clin Ultrasound 1996; 24: 305–8.

9. Bessis R, Papiernik E. Echographic imagery of amniotic membranes in twin pregnancies. In: Gedda K, Parisi P, eds. Twin Research Vol 3: Twin Biology and Multiple Pregnancy. 1981; 11: 571–7.

10. Finberg H. The twin peak sign: reliable evidence of dichorionic twinning. J Ultrasound Med 1992; 11: 571–7.

11. Overton TG, Denbow ML, Duncan KR, Fisk NM. First trimester cord entanglement in monoamniotic twins. Ultrasound Obstet Gynecol 1999; 13: 140–2.

12. Copperman AB, Kattenbacher L, Walker B et al. Early first-trimester ultrasound provides a window through which the chorionicity of twins can be diagnosed in an in vitro fertilization (IVF) population. J Assist Reprod Genet 1995; 12: 693–7.

13. Monteagudo A, Timor Tritsch IE, eds. Ultrasound and Multifetal Pregnancy. Carnforth, UK: Parthenon Publishing, 1988.

14. Bronshtein M, Rottem S, Yoffe N, Blumenfeld Z, Brandes JM. Early determination of fetal sex using transvaginal sonography: technique and pitfalls. J Clin Ultrasound 1990; 18: 302–6.

15. Shalev E, Weiner E, Zuckerman H. Ultrasound determination of fetal sex. Am J Obstet Gynecol 1981; 141: 582–3.

16. Scardo JA, Ellings JM, Newman RB. Prospective determination of chorionicity, amnionicity, and zygosity in twin gestations. Am J Obstet Gynecol 1995; 173: 1376–80.

17. Monteagudo A, Timor-Tritsch IE. Second- and third-trimester ultrasound evaluation of chorionicity and amnionicity in twin pregnancy. A simple algorithm. J Reprod Med 2000; 45: 476–80.

18. Birnholz JC. Determination of fetal sex. N Engl J Med 1998; 309: 942–4.

19. Mahoney BS, Filly RA, Callen PW. Amnionicity and chorionicity in twin pregnancies: prediction using ultrasound. Radiology 1985; 155: 205–9.

20. Westover T, Perry R, Dunh T, Fischer R. Prospective assessment of placental cord insertion in twin gestation. Am J Obstet Gynecol 1997; 176: S74.

21. Hertzberg BS, Kurtz AB, Choi HY, Kaczmarczyk JM. Significance of membrane thickness in the sonographic evaluation of twin gestations. Am J Radiol 1987; 148: 151–3.

22. Winn HN, Gabrielli S, Reece EA, Roberts JA, Salafia C, Hobbins JC. Ultrasonographic criteria for the prenatal diagnosis of placental chorionicity in twin gestations. Am J Obstet Gynecol 1989; 161: 1540–2.

23. Tessen JA, Zlatnik FJ. Monoamniotic twins: a retrospective controlled study. Obstet Gynecol 1991; 77: 832–4.

6

Approach to genetic counseling

INTRODUCTION

The goal of genetic counseling is to provide accurate, up-to-date, and comprehensive information related to inherited diseases in patients, their offspring, or family members. Such information should be presented in a non-directive manner and in an empathic atmosphere using the simplest possible terminology. At the end of this process, the patient and the counselor should both be able to reach mutual informed management decisions. To achieve this objective, relevant family, pregnancy, and medical histories are initially obtained. Thereafter, appropriate genetic testing, and other indicated diagnostic modalities or therapeutic means, should be offered to the patient. Although most genetic counselors act accordingly, it is nonetheless surprising how differently information is given to the patient and how often, despite all efforts, significant parts of the information are either misunderstood, misinterpreted, or forgotten.

The most common situations discussed in the context of multiple pregnancies are screening and diagnostic measures to detect aneuploidy, genetic counseling when a structural anomaly is detected, and circumstances with increased risk for specific inherited conditions. The basic rules of genetic counseling in singletons are also applicable in multiples; however, there are specific facets in multiple gestations that need special attention, which makes counseling more complex. Indeed, it is the combination of the medical and ethical aspects of counseling that makes it so complicated. The basic difference between counseling singletons and multiples is the fact that, as opposed to singletons, any decision in multiples should take into consideration the implication of that decision for the remaining sib(s) if only one is affected. This includes both diagnostic and therapeutic measures.

Before any prenatal diagnostic procedure is performed, numerous medical, emotional, and moral issues must be addressed with parents with multiple gestations. There must be a favorable cost:benefit ratio, i.e. the reproductive risk of a genetic disorder in one or more gestations must significantly exceed the risk of serious obstetric complications of the diagnostic procedure, particularly the loss of one or more fetuses as a direct consequence of the procedure itself. As an initial part of the genetic counseling, prospective parents must be informed that there are no cures for the genetic disorder in question, and if a genetic abnormality is detected, there are only two choices: either to continue the pregnancy recognizing that one or more infants will be compromised physically and functionally for their entire life, or to terminate the pregnancy. In the case where only one fetus is genetically affected, selective termination with all of its medical, emotional, and ethical implications must be discussed as an option. It has been recommended that no diagnostic procedure should be performed if a multiple gestation is observed during the course of an ultrasound examination prior to an anticipated singleton prenatal diagnostic procedure.[1] Rather, the patient should be removed from the examining room, undergo with her partner additional genetic counseling pertinent to all aspects of diagnostic testing in the case of multiple gestations, and then be given sufficient time to process the additional information such that an informed decision for which they share responsibility can be reached by the prospective parents.

This chapter describes specific medical situations that require the attention of the genetic counselor. Detailed accounts of non-invasive and invasive genetic diagnosis in multiple pregnancies are described elsewhere in this volume.

CHORIONICITY

Chorionicity is undoubtedly one of the most important factors in genetic counseling in multiples. As discussed in Chapter 5, the diagnostic accuracy of chorionicity approaches 100% in the first trimester (Figure 6.1). However, accuracy is reduced when chorionicity assessment is performed later in pregnancy. From the genetic point of view and excluding the rare cases of heterokaryotypic monochorionic (MC) twins, monochorionicity implies monozygosity and high genetic resemblance. On the other hand, unlike-sexed dichorionic (DC) twins are 100% dizygotic (DZ), but zygosity is unknown in all like-sex DC twins unless specific testing is done. Uncertainty about zygosity is even greater in iatrogenic conceptions because the proportion of DZ to monozygotic (MZ) twins (about 15:1) is different from that of spontaneous conceptions. The proportion of DC to MC twins in the subpopulation of MZ twins is unknown and adds to the uncertainty.

When chorionicity is unclear and management decisions might be altered by determination of zygosity, prenatal DNA studies should be considered. An example of the difficulty arising from inconclusive chorionicity determination in the later parts of pregnancy is presented by a case of twin pregnancy discordant for hydrocephaly and oligohydramnios, in which sonographic evaluation could not exclude MC twinning. Before considering selective feticide, blood samples from both fetuses were examined by DNA 'fingerprint' analysis. The different banding patterns of the

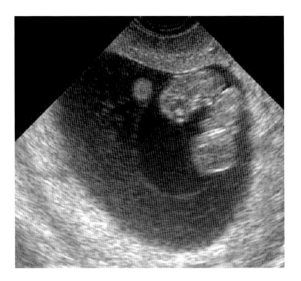

Figure 6.1 A single yolk sac and two fetuses were observed within a single amniotic sac. This sonographic scan at 9 weeks led to the diagnosis of monoamniotic twins. Image courtesy of B. Caspi, MD, Kaplan Medical Center, Israel

blood samples established dizygosity.[2] Similarly, DNA zygosity studies were performed on amniocytes to guide management of four such pregnancies.[3] In this series, DNA zygosity analyses provided > 99% likelihood of MZ twins in two cases, a fact that altered counseling regarding selective termination options.[3] In the other two cases, DNA studies were used to assess risk to the normal twin in the event of the co-twin's demise, based upon the differentiation of twin–twin transfusion syndrome (TTTS) from discordant severe intrauterine growth restriction (IUGR) and oligohydramnios.[3]

MZ twins have a 2–3-fold increased risk of structural anomalies (see Chapter 8). The patient should be informed about this risk when an MC gestation comes to the attention of the genetic counselor. She should be referred for a comprehensive sonographic scan, including detailed echocardiography. When a discordant structural anomaly is found, discussion of management options should consider the vascular anastomoses between the circulations of the twins. This circumstance precludes termination of the anomalous twin by intracardiac KCl injection, which may lead to the so called 'embolization' syndrome. Selective termination of the malformed twin can be carried out by one of the cord occlusion techniques. Similarly, single fetal demise of an MC twin may indicate appropriate counseling regarding the potential damage to the survivor.

When a case of MC twins is referred early enough, there seems to be a clear benefit of nuchal translucency (NT) measurement. Although NT assessment may be indicated in all twins in order to detect chromosomal aberrations and cardiac anomalies, an increased NT in MC twins may also be an early sign of TTTS (see Chapter 13). It should be noted, however, that the risk of TTTS is mainly associated with MC–diamniotic twins and is rarely seen in MC–monoamniotic twins. The fact that utility of biochemical screening in twins is limited and practically not available in higher-order multiples only underscores the importance of performing NT measurements in all multiples.

INDICATIONS FOR PRENATAL DIAGNOSIS IN MULTIPLE GESTATIONS

Indications for prenatal diagnostic genetic testing have become established as standard, routine, and applicable to both single and multiple gestations. These indications include: (1) advanced maternal age; (2) a previous offspring with a chromosome abnormality; (3) a family history of a chromosome abnormality or known carriers of a Mendelian mutation; (4) a previous offspring with an open neural tube defect; (5) a family history of a congenital malformation; and (6) structural abnormalities identified in the course of ultrasound examination.

Maternal age-related risk of aneuploidy in multiple gestations

The most common indication for prenatal genetic diagnosis is advanced maternal age. The well-recognized association of advancing maternal age with increased risk of having a conception with trisomy 21 (Down's) or other autosomal trisomies immediately distinguishes mothers with multiple gestations. In a multiple gestation, the overall risk of an aneuploid fetus is directly determined by zygosity. The theoretic risks of fetal aneuploidy in a twin gestation are listed in Table 6.1. Four risk combinations are presented:

(1) The risk of *both* fetuses being simultaneously chromosomally abnormal;
(2) The risk of *only one* chromosomally abnormal fetus;
(3) The risk of *at least one* chromosomally abnormal fetus;
(4) The risk of *both* fetuses being chromosomally normal.

Table 6.1 Maternal age-related risks of fetal chromosome abnormalities in twin gestations (derived in part from reference 4)

	Monozygotic pregnancy	Dizygotic pregnancy	Zygosity unknown
Risk of both fetuses affected	X	$(X)(X) = X^2$	$X + X^2 \approx X$
Risk of only one affected fetus	0	$X(1 - X) + (1 - X)X$ $= 2X - 2X^2$	approximately same as risk for dizygotic pregnancy
Risk of at least one affected fetus	X	$2X - X^2 \approx 2X$	$1/3X + 2/3(2X) = 5/3X$
Risk of both unaffected	$1 - X$	$1 - X^2$	$(1 - X) + (1 - X^2)$

X, age-related risk of chromosome abnormality; $1 - X$, age-related risk of normal karyotype

The risk of *both* fetuses being simultaneously abnormal in monozygotic twins is the same as the age-related risk for a singleton, ignoring the rare occurrence of discordant chromosome constitutions due to post-zygotic mitotic non-disjunction. For dizygotic twins, since each fetus has an independent risk of an abnormal chromosome constitution, the probability of both fetuses being chromosomally abnormal is the product of their separate probabilities, i.e. this risk is relatively small except for women 45 years of age or older. And, therefore, the risk of both fetuses being chromosomally abnormal for twins of unknown zygosity approximates that of monozygotic twins.

The risk of *only one* affected fetus in the case of a monozygotic pregnancy is essentially zero, with exceptions due to post-zygotic mitotic non-disjunction. In a dizygotic pregnancy, twin A may be chromosomally abnormal (X) and twin B normal (1–X) or vice versa; therefore, the probabilities are added to determine the likelihood of either occurrence. In clinical practice, the risk of only one affected fetus in a dizygotic pregnancy or a pregnancy of unknown zygosity is approximately two times the age-related risk of a singleton pregnancy, since the contribution of the component $-2X^2$ is negligible.

The risk of having *at least one* chromosomally abnormal fetus is the same as the probability of either having both fetuses affected or having one affected. For monozygotic twins, this risk is the same as the risk of both fetuses being affected. For dizygotic twins, this risk is approximately two times the risk of the age-related risk of a singleton pregnancy, since the component X^2 will be insignificant and can essentially be ignored, with the possible exception of women 45 years of age or older. For twins of unknown zygosity, the general assumption is that one-third of twin gestations are monozygotic and two-thirds are dizygotic, and therefore the best overall estimate of having *at least one* chromosomally abnormal fetus is five-thirds of X. However, this last ratio will vary according to race, e.g. African women have a higher risk of DZ pregnancies and Asian women a lower

probability than Caucasian women.[1] It also varies according to maternal age, e.g. the rate of dizygotic pregnancies increases with maternal age, and to form of conception, e.g. monozygosity occurs at higher rates than expected in cases when multiple gestations result from the application of artificial reproductive technologies (ART). The clinical significance of these calculations is illustrated by the choice of maternal age as to when to offer prenatal invasive testing for chromosome aberrations in the case of multiple gestations. There is no internationally accepted, standard criterion for determining at what age a mother with a singleton pregnancy should be offered the option of an invasive prenatal diagnostic test for fetal chromosome analysis. For example, in the United States, this option is generally offered to women 35 years of age and older, whereas in the United Kingdom and France, chorionic villus sampling and amniocentesis are available to women 37 years of age and older. This choice is further complicated by the fact that risk figures at the time of first-trimester chorionic villus sampling, mid-trimester amniocentesis, and delivery differ remarkably because a subset of pregnancies with chromosome abnormalities is spontaneously lost during each of the three trimesters of pregnancy.

The risks of at least one chromosomally abnormal twin at these three periods of gestation are listed in Table 6.2. In general, this table indicates that *diagnostic genetic testing should proceed 3 years earlier* in twin gestations when compared with the maternal entry age for a singleton pregnancy, regardless of which entry age is applied (35, 37, or 38 years), regardless of what type of zygosity is present, and regardless of what gestational age is used as the entry age (risk at first-trimester chorionic villus sampling, at amniocentesis, or at term). The theoretic calculations presented above, however, may be misleading, particularly when rates at birth are applied because of high intrauterine mortality.[6] For example, the birth prevalence of Down's syndrome in twins was estimated by meta-analysis of five cohort studies including a total of 106 Down's syndrome

Table 6.2 Risk of at least one chromosomally abnormal twin by maternal age and zygosity for Caucasian women (derived in part from reference 5)

Maternal age (years)	Chorionic villus sampling (10–12 weeks)			Amniocentesis (~16 weeks)			Term		
	Mono	Di	Unkn	Mono	Di	Unkn	Mono	Di	Unkn
25				1/1533	1/767	1/920	1/476	1/238	1/285
30				1/455	1/228	1/273	1/385	**1/193**	1/231
31				1/357	1/179	1/214	1/385	**1/193**	1/231
32				1/280	**1/140**	1/168	1/322	1/161	**1/193**
33				1/219	1/110	**1/131**	1/286	1/143	1/171
34				1/172	**1/86**	1/103	1/238	**1/119**	1/142
35	1/113*	1/57	1/68	**1/135**	**1/68**	**1/81**	**1/192**	**1/96**	**1/115**
36	1/87	1/44	1/52	1/106		1/63	1/156		**1/93**
37	**1/66**	1/33	1/40	**1/83**			**1/127**		
38	**1/50**	1/25	1/30	**1/65**			**1/102**		

*Bold numbers indicate entry age of 35, 37, or 38 years for singleton pregnancy undergoing diagnostic genetic testing; Mono, monozygotic; Di, dizygotic; Unkn, unknown twins.[7,8] The estimate was only 3% higher than the prevalence in singletons.

None of the studies was stratified for maternal age, and the chance of having twins increases with age. Therefore, the observed small increase in the crude Down's syndrome prevalence rate among twins implies a reduction in the age-specific prevalence. However, until there is a more precise estimate of these rates, it may be reasonable to assume no difference from singletons.[6] A Belgian group recently collected 512 prenatal diagnoses (amniocentesis or CVS) from 278 twin pregnancies.[8] The most frequent indications were maternal age ≥ 35 years (38.8%), assisted procreation (12.3%), and suspicious ultrasound findings (7.2%). Autosomal chromosome aberrations were found in eight twin sets (2.9%): four inherited balanced rearrangements (two Robertsonian translocations and two paracentric inversions of chromosome 11) and four cases of trisomy 18. Surprisingly, the authors did not detect any trisomy 21 in this population.[8]

It follows that there is an urgent need to conduct a multicenter study that documents the actual rates of chromosome aberrations at the time of first-trimester chorionic villus sampling and compare such rates with those at mid-trimester amniocentesis and term. For example, the concordance for Down's syndrome at birth is relatively low, 12% in one study,[9] indicating either a selection pressure against monozygotic Down's syndrome twins over dizygotic Down's syndrome twins during gestation or that the approximation that one-third of pregnancies are monozygotic is in fact an overestimate.

Theoretic risk calculations for karyotypic anomalies in triplet pregnancies also warrant consideration, given the increasing number of multiple gestations beyond twinning particularly as a consequence of *in vitro* fertilization. The theoretic risks of chromosome abnormalities in a triplet gestation are listed in Table 6.3. Four theoretic risk combinations are presented:

(1) *All three* fetuses being chromosomally abnormal;
(2) *One* chromosomally abnormal fetus and two unaffected fetuses;
(3) *Two* chromosomally abnormal fetuses and one unaffected fetus;
(4) *All three* fetuses being chromosomally normal.

At the time of amniocentesis, the risk of one chromosomally abnormal fetus for a 30-year-old woman with a triplet pregnancy is the same as the risk for a 35-year-old with a singleton pregnancy. Thus, the general rule in triplet gestations is that *diagnostic genetic testing should proceed 5 years earlier* when compared with the maternal entry age in a singleton pregnancy.

Counseling the older patient is a very timely issue, and the increased maternal age in multiple pregnancies observed worldwide has led to tailored approaches to these patients. On the one hand, the risk of aneuploidy is age-dependent, placing the older mother at increased risk. On the other, every invasive diagnostic test entails risks of miscarriage, and very rarely infection and/or fetal injury. Given the fact that many of these pregnancies are considered 'premium' because of adverse prior maternal reproductive history, the reluctance for invasive testing in the older patients seems understandable. In such circumstances, and only in countries where late feticide is legally permissible, late amniocentesis may be offered. In a study from Israel, elective third-trimester cytogenetic amniocentesis was performed in 14 women, including five with twin pregnancies.[10] There were no procedure-related complications, and all newborns weighed > 2000 g and exhibited normal development. This study did not attempt to answer the moral and ethical questions surrounding the use of third- (versus second) trimester amniocentesis, but shows that the procedure (late amniocentesis) is safe and may constitute a good alternative for patients who are unwilling to accept the risks of early fetal karyotyping.

Table 6.3   Maternal age-related risks of chromosome abnormalities in triplet gestations

	Monozygotic pregnancy	Dizygotic pregnancy	Zygosity unknown
Risk of all three fetuses affected	X	$(X)(X)(X) = X^3$	$X + X^2 \approx X$
Risk of only one affected fetus	0	$3X(1 - X)^2$	$3X(1 - X)^2$
Risk of two affected fetuses	0	$3(1 - X)X^3$	$3(1 - X)X^3$
Risk of all three fetuses unaffected	$1 - X$	$1 - X^3$	$(1 - X) + (1 - X^3)$

X, age-related risk of chromosome abnormality; 1 − X, age-related risk of normal karyotype

An interesting issue is the case of pregnancies following use of donor oocytes. Intuitively, one may think that the donor's age should be used for aneuploidy risk assessment. However, the donor's age may not always be known or reliable. For example, in a series of established pregnancies from oocyte donation in women aged ≥50 years, the authors found one case of Down's syndrome in 23 infants.[11] Although this single case does not imply an increased risk in pregnancies following oocyte donation, it demands the same attention as all other multiples to markers of aneuploidy.

Previous child with a chromosome abnormality

There are a series of recurrence risk estimates for couples who have had a child with Down's syndrome due to non-disjunction. For women less than 35 years of age, the risk for a subsequent trisomic Down's syndrome singleton pregnancy is usually given as the mother's age-related risk plus 0.5%, and the risk of a subsequent pregnancy for all chromosome abnormalities is usually given as the mother's age-related risk plus 1.0%. Above the age of 35 years, the risk appears to be little different from the general population age-specific risk. For twin and triplet pregnancies, the estimates listed in Tables 6.1–6.3 should be adjusted accordingly for a couple who have one Down's syndrome child and presumably for other aneuploidies as well, although the latter has not been established.

A family history of a chromosome abnormality or known carriers of a mendelian mutation

Familial chromosome rearrangements such as Robertsonian and reciprocal translocations and inversions carry their own specific risk of recurrence, depending on a variety of factors including the chromosome(s) involved, the breakpoints, and the sex of the parent carrying the chromosome rearrangement. Once defined for singleton pregnancies, risks for familial chromosome rearrangements can therefore be easily calculated for multiple gestations by substituting in Tables 6.1 and 6.3, for twin and triplet pregnancies, respectively, the age of the mother (X) for the risk of recurrence for any specific chromosome rearrangement. Such risk calculations can be applied to all aspects of the reproductive risks, e.g. the risk of a spontaneous abortion or the risk of a newborn with congenital malformations as a consequence of an unbalanced chromosome constitution, as well as the risk of an unaffected newborn. For known carriers of a mendelian mutation, the risk in twin pregnancies will depend on whether the mutation is expressed as autosomal dominant, autosomal recessive, X-linked for fetal sexing, or X-linked recessive (Table 6.4).

X-linked disorders

If only fetal sexing is applied in X-linked disorders, the risk of at least one twin being affected, if both males, is approximately two

Table 6.4   Genetic risks in twin pregnancies* for mendelian mutations (derived in part from reference 12)

	Autosomal dominant	Autosomal recessive	X-linked (fetal sexing only)	X-linked (specific diagnostic test)
Risk for singleton pregnancy	—	1/4	1/2	—
Risk of at least one twin being affected	2/3	3/8	2/3	3/8
Risk of both twins being affected	1/3	1/8	1/3	1/8
Twin A normal; risk of only twin B being affected	1/3	1/6	1/3	1/6

*Assumes one-third of twin pregnancies are monozygotic

times higher (66%) than if specific testing is applied (36%) (Table 6.4). Similarly, the risk of both twins being affected is approximately one-third lower if diagnostic testing is applied in known sex (12%), in comparison with the risk when only fetal testing is performed (33%).

Autosomal recessive disorders

In the case of an autosomal recessive trait, the overall risk of at least one twin being clinically affected is 36%, compared with the established 25% recurrence risk for singleton pregnancies (Table 6.4). On the other hand, the risk of only one twin being affected (16%) is less than the risk of recurrence in a singleton pregnancy. In comparison with most other genetic patterns of inheritance, however, the recurrence risk that both twins would be clinically affected with an autosomal recessive disorder is considered high because the risk exceeds 10%.

Autosomal dominant disorders

The recurrence risk figures for an autosomal dominant disorder are the same as those for X-linked disorders when only fetal sexing is performed (Table 6.4). Since the recurrence risk to a singleton pregnancy is extremely high, the recurrence risk of at least one twin being affected is strikingly elevated, 66%, as is the risk of both twins being affected (33%), when zygosity is undetermined.

A previous offspring with an open neural tube defect

The occurrence of an open neural tube defect is based on the interaction of a genetic predisposition, environmental factors (e.g. reduced folic acid intake and geography), and time, i.e. 18–27 days post-fertilization. Hence, open neural tube defects are described as multifactorial in their pattern of inheritance, involving several genes (polygenic) interacting with various environmental factors at a specific time during embryogenesis. The risk of recurrence after an affected conception with an open neural tube defect, therefore, varies between 1 and 4% depending on geography. Table 6.5 lists the genetic risk for an open neural tube defect based on a recurrence risk of either 1 or 4%. The risk of at least one twin being affected with an open neural tube defect is approximately two times that of a singleton pregnancy, whereas the risk of only one twin being affected, if one twin is normal, is the same as the risk to a singleton pregnancy.

A family history of a congenital malformation

Diagnostic testing in the case of a family history of a congenital malformation is determined on the basis of genetic etiology. The issue to be resolved is whether a specific test is available for the diagnosis of the congenital malformation. Such tests can take the form of

Table 6.5 Genetic risk of recurrence in twin pregnancies for an open neural tube defect based upon geography (derived in part from reference 12)

	Recurrence risk 1%	Recurrence risk 4%
Risk for singleton pregnancy	1/100	1/25
Risk for at least one twin being affected	1/50	2/25
Risk of both twins being affected	< 1/100	< 1/100
Risk of only one twin being affected	1/100	1/25

karyotyping for a chromosome analysis, FISH (fluorescence *in situ* hybridization) for specific deletions or duplications of genetic material, a DNA molecular analysis for single gene mutations as well as chromosomal duplications and deletions, or biochemical analysis for inborn errors of metabolism, among others. Each of these technologies has very high efficiencies and accuracies, and therefore the focus of the genetic counseling relates to recurrence risks as outlined in Tables 6.1–6.5. For those birth defects for which the etiology is unknown, multifactorial inheritance is usually invoked. Recurrence risks for multifactorial disorders are influenced by the disease severity, the degree of relationship to the index case, the number of affected close relatives, and, if there is a higher incidence in one particular sex, the sex of the index case. In general, if the empiric recurrence risk for a singleton pregnancy has been determined, then it is possible to utilize the formulae listed in Tables 6.1 and 6.3, substituting the estimated recurrence risk for that of maternal age.

Structural abnormalities identified in the course of ultrasound examination

'Reversed' cytogenetics refers to an indication for cytogenetic analysis following a suspected or a pathognomonic ultrasonographic finding. The literature is replete with such signs in singletons, but, regrettably, only rarely discusses the value of these signs in multiples. The application of genetic testing for multiple gestations in such cases is dependent on the availability of specific laboratory technologies that can appropriately address the issue of differential diagnosis and etiology. Since accurate assessment of the increased risk for a chromosome aberration is available for many anomalies detected on ultrasound in singleton pregnancies, it should be readily possible to determine the level of risk in the case of multiple gestations, using the approaches outlined in Tables 6.1 and 6.3.

Some findings which indicate further assessment in singletons are seen more frequently in twins (i.e. major anomalies such as cardiac malformations, and minor anomalies such as a single umbilical artery, intrauterine growth restriction, polyhydramnios, oligohydramnios, etc.). Regardless, the approach in such cases should be the same as in singletons with the same presentation.

GENETIC COUNSELING BEFORE REDUCTION PROCEDURES

The genetic counselor may be required to enter into discussions about issues related to prenatal diagnosis in cases scheduled for numerical or selective multifetal pregnancy reduction (MFPR) for elective or medical reasons. In the former case, the embryos/fetuses are considered at low risk for genetic problems, and MFPR is carried out only to reduce the risks associated with high-order multiple pregnancies. In the latter, the reduction is performed after the diagnosis of a problem in one or more of the sibs. Even so, the parents may request to know whether the remaining fetus(es) are also affected. When such a question is posed, the most common diagnostic procedure in the second trimester is amniocentesis. In contrast, when this question arises in the first trimester, or in relation to MFPR, the options are chorionic villus sampling (CVS) or early amniocentesis (performed at 11–14 weeks' gestation). Appelman and co-workers performed CVS in five triplet sets before MFPR for a variety of genetic reasons.[13] No sampling failure occurred. A chromosomal mosaic 46,XY/47,XXY was detected in one fetus; in another set, a 47,XXY (Klinefelter's syndrome) was found in one triplet, and in a third set, fragile X syndrome was diagnosed in one fetus. All these affected fetuses were selectively reduced. Brambatti and colleagues[14] offered genetic analysis before fetal reduction to both high- and low-risk pregnant women carrying two or more fetuses after ovulation induction. The use of short-term culture, the polymerase chain reaction (PCR), and fresh tissue enzymatic analyses enabled genetic diagnosis in a few days.[14]

The alternative to CVS, namely early amniocentesis, was evaluated in a recent randomized trial in a predominantly advanced-maternal-age population with singletons. The results show that amniocentesis at 13 weeks carries a significantly increased risk of talipes equinovarus compared with CVS, and also suggest an increase in early, unintended pregnancy loss.[15] These and other studies indicate that first-trimester CVS is a highly efficient, reliable, and relatively safe approach for genetic diagnosis in multiple pregnancies. Although a precise relative risk of CVS compared with amniocentesis in multiples must await randomized controlled studies, the advantages of a first-trimester diagnosis to enable early decision making about selective or numerical fetal reduction are obvious. Care should, however, be exercised, not to abuse the technology for sex selection. A couple, for example, may wish to reduce the male fetus in triplets with two males and one female, in order to have 'one of each'. It is therefore strictly advisable to perform CVS on the two embryos that are selected to remain, and to totally disregard the gender of the embryo destined for reduction.

In the common scenario, and if pre-MFPR genetic diagnosis was not done, patients may wish to determine if the remaining fetuses after MFPR have a normal karyotype. Stephen et al[16] reviewed the obstetric outcomes of women with MFPR who subsequently underwent elective amniocentesis ($n = 91$) and compared them with those who did not undergo amniocentesis. Among patients who subsequently underwent elective amniocentesis the total uncorrected pregnancy loss rate was 9.0% and the early premature delivery rate was 4.5%. These rates were comparable to those of patients with MFPR who did not undergo amniocentesis.

Another option is to postpone MFPR into the mid-second trimester. Geva et al[17] compared 38 and 70 patients who underwent selective second-trimester MFPR and first-trimester MFPR at mean gestational ages of 19.7 ± 3.3 weeks and 11.7 ± 0.7 weeks, respectively. No statistically significant difference was found between the two groups in terms of mean gestational age at delivery, mean birth weight, and the incidence of obstetric complications. The authors concluded that selective second-trimester MFPR is associated with favorable perinatal outcome and may facilitate detection of structural and chromosomal anomalies before the procedure and selective reduction of the affected fetus.

ETHICS

Genetic counseling frequently involves difficult ethical issues. In the antepartum period, a conflict may arise in the case of discordant anomalies, when any form of treatment of the anomalous twin may endanger the well-being of the co-twin. For instance, consider the possibility of a DC twin pregnancy with a suspected discordant chromosomal anomaly. Would it be ethical to perform an invasive procedure to reach the diagnosis, and, at the same time, put the co-twin at risk for potential adverse outcome? Moreover, in the context of multiple pregnancy, these issues are not restricted to prenatal diagnosis only. It may start postpartum with parental requests for zygosity diagnosis of their infants. In the absence of a medical indication, is it ethical to perform any procedure to satisfy the curiosity of the parents to know if their twins are 'identical'? This may go on to adulthood, when one twin of an MZ set is diagnosed with a late-onset genetic disease. Is there an ethical obligation to reveal the patient's disease state to his/her co-MZ twin? In this specific case, one might also ask is it ethical not to perform zygosity diagnosis if for no other reason except to give this information to the parents and their children.

Finally, consider the situation when one twin wishes to know the results of her deceased mother's tests for *BRCA1* mutations (increased risk for breast cancer) and the second twin objects to researchers making this information available.[18] Who is in the position to decide? Obviously, answers are not quickly or easily at hand.[18] This conflict is not uncommon in medicine, as greatly appreciated technical advances frequently precede ethical dilemmas. In this respect, especially in multiple pregnancies, the future does not appear to diminish the potential for ethical conflicts in genetic counseling.

REFERENCES

1. Wapner RJ. Genetic diagnosis in multiple pregnancies. Semin Perinatol 1995; 19: 351–62.
2. Appelman Z, Manor M, Magal N et al. Prenatal diagnosis of twin zygosity by DNA 'fingerprint' analysis. Prenat Diagn 1994; 14: 307–9.
3. Norton ME, D'Alton ME, Bianchi DW. Molecular zygosity studies aid in the management of discordant multiple gestations. J Perinatol 1997; 17: 202–7.
4. Myrianthopoulos NC. An epidemiologic survey of twins in a large prospectively studied population. Am J Hum Genet 1970; 22: 611–29.
5. Wenstrom KD, Syrop CH, Hammitt DG, Van Voorhis BJ. Increased risk of monochorionic twinning associated with assisted reproduction. Fertil Steril 1993; 60: 510–14.
6. Cuckle H. Down's syndrome screening in twins. J Med Screening 1998; 5: 3–4.
7. Wald NJ, Cuckle HS. Recent advances in screening for neural tube defects and Down's syndrome. In: Rodeck CH, ed. Fetal Diagnosis of Genetic Defects. Baillière's Clin Obstet Gynaecol 1987; 1: 649–76.
8. Doyle PE, Beral V, Botting B, Wale CJ. Congenital malformations in twins in England and Wales. J Epidemiol Community Health 1991; 45: 43–8.
9. Mutton D, Alberman E, Hook EB. Cytogenetic and epidemiological findings in Down syndrome, England and Wales 1989 to 1993. National Down Syndrome Cytogenetic Register and the Association of Clinical Cytogeneticists. J Med Genet 1996; 33: 387–94.
10. Shalev J, Meizner I, Rabinerson D et al. Elective cytogenetic amniocentesis in the third trimester for pregnancies with high risk factors. Prenat Diagn 1999; 19: 749–52.
11. Sauer MV, Paulson RJ, Lobo RA. Pregnancy in women 50 or more years of age: outcomes of 22 consecutively established pregnancies from oocyte donation. Fertil Steril 1995; 64: 111–15.
12. Harper P. Practical Genetic Counseling, 5th edn. Oxford: Butterworth Heineman, 1988: 118.
13. Appelman Z, Vinkler C, Caspi B. Chorionic villus sampling in multiple pregnancies. Eur J Obstet Gynecol Reprod Biol 1999; 85: 97–9.
14. Brambatti B, Tului L, Baldi M, Guercilena S. Genetic analysis prior to selective fetal reduction in multiple pregnancy: technical aspects and clinical outcome. Hum Reprod 1995; 10: 818–25.
15. Philip J, Silver RK, Wilson RD et al. NICHD EATA Trial Group. Late first-trimester invasive prenatal diagnosis: results of an international randomized trial. Obstet Gynecol 2004; 103: 1164–73.
16. Stephen JA, Timor-Tritsch IE, Lerner JP, Monteagudo A, Alonso CM. Amniocentesis after multifetal pregnancy reduction: is it safe? Am J Obstet Gynecol 2000; 182: 962–5.
17. Geva E, Fait G, Yovel I et al. Second-trimester multifetal pregnancy reduction facilitates prenatal diagnosis before the procedure. Fertil Steril 2000; 73: 505–8.
18. Green RM, Thomas AM. Whose gene is it? A case discussion about familial conflict over genetic testing for breast cancer. J Genet Couns 1997; 6: 245–54.

Non-invasive screening tests: biochemical markers

7

WHAT ARE SCREENING TESTS AND HOW ARE THEY USED?

Screening is provided for symptom-free individuals who may have a disease in its early stages. In contrast, a diagnostic test is indicated for persons with a possible disease condition. The prevalence of affected cases expected to be identified by a screening procedure is low, and positive results are likely to be false-positive. Hence, the efficacy of a screening test for a population at large is usually measured by its cost-effectiveness, on the one hand, and, on the other, by the ability of a subsequent diagnostic test to reach a diagnosis.

A positive screen can be either true-positive or false-positive (positive when disease is present or false-positive when disease is absent, respectively). Similarly, a negative screen can be either true-negative or false-negative (negative when disease is absent or false-negative when disease is present, respectively). The sensitivity of a test reflects its ability to detect true-positive cases and is calculated by the number of true-positive cases divided by the total number of affected cases (true-positive + false-negative). Clearly, the higher the sensitivity the lower the number of false-negative cases.

On the other hand, the specificity of a test reflects its ability to correctly exclude a disease state and is calculated by the number of true-negative cases divided by the number of unaffected cases (true-negative + false-positive). As with sensitivity, the higher the specificity the lower the number of false-positive test results.

Logically, one would be interested in the 'missed' cases of a screening procedure, i.e.

the probability that a test result is positive when the disease is absent (false-positive) and the probability that a test result is negative when the disease is present (false-negative). These probabilities are directly derived from the specificity and sensitivity of the test, respectively.

When the effectiveness of a screening test is of interest, one should consider the positive and the negative predictive values. The positive predictive value characterizes how good a screening test is, i.e. the probability that a disease is present when the test is positive (either truly or falsely), and increases with increased specificity. Conversely, the ineffectiveness of a screening test is determined by the negative predictive value, i.e. the probability that a disease is absent when the test is negative (either truly or falsely), and increases with increased sensitivity.

In the ideal, the detection of the presence or absence of a disease condition is only possible if the screening test has 100% sensitivity or 100% specificity. Because it is impossible to achieve both, an arbitrary cut-off between normal and abnormal results is set, which determines the trade-off between these parameters. Mathematic considerations may show that when multiple tests are used to detect a possible disease, their combined effect is important. For example, when all tests are normal or abnormal, the combined effect may be helpful to exclude or confirm the presence of disease. However, when the results are at variance (i.e. one positive and the other negative), multiple tests are least helpful.

Table 7.1 Various characteristics of a screening test

True-positive	positive screen when disease present
True-negative	negative screen when disease absent
False-positive	positive screen when disease absent
False-negative	negative screen when disease present
Sensitivity	true-positive/(true-positive + false-negative) false-negative)
Specificity	true-negative/ (true-negative + false-positive)
False-positive rate	100% minus the specificity (%)
False-negative rate	100% minus the sensitivity (%)
Positive predictive value	true-positive cases/ (true-positive + false-positive)
Negative predictive value	true-negative cases/ (true-negative + false-negative)

Table 7.2 Complex issues associated with screening for chromosomal anomalies in twin pregnancies

- Interpreting the marker values
- Paucity of data in abnormal pregnancies
- Dilemmas regarding which invasive test to offer
- The perceived increased risk of invasive procedures in twins
- Ensuring fetal tissue is obtained from each fetus
- Ensuring that each fetus can be clearly identified later
- Management of fetal reduction
- Potential increased risk to the unaffected co-twin

As noted above, a positive result for a given disease condition is more likely to be false-positive if the risk of having this condition in the evaluated population is low. Therefore, the prevalence of a rare condition determines the predictive value of the test to detect it. Although the actual *a priori* prevalence of a disease is frequently unknown, one may use an estimate of the prevalence and the rather complex Bayes' theorem to calculate the quantitative effect of the prevalence on predictivity. Table 7.1 summarizes the various characteristics of a screening test used in this chapter.

PRENATAL SCREENING: GENERAL PRINCIPLES

Prenatal screening is used to identify fetuses with neural tube defects (NTDs) or chromosomal abnormalities. It is practiced worldwide. As discussed in the preceding section, the aim is to identify a subset of women within the general pregnant population whose pregnancy may be at increased risk of being affected with such a problem, and subsequently, to offer these women a diagnostic test. Whereas the diagnosis of an NTD is currently accomplished using a detailed ultrasound scan, fetal chromosomal abnormalities can only be diagnosed from cultured amniotic fluid cells or chorionic villi, using either conventional techniques, the recently advocated more rapid techniques of fluorescent *in situ* hybridization (FISH), or the quantitative polymerase chain reaction (Q-PCR).

At present, the only method of diagnosis for chromosomal abnormalities is an invasive test. Such procedures, as carried out in singleton pregnancies, carry risks to both the fetus and the mother. In particular, the fetal loss rate is 0.5–1.0% and some 1–2% above the background rate following amniocentesis and chorionic villus sampling (CVS), respectively. Fetal loss rates vary between operators, and depend on skill, training, and experience.

Twin pregnancies are associated with a higher risk for chromosomal abnormalities,[1] although the available evidence for trisomy 21 is questionable.[2] Some complex issues associated with screening for chromosomal anomalies in twin pregnancies are shown in Table 7.2 and form the basis of arguments that screening in twins poses such a serious clinical, ethical, and moral dilemma[2,3] that it should be discouraged.[4] Despite these reservations, screening programs for twin pregnancies have been proposed and successfully implemented in both the second and first trimesters, especially in units that have links with specialized fetal medicine centers capable of dealing with the clinical management of invasive testing and selective fetal reduction in twin pregnancies.

SCREENING FOR NEURAL TUBE DEFECTS

In the presence of an open NTD, either anencephaly or open spina bifida, fetal proteins pass into the amniotic fluid and concentrate at an increased rate. One important substance – α-fetoprotein (AFP) – is a 69-kDa single-chain glycoprotein produced initially in the embryonic yolk sac, and subsequently, nearly all AFP is synthesized in the liver by the end of the first trimester. Normally, only a small amount of AFP escapes and appears in fetal urine, and eventually, by micturition, in the amniotic fluid. Early in gestation, AFP also enters the amniotic fluid via transudation across the fetal immature epithelium. Diffusion of AFP from the fetal to the maternal compartment is across the fetal membranes as well as at the placental level. As a consequence, the relative levels of AFP in the three compartments (i.e. fetal serum, amniotic fluid, and maternal serum) differ markedly, with levels in fetal serum reaching a peak of about 3000 ng/ml at around 13 weeks, followed by a decline. Levels in amniotic fluid follow a similar pattern, with a peak concentration of about 30 ng/ml. In contrast, levels in maternal serum increase to a peak of about 1 ng/ml only at around 32 weeks of gestation, falling slightly towards delivery. Because concentrations of AFP in the fetal serum are approximately 100 000 times those in maternal serum in the second trimester, it is easy to understand how even small amounts of fetal blood may cause increased levels of amniotic fluid AFP and subsequently elevated levels in maternal serum. As AFP levels change with gestational age (in both amniotic fluid and maternal serum), accurate pregnancy dating is important for interpretation of levels. AFP concentrations are usually expressed as the multiple of the normal median (MoM) for a gestation of the same duration.

The relationship between maternal serum AFP and fetal NTDs was comprehensively examined in a large collaborative study of 301 affected cases and 18 684 unaffected pregnancies.[5] Using a cut-off of 2.50 MoM in singleton pregnancies at 16–18 weeks, 88% of pregnancies with anencephaly and 79% of cases with open spina bifida could be identified, with a false-positive rate of 3%. These findings formed the basis of a screening program in which women with levels above 2.49 MoM could be offered amniocentesis and further testing of the amniotic fluid for AFP. The second report of the UK collaborative study[6] provided the definitive diagnostic criteria for anencephaly and open spina bifida by showing that at 16–18 weeks and using a cut-off of 3.0 MoM, 99% of cases with anencephaly as well as 95% of cases with open spina bifida could be identified with a false-positive rate of 0.42%.

Further improvements to the diagnostic accuracy of NTDs were shown with electrophoresis of the amniotic fluid for the presence of cerebrospinal fluid (CSF)-derived acetylcholinesterase.[7] Studies of this secondary test in cases with a high amniotic fluid AFP (≥ 3.0 MoM) initially allowed the same level of detection, but at a much reduced false-positive rate.[8] These same studies subsequently suggested that an AFP level of 2.0 MoM was a more appropriate cut-off to select for acetylcholinesterase measurement and, in such instances, the false-positive rate could be reduced to 0.14%.[9] However, since the early 1990s, detailed ultrasound scanning has largely replaced amniocentesis and biochemical analysis as the diagnostic test of choice. The reliability of ultrasound diagnosis in high-risk populations is judged to be of the order of 97% sensitivity and 100% specificity.[10] When used as a primary screening test, however, it is somewhat more variable, with results for spina bifida varying from 70 to 98%.

Table 7.3 Summary of the median multiple of the normal median (MoM) α-fetoprotein (AFP) in unaffected twin pregnancies in published series

Study	Twins (n)	Median AFP MoM
Wald[4]	1892	2.23
Thom[11]	100	1.9
Crossley[47]	81	1.91
Raty[30]	145	2.18
Raty[30]	30	2.3
Muller[13]	3043	2.1
Barnabei[46]	225	1.91
O'Brien[44]	4443	2.02
Total	9959	2.081

Maternal serum AFP levels in normal twin pregnancies are approximately twice those observed in normal singleton pregnancies. In a meta-analysis of 1892 published cases, the overall median MoM was 2.23.[4] When a further series of published cases is added to this series, the median MoM from 9959 cases is now 2.081, as summarized in Table 7.3.

Although in small studies[11,12] monozygotic twin pregnancies are reported to have higher levels of AFP, one large study[13] looking at chorionicity has found no difference in maternal serum AFP levels between monochorionic and dichorionic twin pregnancies in the second trimester.

In second-trimester normal twin pregnancies, amniotic fluid AFP levels do not appear to be elevated[6] compared with singleton pregnancies. Despite this, at least two reports show increased amniotic fluid AFP levels in cases with twins concordant or discordant for NTD,[6,14] although the diffusion of AFP and acetylcholinesterase between adjacent sacs in both normal and abnormal pregnancies makes the interpretation of amniotic fluid biochemistry difficult in cases when only one twin is affected.[14,15]

In a proportion of twin pregnancies in which one or both twins are affected by NTD, maternal serum levels of AFP are elevated when compared with the levels in normal, unaffected twins. In a report of 11 cases of twins discordant for an open NTD, Ghosh and colleagues[16] found maternal serum AFP levels over 5.00 MoM in each instance. In extending this series to 46 cases (22 with anencephaly, 24 with open spina bifida), Cuckle and co-workers[17] found that the median MoM in anencephalics was 7.5 times the MoM in unaffected singleton pregnancies, whereas that for open spina bifida was only 4.4 times higher. To achieve a similar false-positive rate in twin pregnancies equivalent to singleton pregnancies at 16–18 weeks, the cut-off level would need to be raised to 5.0 MoM (false-positive rate 3.3%). In this circumstance the detection rate for anencephaly would be 83% and that for open spina bifida 39%. This is a considerably lower detection rate for open spina bifida compared with the 79% in singleton pregnancies. To achieve a similar open spina bifida detection rate in twins, the cut-off level would need to be 3–3.5 MoM with the consequent increase in the false-positive rate to 15–20%.

SCREENING FOR DOWN'S SYNDROME AND OTHER ANEUPLOIDIES

The natural frequency of chromosomal abnormalities at birth in an unscreened population is estimated at 6/1000 births. The most common is trisomy 21 (Down's syndrome), the risk of which increases dramatically with advancing maternal age. In the United States, for example, in parallel with the shift in the past 20 years to women having babies at an older age, the general prevalence of trisomy 21 during the second trimester increased from 1 in 740 in 1974 to 1 in 504 by 1997.[18] The other common autosomal trisomies including trisomy 18 (Edwards' syndrome) and trisomy 13 (Patau's syndrome) occur with birth incidences of 1 in 6500 and 1 in 12 500, respectively. The commercial software developed by Cuckle and associates[19] is commonly used to provide regressed maternal age risks at individual maternal ages based on data from eight published surveys. This background risk is the starting point for calculating any posterior risk based on previous history or based on prenatal screening tests.

MARKERS OF ANEUPLOIDY

Maternal age

The first prenatal screening test for trisomy 21 was based on using a specific maternal age to select women for an invasive test such as amniocentesis. In the USA and UK during the 1970s and 1980s, a cut-off of 35 years was used to select women for amniocentesis, which would identify some 30% of cases for an invasive testing rate of around 6%. However, as the predictive value of screening by maternal age alone is poor, with about one abnormal case being identified for every 125 invasive procedures, and because the uptake of amniocentesis amongst this group was low, a much lower detection rate was found than the 30% predicted. Of perhaps greater importance, the changing demographics of pregnant populations in the Western world show that the proportion of pregnant women over age 35 is now in excess of 15%. Using a maternal age cut-off of 35 in today's populations would identify some 50% of cases with a 15% false-positive rate. Assuming a fetal loss rate of 1% due to the invasive procedure, such screening would result in the loss of three normal, unaffected fetuses for every two cases with trisomy 21 identified – a loss rate that cannot be considered acceptable.

Maternal serum AFP

The association of low second-trimester maternal serum AFP in pregnancies complicated with fetal aneuploidy was first reported in 1984, and the significant reduction of AFP in cases with trisomy 21 and trisomy 18 was confirmed in the same year,[20] and subsequently in many other studies. The initial screening proposal to use specific maternal age-related AFP MoM cut-offs to select women for amniocentesis revealed that AFP alone was a poor marker for trisomy 21.[21]

A potential complication of the screening algorithm using maternal serum AFP exists in cases of fetal reduction, because elevated mid-gestation levels are present following this procedure. Grau and co-workers[22] reviewed maternal serum and amniotic fluid levels of AFP from 40 women who underwent fetal reduction at approximately 12 weeks of gestation. Respectively, 95% and 25% of the patients had elevated levels of AFP in maternal serum and amniotic fluid. Fortunately, none of those abnormal levels were associated with neural tube defects, although two structural defects were detected by other means. The difference between serum and amniotic fluid AFP was attributed to either one or several mechanisms. All pregnancies were reduced to twins and one to triplets, and it is not uncommon to find elevated maternal serum AFP in such pregnancies. Alternatively, fetal AFP could have been released from the dead fetuses because of autolysis.[23] In such circumstances, the transport of AFP across fetal membranes and the placenta may be enhanced by the remaining live co-twin(s).[22] Lynch and Berkowitz[23] reported similar findings, and concluded that mid-gestation maternal serum AFP is always elevated after multifetal pregnancy reduction, and thus is not necessarily indicative of fetal defects. In contrast, Groutz and colleagues[24] found elevated AFP maternal serum in only two of 28 cases studied, both having adverse perinatal outcomes. Other groups[23–25] studied the effect of first-trimester fetal reduction on triple test results (AFP, unconjugated estriol (uE_3), and human chorionic gonadotropin (hCG)), and confirmed the elevation of maternal serum AFP. Rotmensch and associates[25] reported mid-gestation triple serum screening results from 27 high-order multiple gestations reduced to twins. About 90% of women exhibited maternal serum AFP levels > 2 MoM, but only one of the newborns had structural anomalies. In their experience, this marker did not correlate with either the number of reduced fetuses or adverse obstetric outcome.

Maternal serum human chorionic gonadotropin

In what proved to be one of the key developments in these types of investigations, Bogart and colleagues[26] reported that levels of maternal serum hCG and its free β-subunit were

Table 7.4 Meta-analysis of published maternal serum biochemical markers in cases with trisomies 21, 18, and 13 in the first and second trimesters. Modified from reference 49

Maternal serum marker	Second trimester				First trimester					
	Trisomy 21		Trisomy 18		Trisomy 21		Trisomy 18		Trisomy 13	
	n	Median MoM	n	Median MoM	n	Median MoM	n	Median MoM	n	Median MoM
AFP	1328	0.75	519	0.65	611	0.80	53	0.91	42	0.92
Total hCG	907	2.06	347	0.32	625	1.33	53	0.38	42	0.74
Unconjugated estriol	733	0.72	263	0.42	210	0.71				
Free β-hCG	562	2.20	145	0.33	846	1.98	126	0.27	45	0.51
Inhibin A	524	1.92	73	0.87	112	1.59	235	1.41	45	0.74
SP-1	448	1.46	25	1.13	246	0.86				
Free α-hCG	239	1.43	12	0.86	162	1.00				
CA125	187	1.01			34	1.14				
PAPP-A	159	0.97	90	0.11	777	0.45	119	0.20	42	0.25
Activin	82	1.23			45	1.36	45	1.23		
HPL	81	1.29	12	0.55						

MoM, multiple of the normal median; AFP, α-fetoprotein; hCG, human chorionic gonadotropin; SP-1, Schwangerschafts protein 1; PAPP-A, pregnancy- associated plasma protein-A; HPL, human placental lactogen

altered in the late second trimester (18–25 weeks) in pregnancies complicated by fetal aneuploidy. Many subsequent studies confirmed that hCG levels are increased by approximately two-fold in cases with trisomy 21, and reduced in association with trisomy 18. For the free β-subunit, other workers found only small but significant elevation in cases with trisomy 21.

Assays for hCG have varying specificities and, broadly speaking, can be categorized into three types: those detecting intact or dimeric hCG, those detecting total hCG (i.e. dimeric hCG plus free β-hCG) and those detecting specifically free β-hCG only. It is now clear that second-trimester maternal serum levels of the free β-subunit of hCG are elevated in cases with trisomy 21, that the clinical separation between unaffected and trisomy 21 cases is greater than with intact or total hCG, and that in cases with trisomy 18, free β-hCG levels are also reduced.[27]

In the first trimester between 10 and 14 weeks free β-hCG levels in cases with trisomy 21 are on average close to 2.00 MoM,[28] being only slightly less than those seen in the second

trimester. Levels in trisomy 13 and trisomy 8 are also significantly reduced. On the other hand, intact and total hCG are not significantly elevated in trisomy 21, although they are reduced in trisomy 18.

One problem associated with hCG assessment in multiple pregnancies is that levels of this marker are increased in ART pregnancies, leading to a higher false-positive rate in singletons and in twins as well.[29,30]

Maternal serum unconjugated estriol

In 1988, several authors reported that second-trimester maternal serum unconjugated estriol levels were reduced in pregnancies with trisomy 21, as also seen in cases with trisomy 18. Although reduced levels of unconjugated estriol have been confirmed in many studies, the use of this marker in screening programs remains controversial.[31–33]

Inhibin A

In the early 1990s, preliminary studies showed that levels of immunoreactive inhibin were increased in pregnancies with trisomy 21. Inhibin is a dimer composed of an α-subunit and one of two similar but distinguishable β-subunits. When more specific assays allowing the measurement of dimeric inhibin A were developed, they became a useful second-trimester marker, because levels are increased in trisomy 21. There is a strong correlation with inhibin A and hCG, but an evolving assay methodology, variable standardization, lack of stable and robust commercially developed assays, and poor comparability from center to center all served to delay the appearance of prospective data using this marker. In the first trimester, this marker appears to have little if any clinical discrimination for trisomy 21.

Pregnancy-associated plasma protein-A (PAPP-A)

In cases with trisomy 21, 13, or 18 at 10–14 weeks, levels of PAPP-A – a placental product – are reduced to around 0.45 MoM for trisomy 21[28] and to around 0.20 MoM for trisomies 13 and 18. In cases with trisomy 21 and, possibly, trisomy 18, the clinical discrimination with PAPP-A changes across the first trimester and into the second trimester.[34-36] In the case of trisomy 21, better clinical discrimination is achieved earlier (at around 8 weeks) but declines as gestation progresses, such that by the 17th week there is no difference in PAPP-A between normal pregnancies and those with trisomy 21.[34] In contrast, the clinical discrimination with free β-hCG prior to 10 weeks gets worse.[34] These balancing temporal changes mean that across the 9–14-week period, detection rates using these two biochemical markers remain relatively constant.[35] Table 7.4 summarizes a meta-analysis of the various biochemical markers that have been investigated in the first and second trimesters in cases with trisomies 21, 18, and 13.

Calculation of risk

Many of the biochemical observations in pregnancy vary with the duration of pregnancy. To remove gestational age-variation effects, many

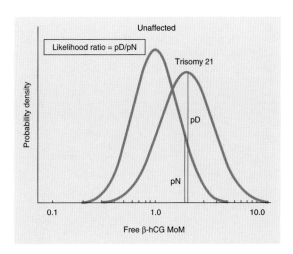

Figure 7.1 Probability density distribution of free β-human chorionic gonadotropin (hCG) in unaffected and pregnancies with trisomy 21 (Down's syndrome). pD represents the probability of trisomy 21 and pN the probability of being unaffected at a given free β-hCG multiple of the normal median (MoM) level

biochemical parameters are expressed as MoMs in a screening context, i.e. the observed result is expressed as a ratio of the median value observed in a normal pregnancy of the same gestational age. When expressed as MoMs, the majority of biochemical markers follow a Gaussian distribution in both normal and affected populations only when the MoM is log transformed. Figure 7.1 shows the distribution of free β-hCG in normal and trisomy 21-affected pregnancies. Unfortunately, there is a significant overlap of the two populations with all markers. In order to better utilize the marker information, Cuckle and colleagues[19] proposed the use of Gaussian statistics to derive a probability or likelihood ratio that a particular marker concentration was associated with an affected pregnancy. In Figure 7.1, the ratio of the heights of the distributions in the affected and unaffected pregnancies at a given marker MoM is the likelihood ratio of the result from the trisomy 21 population. To calculate the patient-specific risk, the *a priori* maternal age risk is then multiplied by the likelihood ratio.

Table 7.5 Mahalanobis distance of the prime candidate markers in second- or first-trimester screening for trisomy 21: the greater the value the more discriminatory

Marker	Second trimester	First trimester
AFP	0.69	0.23
Unconjugated estriol	1.20	0.68
Intact/total hCG	1.86	0.38
Free β-hCG	2.04	1.45
Dimeric inhibin A	1.65	0.35
PAPP-A	0.15	2.08
NT		6.46

AFP, a-fetoprotein; hCG, human chorionic gonadotropin; PAPP-A, pregnancy-associated plasma protein-A; NT, nuchal translucency

Two important features of the marker distribution dictate how good the marker is in discriminating between unaffected and affected populations. These are, first, the difference in the median values between the two populations, sometimes referred to as the median shift, and second, the width of the distributions or the standard deviations. These two features jointly define the extent of the overlap of the two populations. Expressing these features as the Mahalanobis distance, calculated from (mean [unaffected] − mean [affected]/SD [unaffected]),[37] where the mean and standard deviation (SD) are in the log domain, allows markers to be ranked in a scale of clinical effectiveness. Table 7.5 indicates the Mahalanobis distance for the commonly used first- and second-trimester markers, indicating that the most effective markers in the first trimester are nuchal translucency, PAPP-A, and free β-hCG, whereas in the second-trimester free β-hCG, total hCG, and dimeric inhibin A are the most effective.

No individual marker alone has sufficient clinical discrimination; a more efficient screening program can be obtained in practice by combining information from more than one marker. If markers have no interdependence then the likelihood ratios for each marker can simply be multiplied together to obtain the combined likelihood ratio. In practice, markers are correlated to a varying extent (i.e. providing similar information), and this needs to be corrected for. The basis behind multi-marker risk assessment is effectively an extension of that used for the single-marker case, with the addition of marker correlation information. The detailed mathematics behind this approach is beyond the scope of this chapter as is the detailed discussion for each marker or marker combination.

SCREENING IN MULTIPLE PREGNANCY

The preceding discussion focused on singleton pregnancy in order to provide sufficient background for the reader to understand some of the complexities associated with screening in multiple pregnancy. One of the major factors that alters biochemical marker levels is the presence of more than one fetus.

Background rates

Age-specific trisomy 21 prevalence rates for twin pregnancies were derived by Rodis and colleagues.[1] The authors made theoretic calculations of prevalence based not on direct observations but rather on the assumption that 80% of twins were dizygotic. In such cases the trisomy 21 risk for each twin is that in a singleton. Meyers and associates[38] updated these figures based on age-specific dizygosity rates. However, these theoretic rates do not match those observed in birth prevalence studies. A meta-analysis of 106 cases with trisomy 21 in twins showed that the prevalence was only 3% greater than for singletons.[2] Although it is possible that intrauterine lethality for affected twins may suppress birth prevalence, making first-trimester risk much higher, current thinking suggests that the safest assumption is that the prior risk in twins is the same as in singletons.

Pseudo-risk

Wald and colleagues[39] proposed that it should be possible to specify a screening policy for

Table 7.6 Published studies of maternal serum biochemical marker levels in unaffected twins in the second trimester

Study	AFP		Total hCG		Free β-hCG		Dimeric inhibin		uE$_3$	
	n	Median	n	Median	n	Median	n	Median	n	Median
Wald[4]	1892	2.23	1211	2.01	619	2.08	199	1.99	739	1.65
O'Brien[44]	4443	2.02	2101	1.806					830	1.575
Thom[11]	100	1.90								
Crossley[47]	81	1.91			81	1.85				
Raty[30]	175	2.22			68	1.98				
Muller[13]	3043	2.10			3043	2.11				
Barnabei[46]	225	1.91			225	1.99				
Total	9959	2.081	3312	1.878	4036	2.091	199	1.99	1569	1.610

AFP, α-fetoprotein; hCG, human chorionic gonadotropin; uE$_3$, unconjugated estriol

Table 7.7 Published studies of maternal serum biochemical marker levels in unaffected twins in the first trimester

Study	PAPP-A		Free β-hCG	
	n	Median	n	Median
Spencer[50]	159	1.87	159	2.11
Niemimaa[51]	67	2.36	67	1.85
Orlandi[52]	150	1.52	150	2.01
Brambati[41]	39	1.50	39	1.94
Noble[53]			136	1.94
Bersinger[54]	68	1.87		
Berry[55]			50	1.97
Spencer[42]	224	1.98	224	2.15
Total	707	1.826	825	2.035

PAPP-A, pregnancy-associated plasma protein-A; hCG, human chorionic gonadotropin

twins that would be expected to yield a false-positive rate similar to that in singleton pregnancies. These authors suggested that, because the width of the distribution of the maternal serum second-trimester biochemical markers was similar in both singleton and twin pregnancies, it should be possible to calculate a risk in twins by dividing the appropriate analyte MoM value by the corresponding median MoM value for twin pregnancies, and then treating the risk calculation as for a singleton pregnancy.[39] Table 7.6 is a meta-analysis summary of published cases of twins for which biochemical marker levels were measured in the second trimester. A similar summary is given in Table 7.7 for the first-trimester biochemical markers. In the first trimester, the width of the marker distributions is similar to that in singleton pregnancies.[40,41]

The pseudo-risk approach was introduced because it was impossible to establish, by observation, the median MoM in cases of twins in which both were affected with trisomy 21, or indeed in cases of twins discordant for trisomy 21. In only one study in eight cases discordant for trisomy 21 have marker values been published.[42] This observation has been supported by 11 cases in which seven were discordant and

four concordant for trisomy 21.[13] Detection rates have been modeled using the pseudo-risk approach for the double marker combination of AFP and free β-hCG.[42] With a 5% false-positive rate, a detection rate of 51% was expected in twins discordant for trisomy 21, some 15–20% lower than can be achieved in singleton pregnancies. For the triple marker approach, Neveux and colleagues[43] also found a similar detection rate of 53% with a false-positive rate of 5%, based on modeling after taking zygosity into account. Other authors, however, challenge the assumption that the pseudo-risk procedure is valid for estimating risks in twin pregnancies,[44] because maternal serum levels are an integration of what is happening in both twins, and because in discordancy the altered marker levels expected in a trisomy 21 pregnancy are diluted or potentially masked by the marker output from the normal twin.

Very little prospective second-trimester screening performance has been published with respect to twins. One case of twins concordant for trisomy 21 was identified as a result of screening using the pseudo-risk approach.[45] However, the more recently reported series of cases observed in second-trimester prospective screening[13] confirmed that if a pseudo-risk approach had been used with this two-marker (AFP and free β-hCG) protocol, then 54.5% of cases would have been identified with an 8% false-positive rate. Table 7.8 summarizes the values in a total of 20 published cases with trisomy 21 in the second trimester. The median MoM AFP in cases discordant for trisomy 21 appears to be higher than in singleton pregnancies (0.81 vs. 0.75), and the median free β-hCG lower than in singleton pregnancies (1.44 vs. 2.20). These observed values are very similar to what might be expected based on a normal fetus producing 1.00 MoM and an affected fetus producing the expected median in a singleton pregnancy, and the measured value being an average of the two. The standard deviations of the twin-corrected log MoM are very similar to those observed in singleton pregnancies, with perhaps the free β-hCG MoM being

Table 7.8 Summary of second-trimester marker levels in published cases of twins affected by trisomy 21 (T21)

Case (study)	Author-stated chorionicity or zygosity	AFP MoM	Free β-hCG MoM	AFP twin-corrected MoM	Free β-hCG twin-corrected MoM	T21-affected (n)
1[37]	dizygotic	2.01	2.92	0.88	1.35	1
2[37]	dizygotic	0.79	5.26	0.35	2.44	1
3[37]	dizygotic	0.71	3.97	0.31	1.84	1
4[37]	dizygotic	1.42	2.74	0.62	1.27	1
5[37]	dizygotic	1.96	2.89	0.86	1.34	1
6[37]	dizygotic	1.85	2.02	0.81	0.94	1
7[37]	dizygotic	1.19	3.75	0.52	1.74	1
8[37]	dizygotic	1.81	4.62	0.79	2.14	1
9[13]	dichorionic	2.04	30.1	0.97	14.27	1
10[13]	dichorionic	2.06	1.57	0.98	0.74	1
11[13]	dichorionic	2.18	3.00	1.04	1.42	1
12[13]	dichorionic	1.78	2.36	0.85	1.12	1
13[13]	dichorionic	0.99	3.04	0.47	1.44	1
14[13]	dichorionic	1.51	15.25	0.72	7.23	1
15[13]	dichorionic	1.99	5.86	0.95	2.78	1
16[13]	dichorionic	2.31	4.20	1.10	1.99	2
17[13]	monochorionic	1.97	1.14	0.94	0.54	2
18[13]	monochorionic	1.85	16.22	0.88	7.69	2
19[13]	monochorionic	2.10	3.69	1.00	1.75	2
20[45]	monochorionic	1.66	0.72	6.05	2.80	2
Median discordant		1.81	3.04	0.81	1.44	1
Log mean		0.1855	0.6124	−0.1560	0.2830	
SD		0.1588	0.3329	0.1659	0.3345	

SD, standard deviation; AFP, α-fetoprotein; MoM, multiple of the normal median; hCG, human chorionic gonadotropin slightly more widely dispersed than in singleton pregnancies.

Screening in twins clearly results in a lower detection rate than in singletons. However, such detection rates are better than using maternal age alone, and should provide women with twins some chance of determining whether their pregnancy is complicated by trisomy 21. Whether improvements can be made to detection rates by taking into account observed differences in marker levels based on zygosity or chorionicity remains to be seen, as currently few data exist to make a satisfactory conclusion. Wald and colleagues[12] showed significantly higher MoM levels of AFP in monozygotic twins (2.57) compared with dizygotic twins (2.06). On the other hand, in a much larger study with respect to chorionicity, Muller and associates[13] found no difference in AFP MoMs between mono- (2.10) and dichorionic (2.10) twins, although they did find significant difference for free β-hCG (monochorionic 2.16, dichorionic 2.07).

Higher-order multiples

For higher-order multiples, the data to examine marker distributions in normal pregnancies are even rarer, let alone in cases with chromosomal anomalies. In the second trimester, Barnabei and colleagues[46] published a series of 39 cases of high-order multiples with a median AFP of 2.68 and a median free β-hCG of 2.78. Spencer and associates[42] showed an AFP median of 3.77 and a median free β-hCG of 3.75 in 19 cases. The combined series of 57 cases produced a median AFP MoM of 2.997 and of 3.066 for free β-hCG. Brambati and co-workers[40] showed a median MoM for free β-hCG of 2.77 and of 2.22 for PAPP-A in a series of 17 cases

in the first trimester. In a similar unpublished series (Spencer 2003, unpublished) of 17 cases, the median MoM free β-hCG was 2.74 and was 3.26 for PAPP-A. The combined series of 34 cases suggests that the median MoM free β-hCG is 2.755, and for PAPP-A is 2.744. Much larger studies are required before such data could be used in triplet pregnancy screening. At present, the best approach would be to use sonographic markers (nuchal translucency) alone in higher-order multiple pregnancies.

CONCLUSIONS

First- or second-trimester screening in twin pregnancies is feasible using either a combination of ultrasound and maternal serum biochemistry in the first trimester or maternal serum biochemistry in the second trimester. Retrospective modeling studies suggest that detection rates will be of the order of 50–55% in the second trimester, some 20% lower than in singleton pregnancies. Limited prospective data suggest that these modeling figures are realistic. In the first trimester, combined screening appears to achieve detection rates of around 80% using modeling, and in limited prospective practice this has been achieved. Nevertheless, detection rates are some 10% lower than in singletons.

Although studies find that neither hCG nor E3 are altered after fetal reduction, the effect of first-trimester reduction on screening efficacy of trisomy 21 remains undetermined, and amniocentesis is not indicated in these cases. Moreover, ultrasonography for evaluation of fetal anatomy should be considered, mainly because the elevated maternal serum AFP levels after fetal reduction cannot be used to screen for fetal abnormalities.

REFERENCES

1. Rodis JF, Egan JFX, Craffey A et al. Calculated risk of chromosomal abnormalities in twin gestations. Obstet Gynecol 1990; 76: 1037–41.
2. Cuckle H. Down's syndrome screening in twins. J Med Screen 1998; 5: 3–4.
3. Reynolds TM. Down's syndrome screening in twin pregnancies. Prenat Diagn 1995; 15: 386–7.
4. Wald NJ, Kennard A, Hackshaw A, McGuire A. Antenatal screening for Down's syndrome. Health Technol Assess 1998; 2(1).

5. Report of the UK Collaborative Study of α-Fetoprotein in Relation to Neural Tube Defects. Maternal serum α-fetoprotein measurement in antenatal screening for anencephaly and spina bifida in early pregnancy. Lancet 1977; 1: 1323–32.

6. Second report of the UK Collaborative Study on α-Fetoprotein in Relation to Neural Tube Defects. Amniotic fluid α-fetoprotein measurement in antenatal diagnosis of anencephaly and open spina bifida in early pregnancy. Lancet 1979; 2: 652–62.

7. Smith AD, Wald NJ, Cuckle HS et al. Amniotic fluid acetylcholinesterase as a possible diagnostic test for neural tube defects in early pregnancy. Lancet 1979; 2: 685–8.

8. Report of the Collaborative Acetylcholinesterase Study. Amniotic fluid acetylcholinesterase electrophoresis as a secondary test in the diagnosis of anencephaly and open spina bifida in early pregnancy. Lancet 1981; 2: 321–4.

9. Second report of the Collaborative Acetylcholinesterase Study. Amniotic fluid acetylcholinesterase measurement in the prenatal diagnosis of open neural tube defects. Prenat Diagn 1989; 9: 813–29.

10. Lennon CA, Gray DL. Sensitivity and specificity of ultrasound for the detection of neural tube and ventral wall defects in a high risk population. Obstet Gynecol 1999; 94: 562–6.

11. Thom H, Buckland CM, Campbell AGM et al. Maternal serum alphafetoprotein in monozygotic and dizygotic twin pregnancies. Prenat Diagn 1984; 4: 341–6.

12. Wald NJ, Cuckle HS, Peck S, Stirrat GM, Turnbull AC. Maternal serum α-fetoprotein in relation to zygosity. BMJ 1979; 1: 455–7.

13. Muller F, Dreux S, Dupoizat H et al. Second trimester Down syndrome maternal serum screening in twin pregnancies: impact of chorionicity. Prenat Diagn 2003; 23: 331–5.

14. Aitken DA. Biochemical screening in twins. In: Ward RH, Whittle M, eds. Multiple Pregnancy. London: RCOG Press, 1995: 171–85.

15. Drugan A, Sokol RJ, Ager FN et al. Clinical implications of amniotic fluid α-fetoprotein in twin pregnancy. J Reprod Med 1989; 34: 977–80.

16. Ghosh A, Woo JSK, Rawlinson HA et al. Prognostic significance of raised serum α-fetoprotein levels in twin pregnancies. Br J Obstet Gynaecol 1982; 89: 817–20.

17. Cuckle HS, Wald NJ, Stevenson JD et al. Maternal serum α-fetoprotein screening for open neural tube defects in twin pregnancies. Prenat Diagn 1990; 10: 71–7.

18. Egan JF, Benn P, Borgida AF et al. Efficacy of screening for fetal Down syndrome in the United States from 1974 to 1997. Obstet Gynecol 2000; 96: 979–85.

19. Cuckle HS, Wald NJ, Thomson SG. Estimating a woman's risk of having a pregnancy associated with Down's syndrome using her age and serum alpha fetoprotein level. Br J Obstet Gynaecol 1987; 94: 387–402.

20. Cuckle HS, Wald NJ, Lindenbaum RH. Maternal serum α-fetoprotein measurements: a screening test for Down's syndrome. Lancet 1984; 1: 926–9.

21. Spencer K, Carpenter P. Screening for Down's syndrome using serum α-fetoprotein: a retrospective study indicating caution. BMJ 1985; 290: 1940–3.

22. Grau P, Robinson L, Tabsh K, Crandall BF. Elevated maternal serum α-fetoprotein and amniotic fluid α-fetoprotein after multifetal pregnancy reduction. Obstet Gynecol 1990; 76: 1042–5.

23. Lynch L, Berkowitz RL. Maternal serum α-fetoprotein and coagulation profiles after multifetal pregnancy reduction. Am J Obstet Gynecol 1993; 169: 987–90.

24. Groutz A, Amit A, Yaron Y et al. Second-trimester maternal serum α-fetoprotein, human chorionic gonadotropin and unconjugated oestriol after early transvaginal multifetal pregnancy reduction. Prenat Diagn 1996; 16: 723–7.

25. Rotmensch S, Celentano C, Shalev J et al. Midtrimester maternal serum screening after multifetal pregnancy reduction in pregnancies conceived by in vitro fertilization. J Assist Reprod Genet 1999; 16: 8–12.

26. Bogart MH, Pandian MR, Jones OW. Abnormal maternal serum chorionic gonadotropin levels in pregnancies with fetal chromosome abnormalities. Prenat Diagn 1987; 7: 623–30.

27. Spencer K, Mallard AS, Coombes EJ, Macri JN. Prenatal screening for trisomy 18 with free β-human chorionic gonadotrophin as a marker. BMJ 1993; 307: 1455–8.

28. Spencer K, Souter V, Tul N et al. A screening program for trisomy 21 at 10–14 weeks using fetal nuchal translucency, maternal serum free β-human chorionic gonadotropin and pregnancy associated plasma protein-A. Ultrasound Obstet Gynecol 1999; 13: 231–7.

29. Maymon R, Dreazen E, Rozinsky S et al. Comparison of nuchal translucency measurement and second-trimester triple serum screening in twin versus singleton pregnancies. Prenat Diagn 1999; 19: 727–31.

30. Raty R, Virtanen A, Kaskinen P et al. Maternal midtrimester serum APF and free β-hCG levels in in vitro fertilization twin pregnancies. Prenat Diagn 2000; 20: 221–3.

31. Reynolds T, John R. A comparison of unconjugated oestriol assay kits shows that the expression of results as multiple of the median causes unacceptable variation in calculated Down syndrome risk factors. Clin Chem 1992; 38: 1888–93.

32. Crossley JA, Aitken DA, Connor JM. Second trimester unconjugated oestriol in maternal serum from chromosomally abnormal pregnancies using an optimised assay. Prenat Diagn 1993; 13: 271–80.

33. Spencer K, Ong C, Skentou H et al. Screening for trisomy 13 by fetal nuchal translucency thickness and

maternal serum free β-hCG and PAPP-A at 10–14 weeks. Prenat Diagn 2000; 20: 411–16.

34. Spencer K, Crossley JA, Aitken DA. Temporal changes in maternal serum biochemical markers of trisomy 21 across the first and second trimester of pregnancy. Ann Clin Biochem 2002; 39: 567–76.

35. Spencer K, Crossley JA, Aitken DA et al. The effect of temporal variation of biochemical markers of trisomy 21 across the first and second trimester of pregnancy on the estimation of individual patient-specific risks and detection rates for Down's syndrome. Ann Clin Biochem 2003; 40: 219–31.

36. Spencer K, Crossley JA, Green K, Worthington DJ, Brownbill K, Aitken DA. Second trimester levels of pregnancy associated plasma protein-A in cases of trisomy 18. Prenat Diagn 1999; 19: 1127–34.

37. Spencer K, Salonen R, Muller F. Down's syndrome screening in multiple pregnancies using α-fetoprotein and free β-hCG. Prenat Diagn 1994; 14: 537–42.

38. Meyers C, Adam R, Dungan J, Prenger V. Aneuploidy in twin gestations: when is maternal age advanced? Obstet Gynecol 1997; 89: 248–51.

39. Wald NJ, Cuckle HS, Wu T, George L. Maternal serum unconjugated estriol and human chorionic gonadotrophin levels in twin pregnancies: implications for screening for Down's syndrome. Br J Obstet Gynaecol 1991; 8: 905–8.

40. Brambati B, Macri JN, Tului L, Hallahan TW, Krantz DA, Alberti E. First trimester aneuploidy screening: maternal serum PAPP-A and free β-hCG. In: Grudzinskas JG, Ward RHT, eds. Screening for Down Syndrome in the First Trimester. London: RCOG Press, 1997: 135–47.

41. Spencer K, Nicolaides KH. Screening for trisomy 21 in twins using first trimester ultrasound and maternal serum biochemistry in a one stop clinic: a review of three years' experience. Br J Obstet Gynaecol 2003; 110: 276–80.

42. Spencer K, Salonen R, Muller F. Down's syndrome screening in multiple pregnancies using α-fetoprotein and free β-hCG. Prenat Diagn 1994; 14: 537–42.

43. Neveux LM, Palomaki GE, Knight GJ, Haddow JE. Multiple marker screening for Down syndrome in twin pregnancies. Prenat Diagn 1996; 16: 29–35.

44. O'Brien JE, Dvorin E, Yaron Y et al. Differential increases in AFP, hCG and uE3 in twin pregnancies:

impact on attempts to quantify Down syndrome screening calculations. Am J Med Genet 1997; 73: 109–12.

45. Verdin SM, Braithwaite JM, Spencer K, Economides DL. Prenatal diagnosis of trisomy 21 in monozygotic twins with increased nuchal translucency and abnormal serum biochemistry. Fetal Diagn Ther 1997; 12: 153–5.

46. Barnabei V, Krantz DA, Macri JN, Larsen JW. Enhanced twin pregnancy detection within an open neural tube defect and Down syndrome screening protocol using free β-hCG and AFP. Prenat Diagn 1995; 15: 1131–4.

47. Crossley JA. Biochemical screening for fetal chromosome abnormalities. PhD Thesis, University of Glasgow, 1993.

48. Aitken DA, Crossley JA, Spencer K. Prenatal Screening for neural tube defects and aneuploidy. In: Rimoin DL, Connor JM, Pyeritz RE, Korf BR, eds. Emery & Rimoin's Principles and Practice of Medical Genetics. London: Churchill Livingstone, 2002: 763–801.

49. Spencer K. Screening for trisomy 21 in twin pregnancies in the first trimester using free β-hCG and PAPP-A, combined with fetal nuchal translucency thickness. Prenat Diagn 2000; 20: 91–5.

50. Niemimaa M, Suonpaa M, Heinonen S et al. Maternal serum human chorionic gonadotrophin and pregnancy associated plasma protein-A in twin pregnancies in the first trimester. Prenat Diagn 2002; 22: 183–5.

51. Orlandi F, Rossi C, Allegra A et al. First trimester screening with free β-hCG, PAPP-A and nuchal translucency in pregnancies conceived with assisted reproduction. Prenat Diagn 2002; 22: 718–21.

52. Noble PL, Snijders RJ, Abraha HD et al. Maternal serum free β-hCG at 10–14 weeks of gestation in trisomic twin pregnancies. Br J Obstet Gynaecol 1997; 104: 741–3.

53. Bersinger NA, Noble P, Nicolaides KH. First trimester maternal serum PAPP-A, SPI and M-CF levels in normal and trisomic twin pregnancies. Prenat Diagn 2003; 23: 157–62.

54. Berry E, Aitken DA, Crossley JA et al. Screening for Down's syndrome: changes in marker levels and detection rates between first and second trimester. Br J Obstet Gynaecol 1997; 104: 811–17.

Non-invasive screening tests: ultrasound

8

At one time, ultrasound was considered invaluable in obstetrics for making the diagnosis of twins or, for that matter, higher-order multiples. It replaced with great efficiency a number of less reliable diagnostic methods including X-ray. An entire literature soon developed on diagnosis and the pitfalls associated with it. Part of the problem lay with proper description of the fetuses; part lay with the description of the membranes and the placenta.

As this literature was maturing, the techniques of ultrasound also matured and various screening techniques became available. Their value was not restricted merely to singletons but also was seen for twins and higher-order multiples. This chapter reviews the major general screening techniques and then discusses their specific applications in multiple pregnancies.

NUCHAL TRANSLUCENCY

An echogenic area of fluid exists in all fetuses between the fetal skin and soft tissue overlying the cervical spine. In 1992, Nicolaides and colleagues[1] first used the term 'nuchal translucency' (NT) to describe this accumulation of fluid. Today, it is the major marker of fetal aneuploidy using the first-trimester ultrasonography marker of fetal nuchal translucency thickness. The early studies of high-risk populations identified a possible association between increased NT and the presence of a fetal chromosomal anomaly in the first trimester.[1] Pandya and associates[2] later developed a protocol for the measurement of NT that formed the basis of the Fetal Medicine Foundation (FMF) approach to training, certification, and ongoing audit of sonographers and obstetricians who perform the 10–14-week scan. In studies for trisomy 21 using the FMF protocol, detection rates of the order of 70–75% with a 5% false-positive rate have been achieved in practice.[3] In contrast, studies which have not used the FMF protocol, and with sonographers/obstetricians who are not FMF-trained, show much lower detection rates – emphasizing that training, attention to detail, following the set protocol, and ongoing audit are all of great importance.

Combining maternal serum biochemistry (see Chapter 7) and NT measurement in the first trimester is an effective screening procedure, because the two modalities do not appear to be correlated.[4] A retrospective study of 210 cases of trisomy 21 and approximately 1000 controls showed that this combined approach could achieve 89% detection with a 5% false-positive rate.[4] Other studies found that such a combination achieved detection rates in excess of 80%.

In addition to identifying fetuses with trisomy 21, combined screening also identifies pregnancies complicated by trisomy 13 and 18, Turner's syndrome, other sex aneuploidies, and triploidy types I and II. In addition to detecting 89% of cases with trisomy 21, 90% of other chromosomal anomalies can be identified with an additional 1% false-positive rate.

ABSENCE OF THE NASAL BONE

A potential new marker for first-trimester screening of trisomy 21 is the absence of the nasal bone at 11–14 weeks as found in about 70% of fetuses with trisomy 21 and in contrast with only 0.5% of chromosomally normal fetuses.[5] In extending their previous study, Cicero and colleagues[6] examined 3788 cases in which 430 cases had an abnormal karyotype; they confirmed that the nasal bone was absent in 67% of cases with trisomy 21 in contrast to 2.8% of cases with a normal karyotype. They also showed that the incidence of absent nasal bone in the normal pregnancy group varied with ethnic origin and that the incidence of absent nasal bone decreased with increasing crown–rump length and increased with increasing NT thickness.[6]

THE ROLE OF DUCTUS VENOSUS FLOW

In recent studies of vascular hemodynamics in fetuses with increased NT at 10–14 weeks' gestation, abnormal flow in the ductus venosus (DV) was more frequently recorded in fetuses with chromosomal anomalies, with or without cardiac defects, and was related to heart dysfunction.[7,8] The combination of increased NT and abnormal flow could thus serve to differentiate cases of preclinical twin-to-twin transfusion syndrome (TTTS) from those with chromosomal aberrations. In a study of 50 monochorionic pregnancies identified in one ultrasound unit during routine assessment at 11–14 weeks' gestation, NT and Doppler blood flow waveforms in the DV were recorded in both twins. In all cases with intertwin discrepant NT thickness and abnormal blood flow in the DV, TTTS eventually developed. In contrast, whenever intertwin discrepant NT thickness was found but the flow in the DV was normal, TTTS did not develop.[9]

Because the experience with DV flow measurements for screening in singletons and in multiples is not large compared with other markers of aneuploidy, more studies are needed before the utility of this relatively sophisticated marker can be recommended.

DISCORDANT GROWTH

As early as 1994, Weissman and co-workers described a clinical significance in discordant twin growth present during the first trimester

of pregnancy.[10] A retrospective survey performed in 1992–93 identified five twin pregnancies in which considerable interfetal size variation was noted in the first trimester (defined as a difference in crown–rump length corresponding to 5 or more days in the estimated gestational age). All had major congenital anomalies in the smaller twin. The authors concluded that the first-trimester growth-discordant twin is at increased risk for congenital anomalies. More recently, Kalish et al[11] evaluated 159 dichorionic twin pregnancies between 11 and 14 weeks of gestation for growth discordance using crown–rump length. Of 159 twin pregnancies, there were 7 fetal structural anomalies, 2 fetal chromosomal anomalies, 5 second-trimester spontaneous abortions, 3 second-trimester fetal deaths, and 1 third-trimester fetal death. Pregnancies that were complicated by fetal structural or chromosomal anomalies had a significantly greater median crown–rump length discordance than pregnancies without fetal anomalies (4.0 mm vs. 2.0 mm; $p = 0.02$). A crown–rump length discordance $>10\%$, which was the 90th percentile for intertwin crown–rump length disparity in the study population, was associated with a significantly higher incidence of fetal anomalies (22.2% vs. 2.8%; $p = 0.01$). The authors concluded that first-trimester crown–rump length disparity in dichorionic twin gestations is associated with an increased risk of fetal structural and chromosomal anomalies.

SCREENING IN TWINS

Whereas screening with maternal serum biochemistry alone cannot specifically identify the fetus at risk in the presence of twins discordant for an anomaly, it may be possible for the combination of biochemistry and NT screening results to improve the detection rate, yet still retain the benefits of using NT to identify the fetus.[12] A screening protocol in twins based on the calculation of pseudo-risk from NT and maternal serum biochemistry was proposed by Spencer.[12] In this modeled study, it was expected that maternal serum biochemistry would add a further 5% to the detection rate using NT alone, thus bringing the detection rate up to 80% compared with the 90% in singleton pregnancies.

As is the case in the second trimester, first-trimester distribution data for biochemical results on twins concordant or discordant for trisomy 21 are rare. Noble and colleagues[13] published a series of 12 twin pregnancies (10 discordant and 2 concordant for trisomy 21), along with free β-human chorionic gonadotropin (hCG) levels. Brambati and associates[14] published three cases discordant for trisomy 21, along with both pregnancy-associated plasma protein A (PAPP-A) and free β-hCG levels. A further four cases were observed in prospective screening[15,16] using combined ultrasound and biochemical screening. Bersinger and co-workers[17] also published PAPP-A levels in a further 10 cases (6 discordant and 4 concordant for trisomy 21).

In prospective screening in the first trimester over a 3-year period using combined ultrasound and biochemical screening, Spencer and Nicolaides[15] offered screening to 230 women with twins. Screening was accepted in 97% of cases. In this group of women, four cases were observed with twins discordant for trisomy 21. In three of these, combined screening identified the affected pregnancy. In all three instances, the affected twin was reduced, and the normal co-twin was delivered at term. A risk for trisomy 21 was calculated for each fetus based on individual NT values and the maternal serum biochemistry corrected for twin pregnancies. Of the twin fetuses screened, 6.8% had risks greater than the cut-off, and 9.2% of pregnancies had at least one fetus with an increased risk. After counseling, 37% of women declined invasive testing. Of the 63% remaining, chorionic villus sampling (CVS) was chosen by the majority (83%). The uptake of invasive testing was lower than the 77% experienced in singleton pregnancies, reflecting both the added risk and the complexity of the invasive procedure in twins. This study concluded that NT should be the predominant marker upon which women presenting with increased

risk should be counseled regarding invasive testing. As is the case in the second trimester, further studies need to be made of chorionicity and its impact on marker levels. Spencer[18] showed that PAPP-A in monochorionic twins may be lower (0.89 vs. 1.01) than in dichorionic twins after applying the twin correction, whereas free β-hCG levels were not different.

Wald and colleagues[19] suggested that it is more appropriate to calculate a pregnancy-specific risk estimate rather than calculate individual fetus-specific risks in the first trimester, arguing that since it is standard clinical practice to sample amniotic fluid or fetal material from both twins, a woman should not be expected to make two separate decisions on whether to have an invasive test with respect to each fetus. For a dizygotic pregnancy, the risk of trisomy 21 for each fetus is independent of the risk for the other, whereas in monozygotic twins the risk for one fetus is the same as for the other. These authors propose that in dizygotic pregnancies the pregnancy-specific risk should be calculated by summing the individual risk estimates for each fetus. In monozygotic twins, on the other hand, the risk can be calculated based on the geometric mean of both NT measurements. Whether this is an acceptable or a desirable procedure remains to be seen, however, as the detection rates modeled using this procedure showed a rate 10% lower than that in singleton pregnancies, as was previously shown by Spencer[12] using the conventional approach.

HIGH-ORDER MULTIPLES

Because NT is perceived as a valuable marker for detecting fetal abnormalities and complications, its importance is clear-cut for multiple pregnancies in which biochemical screening is of limited value. In twin pregnancies, first-trimester ultrasound screening for chromosomal abnormalities is both reliable and feasible. NT screening in twins is the predominant factor underlying the provision of counseling regarding further invasive testing. Moreover, NT measurement may provide additional data

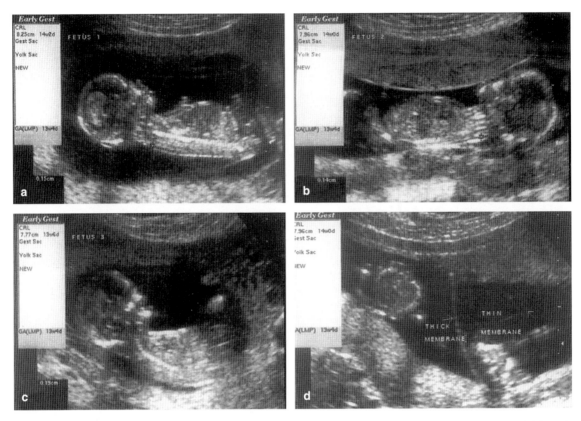

Figure 8.1 Transabdominal nuchal translucency measurement in a dichorionic triplet pregnancy: biamniotic in one chorionic sac and the third triplet in the other chorionic sac. (a, b, c) Adequate nuchal translucency measurements are illustrated. Each fetus is in the mid-sagittal plane, occupying about 75% of the image. The calipers are placed on the inner borders of the hypoechoic area behind the fetal neck (nuchal translucency). The bichorionic triplet pregnancy is demonstrated by a thick membrane of one sac and thin membrane in the monochorionic other sac (d)

about twin pathophysiology, such as underlying hemodynamic changes associated with early onset of TTTS in monochorionic twins.[20]

Caution is appropriate, however, as was shown some years ago by Berkowitz and colleagues,[21] who reported that among 200 patients who underwent fetal reduction, six of the remaining fetuses had either anatomical ($n = 4$) or chromosomal ($n = 2$) abnormalities. Based on this observation, preprocedure genetic counseling and careful scanning was proposed, especially for those patients with an increased risk of karyotype abnormalities.[21]

First-trimester ultrasound screening using NT measurement appears to be the best option to overcome such problems. For example, one group assessed patients who conceived following assisted reproduction and were carrying ≥3 fetuses.[22] Each fetus (Figures 8.1 and 8.2) was ultrasonographically assessed by measuring the crown–rump length and NT thickness using a published protocol.[23,24] Prior to the test, women were provided with a leaflet explaining the nature and implications of the test. Upon completion of the scanning, they were counseled regarding risks, and asked to sign a written NT-informed consent form. Study group patients were scanned by two examiners who showed intra-observer repeatability coefficients of 0.34 mm and 0.28 mm and an inter-observer repeatability coefficient of 0.36 mm.[25] The individual sonographer's and the unit

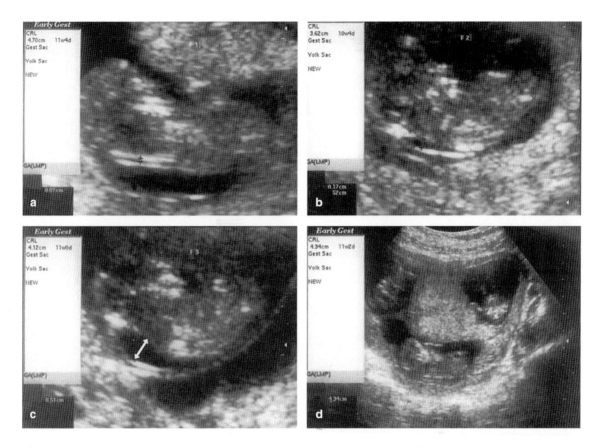

Figure 8.2 Transabdominal nuchal translucency measurement in a triplet pregnancy. (a, b) Adequate nuchal translucency measurements are illustrated (same as in Figure 8.1). Increased nuchal translucency (marked by the arrow heads) in the third fetus is presented (c). This fetus was chosen for reduction because of the increased nuchal area. The three fetuses in three separate sacs are presented (d)

measurements were subject to regular internal audit to check quality control of standardization and distribution of measurements and performance.[25,26] With results that corresponded well with previous reports,[27] the data obtained were used for counseling prior to any invasive procedure.

In this study, 24 pregnant patients, initially carrying 79 fetuses aged between 10 and 14 weeks of gestation, were compared with consecutively matched, singleton controls.[22] NT measurements were feasible for both study and control fetuses, which exhibited similar NT measurements for the 5th, 50th, and 95th centiles. Also, mean NT thicknesses (mm or MoM) were similar for both groups (1.41 ± 0.41 mm and 1.35 ± 0.39 mm, respectively, and 0.87 ± 0.23 MoM and 0.83 ± 0.25 MoM, respectively). No instances of chromosomal abnormalities were detected in either group, and of those infants who had no karyotyping, no traits were observed postnatally that warranted chromosomal analysis.

As there is no other effective screening modality for higher-order multiple pregnancies, it is reasonable to recommend NT measurement for antenatal screening services.[22,28] Moreover, in contrast with others who have

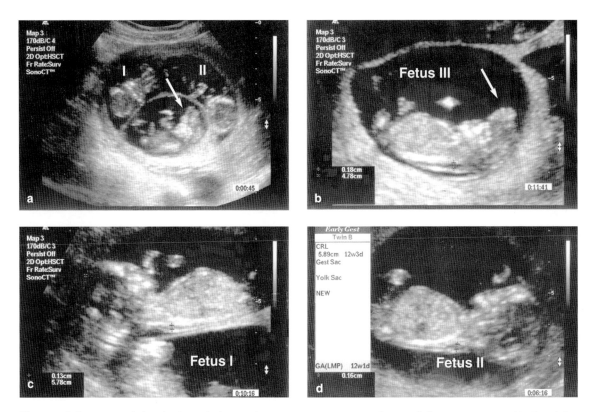

Figure 8.3 Transabdominal nuchal translucency measurement in a triplet pregnancy. (a) A triplet gestation. The arrow head is pointing to a fetus with acrania; (b) an image magnification. This fetus was chosen for reduction because of the severe brain defect. (c, d) Adequate nuchal translucency measurements are illustrated

reported obtaining an NT thickness in only about 83% of assessed singletons,[29] Maymon et al succeeded in measuring it in all of their cases.[22] Regardless, it is premature to draw any conclusions concerning the sensitivity and false-positive rate of the method, as this series is too small, and no other series exist in the English literature. It is believed, however, that these observations[22] validate the use of NT measurements obtained originally in singletons and twins[30–32] in higher-order multiple gestations. Furthermore, this sonographic screening method provides additional data for the identification of an abnormal fetus,[33] thus lowering the complications of leaving an abnormal one after reduction.[21]

Screening before multifetal pregnancy reduction

A critical problem of higher-order multiple gestation management protocols is fetal reduction. Most authorities believe that reducing multifetal pregnancies to twins improves both pregnancy and perinatal outcome. Moreover, this possibility offers an alternative, apart from terminating the entire pregnancy, to those women carrying either a higher number of fetuses than desired or an affected fetus.

Fetal reduction is generally carried out at the end of the first trimester, using a transabdominal intrathoracic introduction of a fine needle under ultrasound guidance, and injection of concentrated potassium chloride solution. Whereas agreement exists as to the number of fetuses to be left (twin pregnancies having the best outcome), the choice as to which fetuses to terminate is governed by a number of variables. Thus, before feticide, careful ultrasonographic assessment of the entire pregnancy is recommended to determine the actual number of living fetuses, their location, the placentation for monochorionic twins (see Figure 8.1), presence of visible fetal anomalies (Figure 8.3) or fetal discordance, as well as slower fetal heart rate. These parameters may indicate an anomaly or poor prognosis for the survival of a particular fetus. Additionally, it seems important to offer preprocedure, non-invasive genetic testing and careful scanning, especially for those patients with a significantly increased risk of karyotypic abnormalities by virtue of their age.[21] In this respect, first-trimester ultrasound screening using NT measurement seems to be a most promising option. Lipitz and colleagues[34] recommend performance of fetal reduction in triplets at 13–14 weeks' gestation rather than at 11–12 weeks, as this allows a more detailed anomaly scan at a slightly more advanced gestational age. According to their experience, pregnancy loss is similar (about 4%) in either group. They conclude that screening before fetal reduction at 13–14 weeks should include NT measurement and ruling out relative intrauterine growth restriction and structural anomalies. At this gestational age, the sex of the fetus can also be determined, a factor which may be of clinical importance for families at risk for chromosomal X-linked disorders. In triplet pregnancies, such an early detailed fetal anomaly scan requires a very experienced sonographer and a modern ultrasound machine with high resolution.

Since transvaginal sonography provides a better picture of the lower fetus, combined transvaginal and transabdominal scan may be required. With such high scanning performance, it seems reasonable to consider additional sonographic markers, or fetal biometric

measurements such as the fetal nasal bone, at the time of an NT scan.[6] For singletons, the corresponding predicted Down's syndrome detection rate for a 5% false-positive rate is 86% for such a sonographic combination.[35] Additional studies are needed to determine the most efficient screening combination by means of ultrasound for the subgroup of high-order multiple gestation.

Brambati and colleagues[36] and Eddleman and co-workers[37] reported performing CVS before multifetal pregnancy reduction. The message from these two studies is that in high-risk groups for chromosomal aneuploidy, CVS should be offered before embryo reduction is employed. Eddleman and co-workers[37] further state that 'rarely, there is a visible anomaly or a smaller than expected crown–rump length that influences the decision about which fetus to remove'. According to their report, however, CVS procedures alone were associated with 1.2% sampling errors, which is actually the primary risk for aneuploidy in this group. Although prereduction CVS has its advantages, primarily in older patients, the following disadvantages hinder the widespread use of this practice: the risk of abortion, the difficulty in carrying out villocentesis in multiple pregnancies, the difficulty in identifying ill fetuses to be eliminated within a few days of taking the sample, and the higher stress level in patients caused by the two invasive procedures carried out within a few days of each other.[38]

The gestational age at which multifetal pregnancy reduction is optimally carried out overlaps with the proper timing for fetal NT measurement.[32] Therefore, during the past few years, several groups[22,38,39] have routinely used NT measurement prior to multifetal pregnancy reduction as the criterion for selecting fetuses at high risk for chromosomal pathology (see Figure 8.2). Maymon and co-workers also showed that screening by NT measurement is feasible and accurate in high-order multiple gestation.[22] This group suggested the following approach, which includes

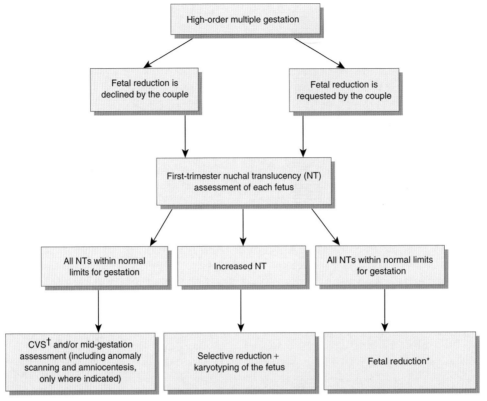

Figure 8.4 Flow chart of first-trimester screening for chromosomal abnormalities in high-order multiple gestation. *Reduction could be postponed until after detailed anomaly scan (around 14 weeks' gestation); †chorionic villus sampling (CVS) is reserved for only very high-risk cases, such as carriers of a single-gene disorder or balanced translocation. Flowchart by Maymon et al.[21,39]

Table 8.1 Categories of structural defects in twins. Adapted from reference 40

Category	Defect
Malformations more common in twins than in singletons	neural tube defects hydrocephaly congenital heart disease esophageal and anorectal atresias intersex genitourinary tract anomalies
Malformations unique to monozygotic twins	amniotic band syndrome twin-reversed arterial perfusion sequence conjoined twins twin embolization syndrome
Placental malformations	single umbilical artery twin–twin transfusion syndrome velamentous cord insertion
Deformations due to intrauterine crowding	skeletal malformations

Table 8.2 Changes in the distribution of congenital malformations/chromosomal anomalies identified at birth between 1989–91 and 1998–2000: United States twin live births

| Congenital malformations and/or chromosomal anomalies | Malformations/anomalies identified at birth | | | | | Adjusted relative risk* (95% confidence interval) |
| | 1989–91 (n = 240 349) | | 1998–2000 (n = 336 258) | | | |
	n	Risk (per 1000)	n	Risk (per 1000)		
No malformation/chromosomal anomaly	237 273	—	332 881	—		—
Any malformation/chromosomal anomaly	3076	128.0	3377	100.4		0.78 (0.74–0.82)
1 malformation/anomaly	2664	111.4	2971	88.2		0.79 (0.75–0.83)
2 malformations/anomalies	347	14.2	366	11.5		0.74 (0.64–0.86)
3 malformations/anomalies	53	2.1	35	1.2		0.46 (0.30–0.72)
≥ 4 malformations/anomalies	12	0.5	5	0.1		0.32 (0.11–0.92)

*Relative risks were adjusted for maternal age, gravidity, maternal education, marital status and maternal race/ethnicity

Table 8.3 Changes in congenital malformations/chromosomal anomalies identified at birth between 1989–91 and 1998–2000: United States twin live births

| Congenital malformations and/or chromosomal anomalies | Malformations/anomalies identified at birth in twin live-borns | | | | Relative risk* (95% confidence interval) |
| | 1989–91 (n = 240 349) | | 1998–2000 (n = 336 258) | | |
	n	Risk (per 10 000)	n	Risk (per 10 000)	
Any malformation/chromosomal anomaly	3076	128.0	3377	100.4	0.78 (0.74–0.82)
Any chromosomal anomaly	311	12.9	271	8.1	0.54 (0.46–0.64)
Down's syndrome	145	6.0	118	3.5	0.48 (0.38–0.62)
Neural tube defect	273	11.4	268	8.0	0.73 (0.61–0.86)
spina bifida	108	4.5	95	2.8	0.65 (0.50–0.86)
anencephaly	172	7.2	177	5.3	0.76 (0.61–0.94)
Hydrocephaly	162	6.7	167	5.0	0.77 (0.62–0.96)
Nervous system anomaly	149	6.2	120	3.6	0.56 (0.44–0.71)
microcephaly[†]	217	9.0	201	5.9	0.68 (0.56–0.83)
Circulatory anomaly	1719	71.5	1903	56.6	0.79 (0.74–0.84)
heart anomaly	721	30.0	817	24.3	0.80 (0.72–0.89)
Renal agenesis	64	2.7	104	3.1	1.25 (0.91–1.71)
Omphalocele/gastroschisis	119	5.0	131	3.9	0.78 (0.61–1.00)
Musculosystem anomaly	545	22.7	659	19.6	0.85 (0.77–0.96)

*Relative risks were adjusted for maternal age, gravidity, maternal education, marital status and maternal race/ethnicity;
[†]microcephaly excludes infants diagnosed with anencephaly

Table 8.4 Trends in infant mortality rates between 1989–91 and 1998–2000: United States twin live births

Congenital malformations and/or chromosomal anomalies	Infant mortality in twin live-borns				Relative risk* (95% confidence interval)
	1989–91 (n = 240 349)		1998–2000 (n = 336 258)		
	n	Risk (per 10 000)	n	Risk (per 10 000)	
Overall	8318	346.1	6547	192.4	0.72 (0.70–0.75)
Any malformation/chromosomal anomaly	538	22.4	472	14.0	0.66 (0.58–0.75)
Any chromosomal anomaly	47	2.0	37	1.1	0.50 (0.33–0.78)
Down's syndrome	14	0.6	8	0.2	0.35 (0.14–0.84)
Neural tube defect	87	3.6	90	2.7	0.81 (0.60–1.09)
spina bifida	18	0.8	15	0.5	0.69 (0.34–1.37)
anencephaly	72	3.0	77	2.3	0.83 (0.60–1.15)
Hydrocephaly	33	1.4	35	1.0	0.85 (0.53–1.38)
Nervous system anomaly	29	1.2	21	0.6	0.51 (0.29–0.90)
microcephaly†	82	3.4	80	2.4	0.76 (0.55–1.04)
Circulatory anomaly	303	12.6	255	7.6	0.63 (0.53–0.75)
heart anomaly	158	6.6	154	4.6	0.73 (0.58–0.91)
Renal agenesis	24	1.0	28	0.8	0.93 (0.54–1.62)
Omphalocele/gastroschisis	32	1.3	25	0.7	0.56 (0.33–0.95)
Musculosystem anomaly	66	2.8	52	1.6	0.62 (0.43–0.90)

*Relative risks were adjusted for maternal age, gravidity, maternal education, marital status and maternal race/ethnicity;
†microcephaly excludes infants diagnosed with anencephaly

NT measurement as part of preprocedure non-invasive genetic testing, before any embryo reduction. This is followed by reducing the fetus exhibiting the highest risk, once detected, and thereby lowering the probability of leaving an affected fetus after the procedure.[21] Using this policy they encountered a triplet pregnancy in which one fetus exhibited an NT of 3 mm (> 95th centile for crown–rump length).[33,39] The other two fetuses had NTs within the normal limit for gestation.[39] Before reducing that fetus and using the same fine needle, a few milliliters of amniotic fluid were aspirated for chromosomal analysis. This test revealed a fetus affected with trisomy 13. Mid-gestation amniocentesis performed later confirmed the euploid karyotype of the remaining fetuses.

A similar experience was reported by Monni et al.[38] The policy advocated by Maymon and co-workers[22,39] is:

(1) Routine NT measurement before any multifetal pregnancy reduction. Patients can be offered postponement of reduction until around 14 weeks, after a detailed anomaly scan.

(2) Reduction and karyotyping of the high-risk fetus (see Figure 8.2) and/or the malformed fetus (see Figure 8.3).

(3) Performance of mid-gestation amniocentesis, where indicated. The performance of genetic amniocentesis after multifetal pregnancy reduction does not increase the risk of pregnancy loss over that observed in association with the reduction itself[39] (Figure 8.4). CVS should be reserved for only highly selected instances, including the presence of balanced translocations or carriers of a single-gene disorder in which prenatal diagnosis is available.

In summary, women who conceive a multifetal pregnancy after assisted conception are naturally wary of any invasive prenatal diagnostic procedure. Because they receive careful antenatal care from the start of their pregnancies, and as serum markers are less discriminative for chromosomal screening, it seems reasonable to offer such women ultrasound assessment including NT measurement, which currently is the only available and highly efficient screening method. This valuable information can contribute to overall management if fetal reduction is planned, and as a screening modality for other structural anomalies associated with increased NT.

Screening for anomalies

The likelihood of a structural anomaly in a given multiple pregnancy is increased, not only because of the increased number of fetuses. Table 8.1 shows the four categories of structural defects in twin gestations. Most of the twinning-specific anomalies are dealt with in other chapters of this book. The diagnostic procedures of other congenital defects are not different from those in singletons and are not discussed in this volume.

There are some changes in the distribution of congenital malformations over time. Table 8.2 shows that the adjusted relative risk of detecting a malformation has decreased from 1989–91 to the period 1998–2000. As Table 8.3 shows, this trend was noted in almost all categories of anomalies. The reduced incidence of detected anomalies at birth neatly translated to reduced infant mortality rates (Table 8.4). These observations may be explained by early detection and termination of pregnancies with affected fetuses. However, other factors, such as folic acid supplementation, might be involved.

REFERENCES

1. Nicolaides KH, Azar G, Byrne D, Mansur C, Merks K. Fetal nuchal translucency: ultrasound screening for chromosome defects in the first trimester of pregnancy. BMJ 1992; 304: 867–975.

2. Pandya PP, Snijders RJM, Johnson SP et al. Screening for fetal trisomies by maternal age and fetal nuchal translucency thickness at 10–14 weeks of gestation. Br J Obstet Gynaecol 1995; 102: 957–62.

3. Nicolaides KH. Screening for chromosomal defects. Ultrasound Obstet Gynecol 2003; 21: 313–21.

4. Spencer K, Souter V, Tul N et al. A screening program for trisomy 21 at 10–14 weeks using fetal nuchal translucency, maternal serum free β-human chorionic gonadotropin and pregnancy associated plasma protein-A. Ultrasound Obstet Gynecol 1999; 13: 231–7.

5. Cicero S, Curcio P, Papageorghiou A, Sonek J, Nicolaides KH. Absence of nasal bone in fetuses with trisomy 21 at 11–14 weeks of gestation: an observational study. Lancet 2001; 358: 1665–7.

6. Cicero S, Longo D, Rembouskos G, Sacchini C, Nicolaides KH. Absent nasal bone at 11–14 weeks of gestation and chromosomal defects. Ultrasound Obstet Gynecol 2003; 22: 31–5.

7. Montenegro N, Matias A, Areias JC et al. Increased nuchal translucency: possible involvement of early cardiac failure. Ultrasound Obstet Gynecol 1997; 10: 265–8.

8. Matias A, Gomes C, Flack N et al. Screening for chromosomal defects at 11–14 weeks: the role of ductus venosus blood flow. Ultrasound Obstet Gynecol 1998; 12: 380–4.

9. Matias A, Montenegro N, Blickstein I. Down syndrome screening in multiple pregnancies. Obstet Gynecol Clin North Am 2005; 32: 81–96.

10. Weissman A, Achiron R, Lipitz S, Blickstein I, Mashiach S. The first-trimester growth-discordant twin: an ominous prenatal finding. Obstet Gynecol 1994; 84: 110–14.

11. Kalish RB, Gupta M, Perni SC, Berman S, Chasen ST. Clinical significance of first trimester crown–rump length disparity in dichorionic twin gestations. Am J Obstet Gynecol 2004; 191: 1437–40.

12. Spencer K. Screening for trisomy 21 in twin pregnancies in the first trimester using free β-hCG and PAPP-A, combined with fetal nuchal translucency thickness. Prenat Diagn 2000; 20: 91–5.

13. Noble PL, Snijders RJ, Abraha HD, Sherwood RA, Nicolaides KH. Maternal serum free β-hCG at 10–14 weeks of gestation in trisomic twin pregnancies. Br J Obstet Gynaecol 1997; 104: 741–3.

14. Brambati B, Macri JN, Tului L et al. First trimester aneuploidy screening: maternal serum PAPP-A and free β-hCG. In: Grudzinskas JG, Ward RHT, eds. Screening for Down Syndrome in the First Trimester. London: RCOG Press, 1997: 135–47.

15. Spencer K, Nicolaides KH. Screening for trisomy 21 in twins using first trimester ultrasound and maternal serum biochemistry in a one stop clinic: a review of three years' experience. Br J Obstet Gynaecol 2003; 110: 276–80.

16. Spencer K, Nicolaides KH. First trimester prenatal diagnosis of trisomy 21 in discordant twins using fetal nuchal translucency thickness and maternal serum free β-hCG and PAPP-A. Prenat Diagn 2000; 20: 683–4.

17. Bersinger NA, Noble P, Nicolaides KH. First trimester maternal serum PAPP-A, SP1 and M-CF levels in normal and trisomic twin pregnancies. Prenat Diagn 2003; 23: 157–62.

18. Spencer K. Screening for trisomy 21 in twin pregnancies in the first trimester: does chorionicity impact on maternal serum free β-hCG or PAPP-A levels? Prenat Diagn 2001; 21: 715–17.

19. Wald NJ, Rish S, Hackshaw AK. Combining nuchal translucency and serum markers in prenatal screening for Down syndrome in twin pregnancies. Prenat Diagn 2003; 23: 588–92.

20. Sebire NJ, D'Ercole C, Hughes K et al. Increased nuchal translucency thickness at 10–14 weeks of gestation as a predictor of severe twin to twin transfusion syndrome. Ultrasound Obstet Gynecol 1997; 10: 86–9.

21. Berkowitz RL, Lynch L, Lapinski R et al. First trimester transabdominal multifetal pregnancy reduction: a report of two hundred completed cases. Am J Obstet Gynecol 1993; 169: 17–21.

22. Maymon R, Dreazen E, Rozinsky S et al. The feasibility of nuchal translucency measurement in higher order multiple gestation achieved by assisted reproduction. Hum Reprod 1999; 14: 2102–5.

23. Hsu T, Hsu CY, Ou JJ et al. Maternal serum screening for Down syndrome in pregnancies conceived by intrauterine insemination. Prenat Diagn 1999; 19: 1012–14.

24. Snijders RJM, Noble PL, Sebire NJ et al. UK multicenter project on assessment of risk of trisomy 21 by maternal age and nuchal translucency thickness at 10–14 weeks of gestation. Lancet 1998; 352: 343–6.

25. Herman A, Maymon R, Dreazen E et al. Image magnification does not contribute to the repeatability of caliper placing in measuring nuchal translucency thickness. Ultrasound Obstet Gynecol 1998; 11: 266–70.

26. Herman A, Maymon R, Dreazen E et al. Nuchal translucency audit: a novel image screening method. Ultrasound Obstet Gynecol 1998; 12: 398–403.

27. Pandya PP, Altman DG, Brizot ML et al. Repeatability of measurement of fetal translucency thickness ultrasound. Obstet Gynecol 1995; 5: 334–7.

28. Maymon R, Jauniaux E. Down's syndrome screening in pregnancies after assisted reproductive techniques: an update. Reprod Bio Med Online 2002; 4: 285–93.

29. Haddow JE, Palomaki GE, Knight GJ et al. Screening of maternal serum for fetal Down's syndrome in the first trimester. N Engl J Med 1998; 338: 955–61.

30. Pandya PP, Hilber F, Snijders RJM et al. Nuchal translucency thickness, crown–rump length in twin pregnancies with chromosomally abnormal fetuses. J Ultrasound Med 1995; 14: 565–8.

31. Sebire NJ, Snijders RJM, Hughes K et al. Screening for trisomy 21 in twin pregnancies by maternal age and fetal nuchal translucency thickness at 10–14 weeks of gestation. Br J Obstet Gynaecol 1996; 103: 999–1003.

32. Sebire NJ, Souka A, Skenton H et al. Early prediction of severe twin-to-twin transfusion syndrome. Hum Reprod 2000; 15: 2008–10.

33. Nicolaides KH, Sebire NJ, Snijders RJM. The 11–14 Week Scan: the Diagnosis of Fetal Abnormalities. Carnforth, UK: Parthenon Publishing, 1999.

34. Lipitz S, Shulman A, Achiron R et al. A comparative study of multifetal pregnancy reduction from triplets to twins in the first versus early second trimesters after detailed fetal screening. Ultrasound Obstet Gynecol 2001; 18: 35–8.

35. Cuckle HS. Growing complexity in the choice of Down's syndrome screening policy. Ultrasound Obstet Gynecol 2002; 19: 323–6.

36. Brambati B, Tului L, Baldi M et al. Genetic analysis prior to selective fetal reduction in multiple pregnancy.

Technical aspects and clinical outcome. Hum Reprod 1995; 10: 818–25.

37. Eddleman KA, Stone JL, Lynch L et al. Chorionic villus sampling before multifetal pregnancy reduction. Am J Obstet Gynecol 2000; 183: 1078–81.

38. Monni G, Zoppi MA, Cau G et al. Importance of nuchal translucency measurement in multifetal pregnancy reduction. Ultrasound Obstet Gynecol 1999; 13: 377–8.

39. Maymon R, Herman A. Multifetal pregnancy reduction. Am J Obstet Gynecol 2001; 185: 772–4.

40. Blickstein I, Smith-Leuitin M. Multifetal pregnancy. In: Petrikovsky BM, ed. Fetal Disorders: Diagnosis and Management. New York: John Wiley and Sons, 1998: 223–47.

9

Invasive diagnostic genetic testing

Compared with singleton pregnancies, diagnostic genetic testing in multiple gestations presents unique and unmatched challenges. Prenatal genetic diagnoses require invasive procedures including first-trimester chorionic villus sampling (CVS) or mid-trimester amniocentesis. The genetic and counseling issues posed by multiple gestations are highlighted in the case of the pregnancy following assisted reproductive technologies (ART) where the likelihood of multiple gestations is increased. In such circumstances, previously infertile couples may not only have to consider the necessity of invasive genetic testing with all of its attendant risks including pregnancy loss, but also must be counseled concerning the unique ethical and moral issues that arise in cases of multiples discordant for anomalies.

This chapter reviews prenatal genetic diagnosis in multiple gestations and describes the risks, benefits, and consequences of diagnostic genetic testing in multiple gestations from a genetic perspective.

AMNIOCENTESIS AND CHORIONIC VILLUS SAMPLING

Diagnostic genetic testing involves several invasive procedures that must be as safe and accurate as possible and, in addition, must ensure that the sampling process represents the genotype of all fetuses. The standard, conventional approaches involve using either second-trimester amniocentesis or first-trimester CVS. The technical skills required to perform either procedure in the case of multiple gestations are not a simple extension of those skills required in the case of singleton pregnancies, primarily because multiple gestations are regarded as at increased risk for spontaneous as well as procedure-related losses when compared with singleton pregnancies. If the fetuses are discordant either by gender or major structural anomaly, accurate labeling generally does not pose a problem. However, in apparently concordant pairs, a high level of technical expertise is essential, because the uterine content has to be meticulously 'mapped' by the operators to ensure separate sampling from each fetus and to minimize the risk of potential chromosomal abnormality being incorrectly assigned to the wrong twin.[1] It follows that invasive procedures in multiple pregnancy should only be performed by specialists who are able to proceed to selective termination of pregnancy if this be necessary or desirable.[1]

Knowledge of the background risk of pregnancy loss in multiple gestations and of the procedural risks following amniocentesis or CVS is essential for prospective patients, as well as their health providers, to make informed decisions concerning diagnostic genetic testing. The descriptions of the techniques of amniocentesis and CVS that follow are based on the premise that the experience and technical skills of the operator performing these procedures are paramount, and more important than the different techniques *per se*.

The techniques of amniocentesis in multiple gestations

Ultrasound evaluation is first undertaken to determine fetal age, position, anatomy, and gender, placental sites, and the presence, locations, and characteristics of the dividing membranes. Meticulous written documentation including diagrams of each of these characteristics is essential, followed by similar painstaking attention to correct labeling of samples. Failure to sample or label correctly has potentially catastrophic consequences if selective reduction should follow diagnostic genetic testing. Amniocentesis is routinely performed after 15 weeks' gestation, based on the first day of the last menstrual period. Despite technical feasibility to perform the so-called early amniocentesis (at 11–14 weeks) in twins, there is no agreement on the safety of this procedure, in general, and in multiple gestation, in particular.

The standard approach in performing amniocentesis in multiple gestations is to sample each amniotic sac separately and sequentially.[2-7] Under continuous ultrasound visualization, a 22-gauge spinal needle is guided to the amniotic sac and 20 ml of amniotic fluid is aspirated; this procedure is then repeated depending on the number of fetuses present. A variant of this approach, and limited in application to twin pregnancies, is to introduce two needles separately but then simultaneously visualize on either side of the septum to document correct sampling of each sac. This approach not only requires more than one operator but appropriate positioning of the septum. Although use of the single-needle ultrasound-guided technique has been reported, this approach is also essentially limited to twin pregnancies, and its worldwide

use has been rather limited.[5-7] There is a real possibility of fetal cell contamination as well as cord entanglement through the creation of pseudo-monoamniotic twins with the single-needle technique. Although no instance of either possibility has been reported in three series, the number of twin pregnancies undergoing the single-needle technique only totals a few hundred cases (Table 9.1).

In the past, following amniocentesis of one sac, dye or sterile air was injected to ensure accurate sampling of the remaining sacs. After fluid was collected, the sac was 'marked' with dye, and a second needle was inserted to sample the other sac(s). When higher-order multiples were sampled, each sac could be marked in series. Dye-free amniotic fluid ensures sampling of different amniotic cavities.

The use of intra-amniotic dye is, however, no longer recommended. Besides the theoretic possibility of introducing infective agents, injections of methylene-blue dye[8] have been associated with a marked increase in intestinal atresia and fetal death; the use of an alternative dye, indigo carmine, or more recently toluidine blue,[9] is contraindicated because of its vasoconstrictive and teratogenic potentials. Given the resolution qualities of current ultrasound technology combined with an experienced operator, the use of any dye, or injecting sterile air, should be discouraged. Nevertheless, even in experienced centers, misdiagnoses have been reported, with inadvertent sampling of the same sac as high as 3.5%.[8] Consequently, and because of insufficient evidence regarding

Table 9.1 Loss rates following amniocentesis in twin pregnancies based on studies reported since 1991

Study	Single-needle technique (n)	Double-needle technique (n)	Loss to 20 weeks (%)	Loss to 28 weeks (%)
Pruggmayer et al[4]	—	529	2.3	3.7
Wapner et al[2]	—	72	1.4	2.8
Ghidini et al[3]	—	101	0	3.0
Sebire et al[5]	176	—	1.1	2.3
Buscaglia et al[6]	55	—	0	0
van Vugt et al[7]	27	—	0	0

the risk or the lack thereof from indigo carmine, some centers continue to employ such dyes as indigo carmine unless the amniotic sacs are clearly distinguishable from each other and there is no doubt of separate samplings.

It goes without saying that careful mapping of the locations of the fetuses and placentas should be undertaken to minimize confusion, and it is advisable that the sample label should include the same description. The possibility of discordant results should be discussed with the couple before any testing, including the options available if a disorder is detected.

Three other points should be mentioned in the context of amniocentesis. First, amniocentesis can be performed any time after 15 weeks' gestation. This may be of importance if a third-trimester test is considered to reduce the risks of miscarriage, very preterm rupture of the membranes, and extremely preterm birth. In one study, 14 women with extremely high-risk ('premium') pregnancies, 5 with twins, underwent elective third-trimester cytogenetic amniocentesis. There were no procedure-related complications, and all newborns weighed more than 2000 g and showed normal development. This preliminary work, however, does not attempt to answer the moral and ethical questions surrounding the use of third- (versus second) trimester amniocentesis in either 'premium' or normal pregnancies. Rather, it showed that the procedure is safe and may constitute an alternative for patients who are unwilling to accept the risks of early fetal karyotyping, and where this practice (and subsequent feticide) is accepted by the law.[10]

The second point relates to rapid assessment of chromosomal anomaly. This can be achieved in multiples in the same manner as in singletons, using quantitative fluorescent polymerase chain reaction (QF-PCR) amplification of highly polymorphic microsatellite markers. A recent study[11] described this method in 52 multiple pregnancies (47 twins, 5 triplets) and where 108 samples of amniotic fluid were sampled between 12 and 20 weeks of gestation using the single-needle technique and QF-PCR amplification of short tandem repeats

(STRs) on chromosomes X, Y, 21, 13, and 18. Normal and aneuploid fetuses were readily identified by QF-PCR, which enabled fetal reduction for trisomic fetuses to be available without further waiting for completion of fetal karyotyping. Contamination between fetuses due to the sampling procedure with a single puncture was never observed.

Finally, it is still debatable whether to perform single sac amniocentesis in monochorionic twins. As it is well established that monozygotic twins are not 'identical' genetic copies, the potential of heterokaryotypic twins should be excluded, especially in cases with discordant nuchal translucency thickness measurement in twins.[12] The exact frequency of heterokaryotypic monochorionic twins remains largely unknown and is presumably underestimated. For example, 1 in 7 dichorionic same-sex twins are monozygotic and may wrongly be classified as dizygotic, especially if not of different gender. Further, embryonic/fetal death may be the result of a non-viable chromosomal abnormality and will remain unnoticed because karyotyping is usually unavailable for 'vanished' twins.[12]

Loss rates following amniocentesis in multiple gestations

No randomized controlled trials have examined the safety and efficacy of amniocentesis performed in the case of multiple gestations and it is extremely unlikely that such a trial would ever be conducted. Therefore, any evaluation of the procedural risks of amniocentesis performed in multiples must rely on a series of reports from individual operators which, in describing personal experiences and clinical outcomes, may, in fact, have no relevance for any other operator. Worldwide, quality assurance in the performance of prenatal genetic diagnosis in the case of multiple gestations is virtually unheard of, unregulated, and/or unknown. This circumstance emphasizes the necessity for procedures such as amniocentesis and CVS in the case of multiple gestations to be performed in a tertiary referral or academic medical center with specific and documented experience.[1]

Only a limited number of reports discuss pregnancy loss rates following amniocentesis in twin pregnancies. Whereas several series provide passing attention to higher-order multiples, publications specifically relevant to gestations beyond twinning are non-existent. In the past decade, only six publications have described the pregnancy loss rate following amniocentesis in multiple gestations: of these one compares amniocentesis and CVS[2] and one is a case–control study comparing 101 twin amnioceateses with a control group of unsampled twin pregnancies recruited in the second trimester (Table 9.1). Pregnancy loss rates in these studies ranged from 0 to 2.3% up to 20 weeks and from 0 to 3.7% up to 28 weeks. In the case–control study by Ghidini and colleagues,[3] loss rates up to 28 weeks were not significantly different between cases and controls, 3.0% and 2.8%, respectively. Based upon the statistics listed in Table 9.1, it appears that the rate of procedure-related pregnancy loss after amniocentesis in twin pregnancies is not different from that after amniocentesis performed in singleton pregnancies, that is, approximately 1%. A more recent study retrospectively assessed the rate of fetal loss among bichorionic twin gestations undergoing genetic amniocentesis ($n = 476$) compared with singletons ($n = 489$) undergoing this procedure and untested twins ($n = 477$).[13] Spontaneous abortion up to 4 weeks after the procedure occurred significantly more often in twin gestations in the tested group (2.73%) compared with twin controls (0.63%, $p = 0.01$) and post-procedure singleton controls (0.6%, $p = 0.01$), respectively. An abnormal karyotype was discovered in 3% of tested twin pregnancies (all discordant for the chromosomal anomaly) and in 1.23% of singletons. Although the number of studies is small and these procedures were performed by experienced operators, these data suggest an increase in background risk of loss in twin pregnancies, and perhaps an increase in procedure-related loss after amniocentesis.

The most recent study assessed the rate of fetal losses in twin pregnancies undergoing genetic mid-trimester amniocentesis.[14] A retrospective cohort study compared a group of women > 32 years old with twin pregnancies who underwent amniocentesis with a similar group unexposed to amniocentesis. The primary outcome was loss of one or both fetuses prior to 24 weeks' gestation. The rate of fetal losses was thrice among the amniocentesis group (3.0% vs. 0.8%), but the difference was not significant. No losses occurred within 4 weeks of the procedure. A meta-analysis of 2026 women with twin pregnancies found that, compared with women unexposed to the procedure, amniocentesis in women with twin pregnancies increased the risk of fetal losses prior to 20–24 weeks' gestation (OR 2.42; 95% CI 1.24–4.74) with an additional risk of one adverse outcome (1 or 2 fetal losses) for every 64 amnioceateses.[14]

The techniques of CVS in multiple gestations

CVS is a safe and effective prenatal diagnostic approach to multiple gestations. CVS, performed between 11 and 13 weeks, provides results much earlier in pregnancy and, if discordant results are discovered, potentially minimizes the medical (risk of loss) and psychologic difficulties encountered with late selective termination of an anomalous twin.

Ultrasound evaluation prior to performing CVS must be more comprehensive and detailed compared to that performed for amniocentesis. Ultrasound evaluation must be undertaken to determine fetal age, as an accepted standard of care is to perform CVS after 10 weeks' gestation based on crown–rump length, in order to avoid the purported increased risk of limb reduction defects when CVS is performed earlier. Also, a critical assessment is that of the site of placental implantation for each fetus. The site of placental implantation and uterine version both directly influence which of the two CVS methods, transcervical or transabdominal, is the approach to

Table 9.2 Loss rates following chorionic villus sampling in twin pregnancies based on studies published since 1991

Study	n	Loss to 20 weeks (%)	Loss to 28 weeks (%)	Fetal–fetal cell contamination (%)
Brambati et al[15]	65	—	1.7	11.2
Pergament et al[20]	128	2.3	3.1	3.2
Wapner et al[2]	161	3.1	3.1	3.8
De Catte et al[27]	104	2.9	—	3.8

optimize the safety for each gestation. Under these circumstances, CVS is routinely offered after 10 weeks' gestation and before the beginning of the 13th week of gestation. This window of time allows the operator to choose which of the two approaches offers the safest and most effective sampling of the placenta, which is based primarily on placental location. Performing CVS in the case of multiple gestations also demands meticulous written documentation, including diagrams of each of these characteristics, followed by similar painstaking attention to correct labeling of samples.

A major concern when performing CVS in multiple gestations is the failure to correctly sample the genotype of each fetus. In one study,[15] fetal–fetal cell contamination was greater than 10% in twin gestations, but subsequent studies have had rates of less than 4% (Table 9.2). Nevertheless, in the limited number of series published since 1991 and involving a total of 458 cases of twin pregnancies, i.e. 916 chorionic villus samplings, there were no instances where fetal–fetal cell contamination had a negative clinical consequence, nor was the number of such pregnancies recommended to undergo a mid-trimester amniocentesis different from that of singleton pregnancies undergoing CVS. Several strategies have been proposed to minimize this possibility and to ensure reliable sampling from each frondosum, including sampling at the margin of a placenta furthest from all other placentas present, avoiding the intertwin membrane, sampling nearest the insertion of

major blood vessels, and using a mixed technique of transabdominal and transcervical approaches, when appropriate. Otherwise, performing CVS in the case of multiple gestations is basically similar to sampling in singleton pregnancies, with attention being given to the specific ultrasound evaluations listed in the previous paragraph.

One study compared the diagnostic accuracy of amniocentesis and CVS in twins and triplets.[16] In the case of CVS performed in 163 twin pregnancies, uncertain results were present in seven CVS samples, five of which related to the presence of confined placental mosaicism. In the amniocenteses performed in 297 women with twins, no uncertain results and one incorrect result were present, probably a consequence of resampling of a single sac. In 15 triplet pregnancies undergoing prenatal genetic diagnosis, four by CVS and 11 by amniocentesis, two (one from each procedure) required repeat amniocentesis secondary to abnormal results. These authors[16] concluded that clinical diagnostic questions involving fetal–fetal cell contamination and confined placental mosaicism can be kept to a minimum with CVS.

It is mandatory that both an experienced operator and an equally experienced sonographer be present to ensure proper instrument placement, because markers are not available to ensure that each sample has been retrieved from a distinct placenta. Appelman and Furman[17] provided data on CVS in twins and delineated a history of the safety and efficacy of CVS for multiple gestations. However, in such complex testing it is to be expected that a 'learning curve' will take place. For example, a study by Casals et al[18] compared the results of two successive periods of CVS performed in multiple pregnancies by means of a transcervical biopsy forceps. Seventy-five samplings were performed in 38 twin sets and one triplet. A cytogenetic report was obtained in 73% of cases in the first period and in 98% in the second period, with the need for repeat amniocentesis decreasing from 38% to 10%, respectively. The spontaneous fetal loss rate in chromosomally and structurally normal fetuses sampled before the 20th week decreased from 8.7% to 3.3%, and the loss rate after the 20th week decreased from 3.3% to none. Such results strongly suggest that effectiveness and safety improve with increasing experience.[18]

Loss rates following CVS in multiple gestations

First-trimester CVS in multiple gestations appears to have pregnancy loss rates no greater than that following amniocentesis; in the four series reported since 1991, pregnancy loss rates ranged from 2.3 to 3.1% to 20 weeks' gestation and from 1.7 to 3.1% to 28 weeks' gestation (see Table 9.2). Furthermore, these rates are not dissimilar to those from CVS performed in singletons. Only two studies compared the procedure-related loss rates of first-trimester CVS with second-trimester amniocentesis.[2,19] In the first,[2] no difference was seen in the overall risk of pregnancy loss, 3.2% for CVS and 2.9% for amniocentesis. This study, however, found an increased risk of losing at least one fetus in the group sampled by amniocentesis, 4.9% for CVS and 9.3% for amniocentesis. The second study,[19] a retrospective comparison of 347 second-trimester amniocenteses and 69 CVS procedures, found that miscarriage occurred in 4.18% of women after amniocentesis and 4.54% of women after CVS. In the amniocentesis group, the risk of miscarriage was higher

in cases using transplacental entry (4.54%) compared to those with transamniotic entry (2.08%). The rates of preterm delivery <32 weeks and preterm delivery <35 weeks in the amniocentesis group were 11.8% and 32.4% and in the CVS group 16.7% and 23.8%, respectively. The total fetal loss rate was similar in the amniocentesis group (8.8%) and the CVS group (10.2%).

A similar conclusion was reached when the experiences of several centers performing CVS in twin gestations were compared with published studies on pregnancy loss rates following amniocentesis.[20] This would suggest that first-trimester CVS should be preferred over second-trimester amniocentesis for prenatal genetic diagnoses in the case of multiple gestations.

Both amniocentesis and CVS have been used in the evaluation of triplets and higher-order multiple gestations, but no data exist regarding relative or absolute safety and efficacy. The main problem is with CVS, which has no marker to exclude repeated sampling of the same chorion. Thus, CVS in higher-order multiples should be limited to only the most experienced centers.

INVASIVE DIAGNOSIS PRIOR TO OR AFTER MULTIFETAL PREGNANCY REDUCTION

The risk of amniocentesis after multifetal pregnancy reduction (MFPR) has been studied because of the increased maternal age associated with high-order multiple pregnancy. Tabsch and Theroux[21] found a higher loss rate for MFPR pregnancies that subsequently underwent amniocentesis (9.4%). McLean et al[22] in 1998 described 79 pregnancies that underwent amniocentesis after MFPR, reporting a loss rate of 5.1%, which was less than the reported loss rates after MFPR alone (11.9%). Selam et al[23] reported on 127 MFPR procedures followed by amniocentesis in the second trimester. The loss rates between the sampled and unsampled groups were not statistically different (3.1 versus

7.2%). However, a reporting bias exists secondary to the loss of some pregnancies before the time of amniocentesis.

CVS before MFPR in an advanced maternal age patient is favored by many centers as a means to avoid later selective termination and to avoid reduction of normal fetuses. Data from several centers show no significant increased risk of preprocedure diagnosis in terms of fetal loss and obstetrical outcome.[24,25]

An important aspect of pre-MFPR CVS is the potential abuse of the genetic analysis for gender selection. It is therefore recommended that CVS should be done only on the fetuses that are selected to survive. If the results are normal, the other fetuses are submitted to MFPR irrespective of their (unknown) gender.

FETAL BLOOD SAMPLING

At times, it becomes necessary to obtain fetal blood via funipuncture (cordocentesis). In a retrospective study of 84 twin pregnancies that were tested with fetal blood sampling, the loss rates were as follows: miscarriage 3.6%, total fetal loss 13.6%, and fetal loss attributed to the procedure 8.2%.[26] The procedure-related fetal loss rate was dependent on the indication for fetal blood sampling. The rates of preterm delivery at ≤ 32 weeks, preterm delivery at ≤ 35 weeks, perinatal mortality at 28 weeks, perinatal mortality at > 28 weeks, and neonatal mortality were 16.9%, 28.3%, 10.9%, 3.1%, and 7.7%, respectively. These figures are substantially higher than those reported for amniocentesis and CVS. Thus, this procedure should be reserved only for special circumstances such as fetal hydrops and infection.

CONCLUSIONS

Genetic diagnoses in multiple gestations present certain unique features both in terms of genetic counseling and in terms of the estimations of occurrence and recurrence risks. The genetic counseling session for multiple gestations must include an assessment of the genetic risks, the risks of the procedure, and the potential for selective termination. Diagnostic genetic testing in the case of multiple gestations involves the same laboratory technologies as applied to singleton pregnancies, and therefore can be considered accurate and efficacious when performed by those experienced in cytogenetics, biochemical analyses, and recombinant DNA technologies.

REFERENCES

1. Alfirevic Z, Walkinshaw SA. Guidelines and Audit Committee of the Royal College of Obstetricians and Gynaecologists: Amniocentesis and Chorionic Villus Sampling. Guideline No 8; revised January 2005.

2. Wapner RJ, Johnson A, Davis G et al. Prenatal diagnosis in twin gestations: a comparison between second trimester amniocentesis and first trimester chorionic villus sampling. Obstet Gynecol 1993; 82: 49–56.

3. Ghidini A, Lynch L, Hicks C et al. The risk of second trimester amniocentesis in twin gestations: a case–control study. Am J Obstet Gynecol 1993; 169: 1013–16.

4. Pruggmayer MR, Jahoda MG, Van der Pol JG et al. Genetic amniocentesis in twin pregnancies: results of a multicenter study of 529 cases. Ultrasound Obstet Gynecol 1992; 2: 6–10.

5. Sebire NJ, Noble PL, Odibo A et al. Single uterine entry for genetic amniocentesis in twin pregnancies. Ultrasound Obstet Gynecol 1996; 7: 26–31.

6. Buscaglia M, Ghisoni L, Bellotti M et al. Genetic amniocentesis in biamniotic twin pregnancies by a single transabdominal insertion of the needle. Prenat Diagn 1995; 15: 17–19.

7. van Vugt JM, Nieuwint A, van Geijn HP. Single-needle insertion: an alternative technique for early second-trimester genetic twin amniocentesis. Fetal Diagn Ther 1995; 10: 178–81.

8. van der Pol JG, Wolf H, Boer K et al. Jejunal atresia related to the use of methylene blue in genetic amniocentesis in twins. Br J Obstet Gynaecol 1992; 99: 141–3.

9. Dinger J, Autenrieth A, Kamin G, Goebel P, Hinkel GK. Jejunal atresia related to the use of toluidine blue

in genetic amniocentesis in twins. J Perinat Med 2003; 31: 266–8.

10. Shalev J, Meizner I, Rabinerson D et al. Elective cyto-genetic amniocentesis in the third trimester for preg-nancies with high risk factors. Prenat Diagn 1999; 19: 749–52.

11. Cirigliano V, Canadas P, Plaja A, Ordonez E, Mediano C, Sanchez A, Farran I. Rapid prenatal diagnosis of aneuploidies and zygosity in multiple pregnancies by amniocentesis with single insertion of the needle and quantitative fluorescent PCR. Prenat Diagn 2003; 23: 629–33.

12. Lewi L, Blickstein I, Van Schoubroeck D et al. Diagnosis and management of heterokaryotypic monochorionic twins. Am J Med Genet 2006; 140: 272–5.

13. Yukobowich E, Anteby EY, Cohen SM, Lavy Y, Granat M, Yagel S. Risk of fetal loss in twin pregnan-cies undergoing second trimester amniocentesis. Obstet Gynecol 2001; 98: 231–4.

14. Millaire M, Bujold E, Morency AM, Gauthier RJ. Mid-trimester genetic amniocentesis in twin preg-nancy and the risk of fetal loss. J Obstet Gynaecol Can 2006; 28: 512–18.

15. Brambati B, Tului L, Lanzani A et al. First trimester genetic diagnosis in multiple pregnancy: principles and potential pitfalls. Prenat Diagn 1991; 11: 767–74.

16. van den Berg C, Braat AP, Van Opstal D et al. Amniocentesis or chorionic villus sampling in multi-ple gestations? Experience with 500 cases. Prenat Diagn 1999; 19: 234–44.

17. Appelman Z, Furman B. Invasive genetic diagnosis in multiple pregnancies. Obstet Gynecol Clin North Am 2005; 32: 97–103.

18. Casals G, Borrell A, Martinez JM, Soler A, Cararach V, Fortuny A. Transcervical chorionic villus sampling in multiple pregnancies using a biopsy forceps. Prenat Diagn 2002; 22: 260–5.

19. Antsaklis A, Souka AP, Daskalakis G, Kavalakis Y, Michalas S. Second-trimester amniocentesis vs. chori-onic villus sampling for prenatal diagnosis in multiple gestations. Ultrasound Obstet Gynecol 2002; 20: 476–81.

20. Pergament E, Schulman JD, Copeland K et al. The risk of and efficacy of chorionic villus sampling in multiple gestations. Prenat Diagn 1992; 12: 377–84.

21. Tabsch KM, Theroux NL. Genetic amniocentesis following multifetal pregnancy reduction to twins: assessing the risk. Prenat Diagn 1995; 15: 221–3.

22. McLean LK, Evans MI, Carpenter RJ Jr, Johnson MP, Goldberg JD. Genetic amniocentesis following multi-fetal pregnancy reduction does not increase the risk of pregnancy loss. Prenat Diagn 1998; 18: 186–8.

23. Selam B, Torok O, Lembet A, Stone J, Lapinski R, Berkowitz RL. Genetic amniocentesis after multifetal pregnancy reduction. Am J Obstet Gynecol 1999; 180: 226–30.

24. Aytoz A, De Catte L, Camus M et al. Obstetric out-come after prenatal diagnosis in pregnancies obtained after intracytoplasmic sperm injection. Hum Reprod 1998; 13: 2958–61.

25. De Catte L, Camus M, Bonduelle M, Liebaers I, Foulon W. Prenatal diagnosis by chorionic villus sam-pling in multiple pregnancies prior to fetal reduction. Am J Perinatol 1998; 15: 339–43.

26. Antsaklis A, Daskalakis G, Souka AP, Kavalakis Y, Michalas S. Fetal blood sampling in twin pregnancies. Ultrasound Obstet Gynecol 2003; 22: 377–9.

27. De Catte L, Liebaers I, Foulon W. Outcome of twin gestations after first trimester chorionic villus sampling. Obstet Gynercol 2000; 96: 714–20.

10

Assessment of growth by ultrasound

INTRODUCTION

This chapter addresses the following specific aspects of growth in the twin fetus:

(1) The importance of correlating the ultrasound measurements of the head circumference (HC), abdominal circumference (AC), and femur length with those derived from twin rather than singleton pregnancies;

(2) The distinction between estimates of birth weight in twins with dichorionic vs. monochorionic placentation;

(3) Use of the best formula for estimating the *in utero* weight of the twin fetus and subsequently assigning the appropriate weight centile;

(4) The interpretation of antenatal findings in the normal twin relative to the discordant co-twin;

(5) Distinguishing the small-for-gestational-age (SGA) from the intrauterine growth-restricted (IUGR) fetus;

(6) Raising the index of suspicion regarding the possibility of the occurrence of twin–twin transfusion syndrome (TTTS) in any pregnancy with monochorionic placentation.

GROWTH CURVES

In the past, it was thought that intrauterine growth in twin pregnancies began to fall below that of singletons at approximately the 30th week.[1] However, more recent observations indicate that ACs of the twin fall below those of singleton as early as 15 weeks' gestation (Table 10.1). Of importance is the observation that, as pregnancy advances, the differences in ACs between twin and singleton fetuses widen from approximately 1.0 cm to 2.0 cm at 31 and 38 weeks, respectively.[2] Likewise, the differences between the actual birth weights of singleton and twin fetuses increase with advancing gestation, from approximately 150 g to 610 g at 31 and 40 weeks, respectively.[1] Of particular interest is that the 50th weight centile of twin fetuses crosses the 10th weight centile of singleton fetuses at approximately the 37th pregnancy week, and subsequently falls below the 10th centile of singletons (Figure 10.1).

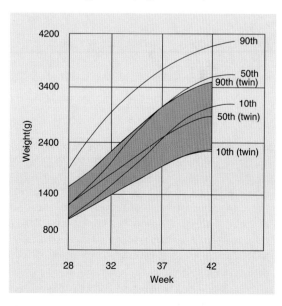

Figure 10.1 Intrauterine growth chart for singleton and twin fetuses. Adapted from reference 1

Table 10.1 Comparison of abdominal circumference (AC) measurements of single and twin fetuses at the 10th centile rank in pregnancies from 14 to 39 weeks' gestation (Sabbagha and colleagues, unpublished data)

GA (weeks)	AC centiles in singletons			AC centiles in twin fetuses		
	5th	50th	90th	5th	50th	90th
14	6.6	9.0	10.8	6.7	9.1	11.0
15	7.7	10.1	11.4	7.3	9.6	11.0
16	8.8	11.1	12.7	8.6	10.9	13.0
17	9.8	12.2	13.7	9.6	12.0	14.0
18	11.5	13.8	14.7	10.6	12.9	15.0
19	12.5	14.8	16.6	12.5	14.9	17.0
20	13.6	15.9	17.4	13.3	15.6	17.0
21	14.5	16.8	18.4	14.3	16.6	18.0
22	15.6	17.9	19.5	15.4	17.7	19.0
23	16.6	18.9	20.8	16.7	19.0	21.0
24	17.7	20.1	21.5	17.4	19.7	21.0
25	18.8	21.1	23.2	19.1	21.4	23.0
26	20.0	22.3	24.2	20.1	22.4	24.0
27	20.9	23.2	25.0	20.9	23.2	25.0
28	22.4	24.7	26.3	22.2	24.5	26.0
29	23.4	25.7	27.2	23.1	25.4	27.0
30	24.4	26.7	28.6	24.5	26.8	29.0
31	25.4	27.7	28.61	24.51	27.82	29.0
32	26.7	29.0	30.1	26.0	28.3	30.0
33	27.6	29.9	30.8	26.7	29.0	31.0
34	28.5	30.9	31.5	27.4	29.7	32.0
35	29.7	32.0	32.5	28.4	30.8	33.0
36	30.9	33.2	33.7	29.6	31.9	34.0
37	31.5	33.8	34.5	30.4	32.7	34.0
38	32.2	34.5	35.3	31.2	33.6	35.0
39	33.0	35.3	36.5	32.4	34.7	36.0

GA, gestational age

Monochorionic and dichorionic twin pregnancies differ in birth weights at varying gestational ages.[3] In a study of 1302 twin gestations, the mean birth weights (one standard deviation, 1 SD) of monochorionic twins (21% of total twin pregnancies) were significantly smaller than those with dichorionic placentation.[3] These differences, as well as the differences in growth curves between twins and singletons, underscore the importance of evaluating antenatal ultrasound measurements in relation to charts derived from twin pregnancies. The use of specific twin growth charts allows for:

(1) More accurate determination of the extent of discordance between twin fetuses;

(2) Better identification of the SGA as well as the IUGR fetus;

(3) Correction of the artefactual increase in the proportion of diagnosed SGA twins, solely because they are compared with the normally larger singleton fetus (see below).

DISCORDANCE IN TWINS

Discordance in the estimated weights of twins is an important contributor to fetal mortality and morbidity.[4] This phenomenon is often defined as at least a 15% difference in the estimated twin weights, calculated according to the larger twin. According to recent studies, however, the more appropriate cut-off difference appears to be 25%.[5] Part of the reason behind this suggestion is that 15% discordance is observed in up to 25% of twin pregnancies, whereas severe discordance (30% or more) is present in only about 5% of twin pregnancies.[4] Moreover, of great clinical importance, a divergence in the estimated twin weights of 25% is associated with a 6.5-fold increase in fetal death risk,[6] but a divergence of 31–40% carries an odds ratio of 5.6 for fetal death.[7] In contrast, the association between birth weight discordance and neonatal mortality is not as clear. Some reports show no significant increase in neonatal mortality,[8] but others point to a significant elevation in neonatal mortality among twins with >30% discordance.[9]

Regardless of such issues, it is useful to emphasize that factors other than mere discordance come into play when assessing divergent intertwin growth. For example, approximately two-thirds of highly discordant twins, that is, those differing in estimated weight by 30% or more, are in fact growth-restricted, weighing at or below the 5th centile for gestational age.[10] Given these circumstances, the presence of IUGR may be a greater contributor to neonatal mortality than is discordance *per se*.[8,11] Other contributors to outcome include, but are not limited to, observations regarding size of the AC, evolution of biometric measurements over time, quantity of amniotic fluid, the biophysical profile, the non-stress test, umbilical Doppler systolic/diastolic ratio, presence of diastolic velocity flow, and occurrence of TTS.

Recently, Blickstein and Keith[10] compared neonatal mortality rates among three groups of discordant twins (>25%), distinguished by the birth weight of the smaller twin being <10th, 10th to 50th, or >50th percentile. Among the 10 683 pairs of twins who were studied, the respective proportions of the three groups were 62.4%, 32.9%, and 4.7%. The neonatal mortality rate was significantly higher among pairs in which the smaller twin weighed <10th birth weight percentile (29.0 vs 11.1 per 1000; OR 2.7; 95% CI 1.3, 5.7). This difference results from the higher mortality rates among the smaller but not among the larger twins. These authors thus defined the subgroup of severely discordant twin pairs at an increased risk of neonatal death. Identification of this group, in other words – defining if the smaller twin of a discordant pair is <10th birth weight percentile – is an imperative step in the management of birth weight discordance in twin gestations.[12]

Unfortunately, the accurate estimation of discordance is quite difficult. This is a direct result of the plus/minus situation that exists in estimated fetal weights. For example, a 2000/2000 g twin pair (0% discordance) can be estimated to be 2200 (+10%, overestimated)/1800 (–10%, underestimated) and to produce a 400/2200 (18.1%) estimated birth weight difference.[13] Blickstein et al[13] compared the efficacies of intertwin difference in AC and estimated fetal weight (EFW) to predict birth weight discordance in 90 twin gestations with sonographic measurements of AC and femur length, performed within 2 weeks before delivery. The authors calculated and compared the rates of false-positive and false-negative prediction of the cut-off values of 15, 20, and 25% intertwin birth weight discordance by the intertwin EFW difference and an intertwin AC difference of ≥18 mm. The two methods were comparable in excluding birth weight differences at 15–25% discordance and at >25% discordance. However, because of the relatively low positive predictive values, birth weight discordance could not be accurately predicted by either method. This view was supported by others.[14] However, some authors still are of the opinion that sonographic prediction of actual intertwin birth weight discordance of 25% or greater,[15] or differences in AC or the ratio between ACs,[16] are valid and reliable methods for clinical use.

THE SGA VERSUS THE INTRAUTERINE GROWTH-RESTRICTED FETUS

The SGA fetus is defined as a small fetus that is not necessarily growth-restricted. Its weight generally falls at or close to the 10th centile rank. It is not associated with markers of growth restriction such as low amniotic fluid level, poor interval growth, and abnormal umbilical Doppler findings – all of which are observed in the IUGR twin. In the twin fetus, the estimated weight, including the centile rank, will be incorrectly low if the comparison is made with charts derived from singleton pregnancies. As a result, the proportion of SGA fetuses will be higher, and poor perinatal outcome will be inappropriately predicted.

Estimating fetal weight

The best estimates of fetal weight by ultrasound are derived from mathematic formulae incorporating measurement of the HC, AC, and femur length (FL). In a large study, Hadlock and colleagues obtained the following formula for estimation of fetal weight:[17]

$$\log_{10}(\text{weight}) = 1.326 - 0.00326\ (\text{AC} \times \text{FL}) \\ + 0.0107\ \text{HC} + 0.0438\ \text{AC} \\ + 0.158\ \text{FL}$$

In this study, the authors showed that the accuracy of estimates of birth weight varied by 14.8% (2 SD). However, they also showed that the accuracy of the estimate deteriorated to 19.4% (2 SD) in smaller fetuses with a birth weight < 1500 g. Further, the formula by Hadlock failed to take into account the specific growth curves of the three recognized fetal populations, namely: the small-, appropriate- or large-for-gestational age groups. Formulae targeted to the specific population in question have a smaller cumulative 2 SD variation (see below).[18]

Targeted weight formulae

In a particular fetus, the estimation of birth weight is more accurate if the formula used is derived from data applicable to the specific fetal population in question. Such formulae are known as targeted formulae and incorporate gestational age (weeks) + HC + 2AC + FL.[18] In targeted formulae, gestational age (in weeks) is included because the HC/AC ratio varies at different intervals in pregnancy.[19] The difference in the HC/AC ratio is noted regardless of whether fetal growth is normal or altered (Table 10.2).

Further, the gestational age used should be based on either dates according to the last menstrual period (LMP) that are confirmed by ultrasound, or ultrasound results obtained by 26 weeks' gestation, because the 2 SD variation in weeks increases, beginning at the 27th pregnancy week. Moreover, targeted formulae doubly weight the AC, a measurement that best correlates with fetal weight.[20] Thus, the AC can be used to determine the specific growth curve of the fetus. When the AC is small (i.e. 5th centile, Table 10.1) the EFW is best derived from a formula targeted to the SGA fetus (Table 10.3).[17] Likewise, when the AC falls in an average centile rank (AC > 5th and < 90th percentiles, see Table 10.1), the EFW is best derived from a formula targeted to the appropriate-for-gestational-age fetus (see Table 10.3).[18] Finally, when the AC is at the 90th centile, the EFW is best derived from a formula targeted to the large-for-gestational-age (LGA) fetus. However, as twins are rarely considered large for gestational age, the EFW in the twin with an AC at the 90th centile can be appropriately derived from the formula targeted to the fetus with an average AC. Compared with the formula by Hadlock and colleagues, formulae targeted to gestational age and fetal AC centile ranks reduce the cumulative absolute 2 SD variation by 21.7%, from 15.6 to 12%.[18]

The addition of Doppler velocimetry of various fetal vessels can help in assessing discordance. This issue is discussed in Chapter 11.

Table 10.2 Dynamic changes in head circumference (HC) and abdominal circumference (AC) measurements in pregnancies with normal and altered fetal growth. Adapted from reference 19

HC/AC ratio is >1.0 prior to 36 pregnancy weeks
HC/AC ratio is <1.0 after 36 pregnancy weeks
HC/AC ratio is <1.0 in the macrosomic fetus
HC/AC ratio is not altered in the LGA fetus
HC/AC ratio is not altered in symmetric IUGR
HC/AC ratio is >1.0 in asymmetric IUGR

IUGR, intrauterine growth restriction; LGA, large for gestational age

Table 10.3 Targeted formulae used in the prediction of fetal weight. Adaped from reference 18

Group	Formula
Appropriate for gestational age	$-55.3 - (16.35 \times SUM) + (0.25838 \times SUM^2)$ $(r = 0.97, r^2 = 0.94)$
Small for gestational age	$1849.4 - (47.13 \times SUM) + (0.37721 \times SUM^2)$ $(r = 0.96, r^2 = 0.92)$ $SUM = GA\ (weeks) + 2AC\ (cm) + HC\ (cm) + FL\ (cm)$

GA, gestational age; AC, abdominal circumference; HC, head circumference; FL, femur length

Assigning *in utero* weight centile

Once the fetal weight is estimated, it should be assigned a centile rank. Ananth and associates published birth weight centiles for both monochorionic and dichorionic twins (Tables 10.4 and 10.5).[3] Interestingly, these investigators found that stratifying the data further relative to parity and gender yielded almost identical curves. The latter finding implies that parity and gender are not significant contributors to differences in the two twin birth weight curves – an important finding, since both parity and gender are implicated as factors influencing birth weight in singleton pregnancies.

A distinct advantage of the birth weight centiles published by Ananth and associates[3] is that the data shown begin at the 23rd pregnancy week and not at the 28th or 32nd pregnancy week, as presented in other reports. Additionally, the data of Ananth and associates are based on accurate estimation of gestational age. Specifically, ultrasound was used either to confirm dates assigned by the LMP or to establish pregnancy dates by early ultrasound.

It is essential, however, to note that differences are present between the twin birth weight centiles published by Ananth and associates and Alexander and co-workers.[3,21] Although such differences are small at the 50th centile level, they are marked both at the 90th and the 10th centile ranks. Specifically, the twin birth weights of Alexander and co-workers are larger at the 90th rank but smaller at the 10th centile rank (Table 10.6). These differences can be explained, in part, by the following factors:

(1) Twin birth weights represent population studies drawn from the 1991–95 Natality Data Files (from the National Center for Health Statistics), and include white and African-American racial groups;

(2) Gestational age in completed weeks is based on the interval between the recorded date of the last menses and the date of birth, but otherwise is not corroborated by ultrasound dating;

(3) Twin birth weights are not stratified by chorionicity, that is, they include both dichorionic and monochorionic twins.

At this stage, it is important to acknowledge the difference between being small for gestational age – a diagnosis that is derived from a point observation in time, and being growth restricted – a diagnosis made from serial (>1) observations. It is true that the likelihood of growth restriction increases if the individual fetus weighs below the 5th or the 3rd centile. For this reason it is important to realize that only the differences observed below the

Table 10.4 Smoothed birth weight centiles for twins with monochorionic placentation. Adapted from reference 3

GA (weeks)	No. of pregnancies	Smoothed birth weight centiles					
		5th	10th	50th	90th	95th
23	3	392	431	533	648	683
24	8	456	501	620	753	794
25	4	530	582	720	875	922
26	2	615	676	836	1017	1072
27	7	713	784	970	1178	1242
28	8	823	904	1119	1360	1433
29	6	944	1037	1282	1559	1643
30	8	1072	1178	1457	1771	1867
31	6	1204	1323	1637	1990	2097
32	15	1335	1467	1814	2205	2325
33	22	1457	1601	1980	2407	2537
34	27	1562	1716	2123	2580	2720
35	30	1646	1808	2237	2719	2866
36	47	1728	1899	2349	2855	3009
37	26	1831	2012	2489	3025	3189
38	27	1957	2150	2660	3233	3408
39	24	2100	2307	2854	3469	3657
40	2	2255	2478	3065	3726	3927
41	2	2422	2661	3292	4001	4217

GA, gestational age

Table 10.5 Smoothed birth weight centiles for twins with dichorionic placentation. Adapted from reference 3

GA (weeks)	No. of pregnancies	Smoothed birth weight centiles				
		5th	10th	50th	90th	95th
23	4	477	513	632	757	801
24	7	538	578	712	853	903
25	13	606	652	803	962	1018
26	10	684	735	906	1085	1148
27	10	771	829	1021	1223	1294
28	18	870	935	1152	1379	1459
29	16	980	1054	1298	1554	1645
30	27	1102	1186	1460	1748	1850
31	39	1235	1328	1635	1958	2072
32	41	1374	1477	1819	2179	2306
33	47	1515	1630	2007	2403	2543
34	86	1653	1778	2190	2622	2775
35	84	1781	1916	2359	2825	2989
36	210	1892	2035	2506	3001	3176
37	139	1989	2139	2634	3155	3339
38	146	2079	2236	2753	3297	3489
39	85	2167	2331	2870	3437	3637
40	46	2258	2428	2990	3581	3790
41	3	2352	2530	3115	3731	3948

GA, gestational age

Table 10.6 Comparison of the 10th birth weight centiles of twin pregnancies. Adapted from references 3 and 21

Pregnancy week	Placentation			
	Dichorionic and monochorionic (Alexander et al)	Dichorionic (Ananth et al)	Monochorionic (Ananth et al)	Average of three charts
23	413	513	431	452
24	454	578	501	511
25	539	652	582	591
26	595	735	676	668
27	680	829	784	764
28	765	935	904	868
29	910	1054	1037	1000
30	1021	1186	1178	1128
31	1183	1328	1323	1278
32	1135	1477	1467	1359
33	1530	1630	1601	1587
34	1695	1778	1716	1729
35	1862	1916	1808	1862
36	2013	2035	1899	1982
37	2155	2139	2012	2102
38	2245	2236	2150	2210
39	2260	2331	2307	2299

10th centile rank have significant clinical implications.

Difficulties may arise. For example, a particular co-twin can be classified as normal if evaluated by the Alexander and co-workers chart, but SGA when compared with the data of Ananth and associates (see Table 10.6). The best practical solution to this issue, at present, is to use the 10th centile data derived from the average of the three twin curves (see Table 10.6). Otherwise, each center would have to obtain the 10th birth weight centile applicable to its own population. Nonetheless, the twin birth weight data of Ananth and associates can be used if the twins in question have similar population characteristics.

Currently, chorionicity can be readily determined antenatally with an accuracy of 94% and 88% in dichorionic and monochorionic placentation, respectively (see Chapter 5). Thus, the ultrasonographer is now capable of utilizing the appropriate birth weight centile chart for the twin fetus in question.

Interpretation of results

Having assigned the estimated birth weight and its centile rank, one is now able to compare the growth status of the twins. The following three examples illustrate the thought process in the interpretation of findings in some twin fetuses.

Interpretation. The twins are discordant in weight (at the 20% level) but twin 1 is not below the 5th or the 10th centile in weight and is thus not considered SGA. Further, the likelihood of being growth restricted is low – although it is smaller in size than twin 2. One has to determine whether the smaller fetus has always been small or whether there has been a recent adverse occurrence. If the decline in weight is not of recent onset, it would be likely that the fetus is SGA rather than growth-restricted. The SGA diagnosis can be further corroborated by:

(1) The finding of normal amniotic fluid (subjectively and by the presence of a vertical pocket of amniotic fluid >2 cm);
(2) Normal umbilical Doppler study (systolic/diastolic, S/D) ratio falling within 2 SD of normal;
(3) The presence of diastolic velocity flow.

Nonetheless, in such cases, close follow-up is still mandatory.

Interpretation. The twins are discordant in weight (at approximately the 30% level). The weight of twin 1 is between the 5th and 10th centile ranks and it is suspected to exhibit

Example 2

Set B twins	Weeks' estimated gestation	Weight (g)	Centile rank for dichorionic pregnancy	Interpretation
Co-twin 1	32	1390	5–10	IUGR twin*
Co-twin 2	32	2000	75	

IUGR. As such, its risk of fetal death is increased and careful evaluation of amniotic fluid level and umbilical Doppler is recommended. Depending on these results, as well as on the attainment of fetal pulmonary maturity, preterm delivery may be indicated. In such cases the administration of steroids to the mother may be a consideration to enhance the development of pulmonary maturity.

Interpretation. The twins are discordant in weight (at approximately the 23% level). However, the centile rank of the smaller twin is considered normal. The likelihood is that

Example 1

Set A twins	Weeks' estimated gestation	Weight (g)	Centile rank for dichorionic pregnancy	Interpretation
Co-twin 1	28	1000	15–20	SGA twin*
Co-twin 2	28	1200	75	

Example 3

Set C twins	Weeks' estimated gestation	Weight (g)	Centile rank for dichorionic pregnancy	Interpretation
Co-twin 1	34	2000	25	Normal twin*
Co-twin 2	34	2600	75–90	

twin 1 is smaller but otherwise normal. The diagnosis should also be corroborated by the finding of normal fetal anatomy, amniotic fluid level, umbilical Doppler study, biophysical profile, and non-stress test.

REFERENCES

1. Leroy B, Lefort F, Neveu P et al. Intrauterine growth charts for twin fetuses. Acta Genet Med Gemellol 1982; 31: 199–206.
2. Socol ML, Tamura R, Sabbagha RE et al. Diminished biparietal diameter and abdominal circumference growth in twins. Obstet Gynecol 1984; 64: 235–8.
3. Ananth CV, Vintzileos AM, Shen-Schwarz S et al. Standards of birth weight in twin gestations stratified by placental chorionicity. Obstet Gynecol 1998; 91: 917–24.
4. Branum AM, Schoendorf KC. The effect of birth weight discordance on twin neonatal mortality. Obstet Gynecol 2003; 101: 570–4.
5. Blickstein I, Kalish RB. Birthweight discordance in multiple pregnancy. Twin Res 2003; 6: 526–31.
6. Erkkola R, Ala-Mello S, Piiroinen O et al. Growth discordancy in twin pregnancies: a risk factor not detected by measurement of biparietal diameter. Obstet Gynecol 1985; 66: 203–6.
7. Hollier LM, McIntire DD, Leven KJ. Outcome of twin pregnancies according to intrapair birth weight differences. Obstet Gynecol 1999; 94: 1006–10.
8. Patterson RM, Wood RC. What is twin birthweight discordance? Am J Perinatol 1990; 7: 217–19.
9. Yalcin HR, Zorlu CG, Lembet A et al. The significance of birth weight difference in discordant twins: a level to standardize? Acta Obstet Gynecol Scand 1998; 77: 28–31.
10. Blickstein I, Keith LG. Neonatal mortality rates among growth-discordant twins, classified according to the birth weight of the smaller twin. Am J Obstet Gynecol 2004; 190: 170–4.
11. O'Brien WF, Knuppel RA, Scerbo JC, Rattan KP. Birth weight in twins: an analysis of discordancy and growth retardation. Obstet Gynecol 1986; 67: 483–6.
12. Fraser D, Picard R, Picard E, Leiberman JR. Birth weight discordance, intrauterine growth retardation and perinatal outcome in twins. J Reprod Med 1994; 39: 504–8.
13. Blickstein I, Manor M, Levi R, Goldchmit R. Is inter-twin birth weight discordance predictable? Gynecol Obstet Invest 1996; 42: 105–8.
14. Caravello JW, Chauhan SP, Morrison JC et al. Sonographic examination does not predict twin growth discordance accurately. Obstet Gynecol 1997; 89: 529–33.
15. Gernt PR, Mauldin JG, Newman RB, Durkalski VL. Sonographic prediction of twin birth weight discordance. Obstet Gynecol 2001; 97: 53–6.
16. Klam SL, Rinfret D, Leduc L. Prediction of growth discordance in twins with the use of abdominal circumference ratios. Am J Obstet Gynecol 2005; 192: 247–51.
17. Hadlock FP, Harrist RB, Sharman RS et al. Estimation of fetal weight with the use of head, body and femur measurements – a prospective study. Am J Obstet Gynecol 1985; 151: 333–7.
18. Sabbagha RE, Minogue J, Tamura R, Hungerford SA. Estimation of birth weight by the use of ultrasound formulas targeted to large, appropriate, and small for gestational age fetuses. Am J Obstet Gynecol 1989; 160: 854–62.
19. Sabbagha RE, Minogue J. Altered fetal growth. In: Sabbagha RE, ed. Diagnostic Ultrasound Applied to Obstetrics and Gynecology. Philadelphia: JB Lippincott, 1994: 187.
20. Landan MB, Mintz MC, Gabbe SG. Sonographic evaluation of fetal abdominal growth: predictor of the large-for-gestational-age infant in pregnancy complicated by diabetes mellitus. Am J Obstet Gynecol 1989; 160: 115–18.
21. Alexander GR, Kogan M, Martin J, Papiernik E. What are the fetal growth patterns of singletons, twins, and triplets in the United States? Clin Obstet Gynecol 1998; 41: 115–25.

Assessing the fetus at risk by Doppler

11

INTRODUCTION

Whereas it is generally recognized that perinatal mortality is higher in multiple than in singleton pregnancies, it is often unappreciated that the incidence of placental insufficiency is also higher in multiples than is the case for singletons, and that this circumstance is associated with the risk of intrauterine growth restriction (IUGR) and intrauterine death of a fetus. The main source of morbidity in multiple pregnancy is prematurity followed by IUGR, manifest in the form of either birth weight below the 10th centile for gestational age or significant discordant.

Growth discordance and overall outcomes

Several studies suggest that discordance and growth restriction are associated with unequal or reduced redistribution of fetoplacental blood flow. In such pregnancies, increased resistance in the umbilical artery (UA) suggests downstream resistance to flow and placental insufficiency.

Many parameters have been used to identify discordant growth patterns, including intrapair differences in biparietal diameter (BPD), abdominal circumference (AC), femoral length (FL), and estimated fetal weight. The most common definitions of growth discordance are based on an intertwin birth weight difference expressed as a percentage of the larger twin weight. The cut-off values for percentage difference of birth weight proposed in the literature vary from 15 to 40%.[1,2]

Numerous investigators report the use of umbilical artery velocimetry for the surveillance of twin pregnancies.[3,4] Abnormal umbilical artery velocity waveforms reflect unequal fetal–placental circulation, a circumstance which is probably a major contributor to growth discordance in twin pregnancies. Saldana and colleagues found that a difference in S/D ratio in the umbilical artery was a better predictor of discordance than a difference in estimated fetal weight.[4] Farmakides and associates used a difference in S/D > 0.4 for identification of discordant growth.[3] Similar results were obtained by Divon and Weiner when applying a difference of S/D ratio > 15%.[1] Perhaps more important, Gerson and colleagues demonstrated in twins and triplets that discordance in S/D ratio was present prior to the development of discordant ultrasound measurements.[5]

Shah and co-workers reported that the S/D ratios for small discordant twins were significantly different from those of normal singleton pregnancies.[6] They found that discordant twin gestations with an SGA fetus had a significant intrapair S/D difference as compared with concordant twins.[6] Degani and colleagues looked for the presence of SGA fetuses, and, by adding the use of the internal carotid artery to the umbilical artery pulsatility index (PI), increased the sensitivity of the diagnosis.[7] Seelbach-Gobel and colleagues, in a study of the pulsatility indices of the fetal aorta and the UA in twin pairs, noted a correlation between aortic and umbilical Doppler differences where there was a greater than 20% weight difference between the twins, and worst outcome with absent diastolic blood flow.[8] Kurmanavicius and associates, on the basis of UA Doppler velocimetry, were able to identify the twin with a reduced growth rate in 77.8% of cases.[9]

Other researchers did not recommend Doppler measurements in the management of unselected twin pregnancies. Faber and co-workers, in a prospective study, assessed the predictive value of Doppler measurements (PI in the umbilical artery, middle cerebral artery (MCA), and aorta) with regard to pregnancy outcome.[10] The prediction of fetal distress (hypoxia, preterm birth, poor fetal growth, acidosis, and disturbed neonatal adaptation) with Doppler had a sensitivity of 25% and a positive predictive value of 63%. These investigators concluded that Doppler screening might be useful even in unselected twin pregnancies.[10]

The potential value of combined Doppler and biometry in assessing discordant fetal growth in twins was studied in 40 sets of twins by Chittacharoen et al,[11] who showed that the diagnostic accuracy provided by ultrasonographic biometry was not significantly different from that provided by umbilical Doppler velocimetry, for overall sensitivity and specificity values of 92% and 70%, respectively. Finally, a recent prospective, randomized, controlled multicenter trial was carried out to assess the value of umbilical artery Doppler ultrasound added to standard ultrasound biometry measurements in the management of twin pregnancies. Women were randomized at 25 weeks' gestation to receive standard ultrasound biometric assessment or standard assessment plus Doppler ultrasound umbilical artery flow velocity waveform analysis.[12] Both groups had close follow-up during pregnancy. Outcome measures were analyzed on intention-to-treat statistics and included mode of delivery, perinatal mortality, hypertension, antenatal admissions, gestational age at delivery, 5 min Apgar scores < 5, admissions to neonatal nursery, and requirements for ventilation. The two groups were similar with respect to demography, antenatal, peripartum, and neonatal outcomes. The perinatal mortality rate in the no Doppler group ($n = 264$, 11/1000 live births) was no different than in the Doppler group ($n = 262$, 9/1000 live births). The authors concluded that close surveillance in twin pregnancy resulted in a lower than expected fetal mortality from 25 weeks' gestation in both the no Doppler and Doppler groups.[12]

Only a few studies evaluated the role of umbilical artery Doppler velocimetry in fetal surveillance of high-order multiple pregnancies.[13-16] Gaziano and colleagues studied twins and triplets and found increased morbidity and mortality in twins when abnormal Doppler values were observed.[14] More recently, Ezra et al[15] evaluated the incidence of abnormal umbilical waveforms in triplet and quadruplet pregnancies and its correlation with adverse pregnancy outcome. Nineteen triplet and 4 quadruplet pregnancies were studied. Of 73 fetuses, 6 had abnormal umbilical artery waveforms (8.2%), characterized by persistent absence of the end-diastolic velocities (AEDV). In comparing the abnormal and normal groups, significant differences were found in birth weights, SGA rate, and perinatal mortality rate. Doppler umbilical artery waveforms in multiple pregnancies fell into either normal or extremely abnormal groups, whereby the latter (i.e. AEDV) was associated with adverse perinatal outcomes.

In summary, unless associated with extremely abnormal results, the umbilical artery velocimetry in multiples has a limited role in assessing birth weight discordance and does not significantly improve the overall perinatal outcome.

Intrauterine growth restriction

Placental insufficiency induces a redistribution of fetal blood flow, with reduced impedance at the cerebral level and increased resistance at the level of peripheral vessels, resulting in preferential perfusion to the brain. Increased impedance in the umbilical artery may be a sign of impaired placental perfusion, and thus reduced diffusion of nutrients and oxygen through the placenta. Compromised fetuses suffer from low oxygen reserves. These fetuses with increased impedance in placental circulation will have little capacity to compensate decreased placental perfusion during uterine contractions. Under such circumstances, fetuses with very high impedance in the umbilical circulation frequently develop signs of distress. However, measurement of umbilical artery impedance is not a good test for acute fetal hypoxia. With progressive fetal compromise, cardiac function deteriorates, resulting in decreased peak velocity at the outflow tracts. As a consequence of a high pressure gradient in the right atrium secondary to the cardiac malfunction, the percentage of reverse flow in the inferior vena cava increases and umbilical vein pulsations may occur.

Rizzo and colleagues evaluated Doppler detectable differences in fetal circulation (PI values in the umbilical artery, MCA, and aorta, and peak velocity from outflow tracts, percentage of reverse flow in the inferior vena cava) in discordant twin growth which resulted from either placental insufficiency or Twin–twin transfusion syndrome (TTTS).[16] Serial recordings in the larger twin showed the absence of any differences, compared with singletons. Conversely, the smaller twin showed progressive changes in Doppler indices similar to those found in growth-restricted singletons secondary to placental insufficiency, characterized by a progressive increase in PI from the UA and descending aorta in the weeks preceding fetal distress, associated with a decrease in PI from the MCA.[17]

It has been suggested that the absolute values of the Doppler indices in the smaller twin, or the intertwin difference between the smaller and the larger twin, may be used for fetal surveillance or for the prediction of fetal distress.[16] Vetter suggested that Doppler velocimetry is a good indicator of placental supply and function, allowing an insight into flow redistribution related to fetal stress.[18] Jensen correlated the intertwin difference in resistance index (RI) of the UA with the oxygen partial pressure (pO_2) difference and

demonstrated that the blood-gas exchange through the placenta is impaired when the impedance level in the UA surpasses a certain threshold value (RI = 76%).[19] He concluded that the absolute impedance level was superior to the difference in impedance between the fetuses. Joern and colleagues found that the results of Doppler sonography are better in predicting growth restriction than fetal outcome.[20] These investigators predicted a 'pathologic outcome' on the basis of Doppler measurements of the fetal aorta, umbilical artery, and MCA, and found low sensitivity and specificity values of 60% and 50%, respectively.[20]

In summary, abnormal UA Doppler results are significantly associated with the birth of an SGA infant in multiple pregnancies. As in singletons, multiple parameter measurements and serial measurements are superior to individual values. Moreover, Doppler examinations supplement biometry and may increase the likelihood of detecting IUGR of multiples.

Extremely abnormal blood flow in the umbilical artery

Absent end-diastolic velocity in the umbilical artery is an uncommon finding, but, if present, the affected fetuses are at increased risk of adverse perinatal outcomes (Figure 11.1). End-diastolic velocities, a normal finding in early pregnancy, first begin to appear at 10 weeks' gestation and are always present by 15 weeks. The absence of end-diastolic velocities is a pathologic finding in the second and third trimesters, at which time the majority of affected placentas show evidence of chronic insufficiency. When AEDV is present, it persists in the majority of cases, and occasionally deteriorates into a pattern of reversed end-diastolic velocity (REDV) flow, the most extreme form of increased vascular resistance in the placental bed. In the absence of intervention, this finding is usually followed by fetal distress and demise (Figure 11.1).

Hastie and colleagues evaluated 89 unselected twin pregnancies and found that persistent

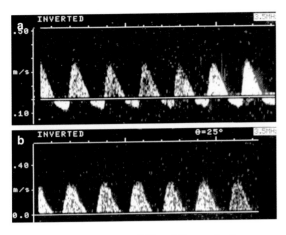

Figure 11.1 Abnormal blood flow velocity waveforms in the umbilical artery. Note (a) the presence of reversed end-diastolic flow; and (b) the absence of end-diastolic flow in the growth-restricted twin

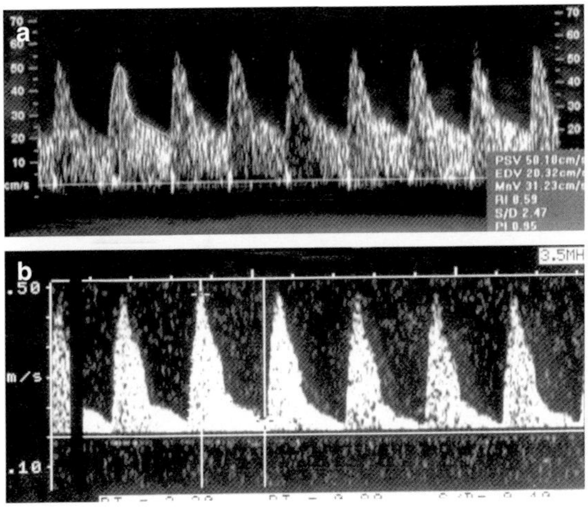

Figure 11.2 Pulsed Doppler waveforms from the middle cerebral artery of a 35-week growth-restricted twin (a) with enhanced diastolic flow and a normally grown twin at 34 weeks' gestation with normal pattern of blood flow (b)

AEDV in the umbilical artery was associated with poor outcome,[21] a finding that should alert the physician about the risk of fetal growth restriction or other adverse perinatal outcome. Rafla also reported increased morbidity in triplets when AEDV was documented,[22] and Giles and co-workers found two stillbirths among 17 fetuses with AEDV in 20 triplet pregnancies.[13]

In the past it was deemed necessary to perform immediate delivery for R/AEDV, but nowadays a much less aggressive approach is advocated. However, even with careful fetal monitoring, it seems unlikely that the duration of pregnancy can be significantly prolonged once this aberration becomes established. Umbilical artery flow velocity waveforms may be altered by betamethasone to enhance lung maturity, to the same extent as in singletons.[23] In nine (50%) of the 18 pregnancies, the administration of betamethasone was associated with return of umbilical artery end-diastolic flow for a median of 5 days. The authors concluded that the maternal administration of betamethasone in multiple pregnancies with umbilical artery absent end diastolic flow is associated with a transient return of end diastolic flow.

CEREBRAL CIRCULATION AND REDISTRIBUTION OF BLOOD

States of chronic fetal deprivation result in blood flow directed preferentially to the brain, myocardium, and adrenal glands. Fetal stress is accompanied by an increase in PI values in the umbilical artery and a reduction of PI values in the MCA. A low PI in cerebral arteries indicates dilatation of downstream resistance vessels (Figure 11.2). The reduced PI in the MCA is thought to reflect the brain-sparing response to inadequate perfusion or oxygenation, and to represent an appropriate compensatory decrease in cerebrovascular impedance, as well as a redistribution of blood flow to the brain. Akiyama and colleagues examined alterations in fetal vascular resistance of fetal peripheral arteries (the MCA, UA, aorta and splenic, renal and femoral arteries) with advancing gestation in appropriate-for-gestational-age (AGA) singleton, twin, and triplet pregnancies, and reported no significant differences for regional

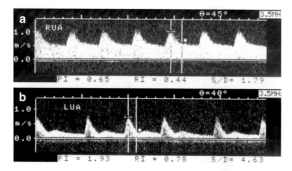

Figure 11.3 Uterine artery flow velocity waveforms. (a) Normal multiple pregnancy, (b) high-impedance pattern with well-defined diastolic notch in twin pregnancy with growth discordance of 1000 g

arterial vascular resistance, irrespective of plurality.[24] Gaziano and co-workers studied fetal growth and blood flow redistribution in monochorionic–diamniotic (MC–DA) compared with dichorionic–diamniotic (DC–DA) twins,[25] finding that the mean cerebral/placental ratio was lower in MC–DA than in DC–DA pairs, indicating a greater blood flow redistribution and brain-sparing effect in the former.

Redistribution of fetal blood flow was also more common in growth-restricted MC–DA twins. This adaptation to fetal stress suggests the differential risk to monochorionic fetuses. MC twins exhibit blood flow redistribution more often, compared with DC twins.[25] Placental vascular connections and the attendant hemodynamic changes in MC fetuses probably account for this difference. Also, brain-sparing events commonly occur without any clinical appearance of fetofetal transfusion in this group.[25] The correlation of MCA peak systolic velocity (MCA-PSV) with fetal anemia is of primary importance in the assessment of TTTS cases, with and without treatment.

UTERINE CIRCULATION

Doppler blood flow velocimetry of the uterine circulation in singleton pregnancies was able to predict to some extent pregnancy complications such as IUGR, pregnancy-induced hypertension (Figure 11.3), and pre-eclampsia. However, no clear evidence supports any indication that Doppler velocimetry of the uterine arteries may be useful for such purposes in multiple pregnancies. Rizzo and colleagues found that the resistance index from both uterine arteries decreases significantly with gestational age, and is lower in singleton pregnancies, suggesting a lower vascular resistance in the uterine circulation.[26] No significant differences were found when the resistance index in all patients with gestational hypertension or pre-eclampsia was compared with that of reference cases. The diagnostic efficacy of the uterine artery resistance index between 20 and 24 weeks of gestation to predict the development of hypertensive disorders was disappointingly low. Chen and associates studied the PI of uterine arteries over the course of pregnancy.[27] The mean values of PI were consistently lower in twins than in singleton pregnancies at any gestational age, declining more rapidly and reaching a plateau earlier in twins. Yu and colleagues reported that Doppler assessment of the uterine arteries at 23 weeks identified a large group of twins at risk of developing adverse outcomes due to placental insufficiency.[28] There were no significant differences in uterine artery PI or notching between monochorionic and dichorionic twins. This may indicate that total placental size may play an essential role in the development of adverse outcome. Geipel et al[29] compared singleton nomograms of the uterine circulation with previously established twin nomograms in the prediction of pre-eclampsia, IUGR, and birth weight discordance ≥ 20% in 256 dichorionic twin pregnancies. The mean uterine artery resistance index was calculated from both sides, and the presence and absence of notching was recorded. Cut-off levels for abnormal flow parameters were the 95th centile of reference ranges of either singleton or twin nomograms. According to twin reference values, 14.0% of patients were screen positive, compared to only 3.1% when singleton reference values were used. The sensitivity of abnormal uterine artery Doppler results defined by twin nomograms vs. singleton nomograms was 36.4% vs. 18.2% for pre-eclampsia, 26.7% vs. 9.7% for IUGR, 28.9% vs. 7.9% for birth weight discordance $\geq 20\%$, and 26.5% vs. 10.3% for any of these adverse outcomes, respectively. It follows that despite using specially constructed twin nomograms, uterine artery Doppler studies in twin gestations had a disappointingly overall low sensitivity in predicting adverse obstetric outcome. Moreover, negative predictive values of uterine Doppler studies in twin gestations are lower compared with those reported in unselected singleton pregnancies.

In summary, gestational hypertension, pre-eclampsia and IUGR may occur in twin pregnancies despite normal uterine artery velocity waveforms. The vascular resistance in the uterine artery is lower in multiple pregnancies than in singleton pregnancies, probably owing to wider invasion of the uterine vessels by the trophoblastic cells originating from a larger placental implantation area. The overall sensitivity for the prediction of pre-eclampsia and IUGR in twins is lower than in singletons. The different physiologic effects of multiple pregnancy on the materno-placental circulation may affect the utility of uterine artery Doppler velocimetry as a screening test.

TWIN–TWIN TRANSFUSION SYNDROME

The use of Doppler in the assessment of twin-twin transfusion syndrome is discussed in Chapter 13.

TWIN REVERSED ARTERIAL PERFUSION SYNDROME

Twin reversed arterial perfusion (TRAP) is a rare anomaly of multiple pregnancy (see Chapter 14). In TRAP, Doppler sonography demonstrates reversed arterial blood flow from the placenta towards the acardiac twin[30] and transvaginal color Doppler ultrasound is able to do so in early pregnancy.[31]

It is essential to stress the role of echocardiography in the diagnosis of congestive heart failure in the 'pump twin' and in the management strategy. Shih and colleagues used Doppler velocimetry to analyze the blood flow pattern in the umbilical arteries.[32] Patterns were classified into one of three categories. The first, the so-called 'collision-summation', is characterized by a pattern of two independent pulsation rates of bidirectional flow (abnormal pulsatile heart in the malformed twin) with cyclic alterations of blood flow. The second, reported as 'twin pulse', shows the flow away from the acardiac twin (with the presence of a primitive heart) with absent diastolic velocity, and the flow pumped into the acardiac twin with a prominent diastolic component. In other words, both flows are constantly pumping in opposite directions and at different rates. The third, the 'pump-in' pattern, demonstrates pulsatile flow towards the acardiac mass in the reverse direction. It was suggested that the flow patterns of acardiac twins are determined by both the existence of a primitive heart and the nature of the vascular anastomosis.[32] Gembruch and colleagues presented a case of TTTS with death of a donor at 25 weeks of gestation and observed reversed flow from the UAs through the aorta, left heart, right heart, inferior vena cava, DV, and back to the placenta through the umbilical vein, similar to the development of the TRAP sequence.[33] This finding suggests that if one fetus dies in an MC pair, the falling blood pressure in the dying fetus may lead to a shift in the pressure gradient and cause an acute transfusion of blood from the surviving twin to the dying one through the superficial A–A or V–V anastomoses.

CORD ENTANGLEMENT

Utility of color flow imaging and Doppler velocimetry in the diagnosis and management of MA twins is discussed in Chapter 15.

REFERENCES

1. Divon MY, Weiner Z. Ultrasound in twin pregnancy. Semin Perinatol 1995; 19: 404–12.

2. Blickstein I, Lancct M. The growth discordant twin. Obstet Gynecol Surv 1988; 43: 509–15.

3. Farmakides G, Schulman H, Saldana LR et al. Surveillance of twin pregnancy with umbilical velocimetry. Am J Obstet Gynecol 1985; 153: 789–92.

4. Saldana RL, Eads MC, Schaefer TR. Umbilical blood waveforms in fetal surveillance of twins. Am J Obstet Gynecol 1987; 157: 712–15.

5. Gerson AG, Wallace DM, Bridgens NK. Duplex Doppler ultrasound in the evaluation of growth in twin pregnancies. Obstet Gynecol 1987; 70: 419–23.

6. Shah YG, Gragg LA, Moodley S, Williams GW. Doppler velocimetry in concordant and discordant twin gestations. Obstet Gynecol 1992; 80: 272–6.

7. Degani S, Paltiely J, Lewinsky R et al. Fetal internal carotid artery flow velocity time waveforms in twin pregnancies. J Perinat Med 1988; 16: 405–9.

8. Seelbach-Gobel B, Kaesemann H, Roos T. Doppler studies in the differential diagnosis in twin pairs. Z Geburtsh Perinatol 1992; 196: 26–32.

9. Kurmanavicius J, Hebisch G, Huch R, Huch A. Umbilical artery blood flow velocity waveforms in twin pregnancies. J Perinat Med 1992; 20: 307–12.

10. Faber R, Viehweg B, Burkhardt U. Predictive value of Doppler velocimetry in twin pregnancies. Zentralbl Gynakol 1995; 117: 353–7.

11. Chittacharoen A, Leelapattana P, Rangsiprakarn R. Prediction of discordant twins by real-time ultra-sonography combined with umbilical artery velocimetry. Ultrasound Obstet Gynecol 2000; 15: 118–21.

12. Giles W, Bisits A, O'Callaghan S, Gill A; DAMP Study Group.The Doppler assessment in multiple pregnancy randomised controlled trial of ultrasound biometry versus umbilical artery Doppler ultrasound and biometry in twin pregnancy. BJOG 2003; 110: 593–7.

13. Giles WB, Trudinger BJ, Cook CM, Connelly AJ. Umbilical artery waveforms in triplet pregnancy. Obstet Gynecol 1990; 75: 813–16.

14. Gaziano EP, Knox GE, Bendel RP et al. Is pulsed Doppler velocimetry useful in the management of multiple-gestation pregnancies? Am J Obstet Gynecol 1991; 164: 1426–33.

15. Ezra Y, Jones J, Farine D. Umbilical artery waveforms in triplet and quadruplet pregnancies. Gynecol Obstet Invest 1999; 47: 239–43.

16. Rizzo G, Arduini D, Romanini C. Cardiac and extracardiac flows in discordant twins. Am J Obstet Gynecol 1994; 170: 1321–7.

17. Arduini D, Rizzo G, Romanini C. Changes of pulsatility index from fetal vessels preceding the onset of late decelerations in growth retarded fctuses. Obstet Gynecol 1992; 79: 605–10.

18. Vetter K. Considerations on growth discordant twins. J Perinat Med 1993; 21: 267–72.

19. Jensen OH. Doppler velocimetry and umbilical cord blood gas assessment of twins. Eur J Obstet Gynecol Reprod Biol 1993; 49: 155–9.

20. Joern H, Schroeder W, Sassen R, Rath W. Predictive value of a single CTG, ultrasound and Doppler examination to diagnose acute and chronic placental insufficiency in multiple pregnancies. J Perinat Med 1997; 25: 325–32.

21. Hastie SJ, Danskin F, Neilson JP, Whittle MJ. Prediction of the small for gestational age fetus by Doppler umbilical artery waveform analysis. Obstet Gynecol 1989; 74: 730–3.

22. Rafla NM. Surveillance of triplets with umbilical artery velocimetry waveforms. Acta Genet Med Gemellol (Roma) 1989; 38: 301–4.

23. Barkehall-Thomas A, Thompson M, Baker LS, Edwards A, Wallace EM. Betamethasone associated changes in umbilical artery flow velocity waveforms in multiple pregnancies with umbilical artery absent end diastolic flow. Aust NZ J Obstet Gynaecol 2003; 43: 360–3.

24. Akiyama M, Kuno A, Tanaka Y et al. Comparison of alterations in fetal regional arterial vascular resistance in appropriate-for-gestational-age singleton, twin and triplet pregnancies. Hum Reprod 1999; 14: 2635–43.

25. Gaziano E, Gaziano C, Brandt D. Doppler velocimetry determined redistribution of fetal blood flow: correlation with growth restriction in diamniotic monochorionic and dizygotic twins. Am J Obstet Gynecol 1998; 178: 1359–67.

26. Rizzo G, Arduini D, Romanini C. Uterine artery Doppler velocity waveforms in twin pregnancies. Obstet Gynecol 1993; 82: 978–83.

27. Chen Q, Izumi A, Minakami H, Sato I. Comparative changes in uterine artery blood flow waveforms in singleton and twin pregnancies. Gynecol Obstet Invest 1999; 45: 165.

28. Yu CKH, Papageorghiou AT, Boli A et al. Screening for pre-eclampsia and fetal growth restriction in twin pregnancies at 23 weeks of gestation by transvaginal uterine artery Doppler. Ultrasound Obstet Gynecol 2002; 20: 535–40.

29. Geipel A, Berg C, Germer U et al. Doppler assessment of the uterine circulation in the second trimester in twin pregnancies: prediction of pre-eclampsia, fetal growth restriction and birth weight discordance. Ultrasound Obstet Gynecol 2002; 20: 541–5.

30. Fouron JC, Leduc L, Grigon A et al. Importance of meticulous ultrasonographic investigation of the acardiac twin. J Ultrasound Med 1994; 13: 1001–4.

31. Schwarzler P, Ville Y, Moscosco G et al. Diagnosis of twin reversed arterial perfusion sequence in the first trimester by transvaginal color Doppler ultrasound. Ultrasound Obstet Gynecol 1999; 13: 143–6.

32. Shih JC, Shyu MK, Hunag SF et al. Doppler waveform analysis of the intertwin blood flow in acardiac pregnancy: implications for pathogenesis. Ultrasound Obstet Gynecol 1999; 14: 375–9.

33. Gembruch U, Viski S, Bagamery K et al. Twin reversed arterial perfusion sequence in twin-to-twin transfusion syndrome after the death of the donor co-twin in the second trimester. Ultrasound Obstet Gynecol 2001; 17: 153–6.

Assessment of the fetal heart by echocardiography

12

INTRODUCTION

Fetal echocardiography presently represents a major part of fetal cardiology, a new and exciting field of perinatal medicine. The use of echocardiography enables confirmation of normal heart anatomy and physiology, detection of structural malformations, follow-up of functional abnormalities, and the monitoring of invasive therapeutic interventions. These diagnostic capabilities are not restricted to singleton gestations; fetal echocardiography also has specific goals when used in multiple pregnancies (Table 12.1). Under normal circumstances, multiple pregnancies are referred for targeted cardiac examination following an obstetric screening examination which detected a cardiac problem. However, numerous maternal and fetal conditions (Table 12.2) also indicate a comprehensive cardiac scan.

The examination duration is much longer in multiple pregnancy than the average 45 min required for a scan in singletons. More important, however, is the timing of the scan. In the first trimester when the size of the heart is 4–6 mm, fetal echocardiography can be misleading with respect to the intrinsic morphology. The optimal gestational age for fetal echocardiography is approximately 20 weeks, when the size of the heart is about 20 mm and large enough for clear and detailed visualization. At this stage cardiac size should be similar in both twins (Figure 12.1). After 30 weeks' gestation, however, when the size of the heart exceeds 30 mm, technical difficulties are more likely and interference with the image quality

Table 12.1 Goals of fetal echocardiography in multiple pregnancy

General
(1) Confirm normal heart anatomy
(2) Diagnose structural anomalies (congenital heart defect, or heart tumor)
(3) Relate neonatal prognosis with fetal cardiac defects
(4) Detect and evaluate functional anomalies such as valvular regurgitations
(5) Evaluate normal or abnormal cardiac rhythms
(6) Evaluate cardiomegaly (regardless of anatomy), myocarditis, or cardiomyopathy
(7) Assess fetal congestive heart failure (imminent or fulminant)
(8) Identify extracardiac malformations
(9) Monitor fetal invasive therapy

Specific to monochorionic twins
(1) Evaluate the twin–twin transfusion syndrome
(2) Assess cardiac pathology in conjoined twins
(3) Assess cardiac function of the 'pump' twin in the TRAP sequence (acardiac twin)

TRAP, twin reversed arterial perfusion

Table 12.2   Indications for fetal echocardiography

Fetal
Abnormal four-chamber view
Increased nuchal thickness
Abnormal heart rhythm
Ascites
Extracardiac malformation
Chromosomal abnormalities
Polyhydramnios
Oligohydramnios
Intrauterine growth restriction
Complicated twin gestation
Invasive fetal therapy

Maternal
Diabetes
Collagen disease
Epilepsy
Hyperthyroidism
Viral infection
Pharmacotherapy
Maternal age > 35 years

Family history
Congenital heart disease in the family
Chromosomal aberrations in the family

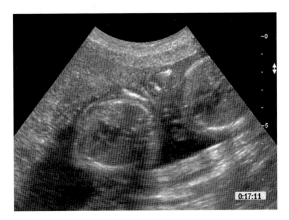

Figure 12.1   Concordant size of fetal hearts in normal twin gestation

is a possibility, owing to fetal presentation and the well-developed rib cage, spine, and lungs. Further, oligohydramnios and a thick maternal abdominal wall represent additional unfavorable conditions that make late fetal echocardiography time-consuming, difficult to perform, hard to interpret, and, consequently, less reliable.

FETAL ECHOCARDIOGRAPHY IN THE TWIN–TWIN TRANSFUSION SYNDROME

This issue is described in Chapter 13. A summary of the echograpic signs follows.

First trimester

The increased risk of developing twin–twin transfusion syndrome (TTTS) in cases with increased nuchal translucency (NT) is discussed in detail in Chapter 13; however, this association at least points to the possibility that increased NT thickness is an early manifestation of fetal congestive heart failure. Recently, Maymon et al[1] reviewed 11 studies reporting on the pregnancy outcome of 2128 euploid fetuses with increased NT (≥ 3 mm or ≥ 95th centile). As many as 2.2 to 10.6% of the fetuses miscarried and 0.5 to 15.8% ended in perinatal death. Importantly, the overall rate of neurodevelopmental problems was 0.5 to 13%, and 2 to 8% of the malformations were undiagnosed before birth, the most common being cardiac anomalies. Thus, these authors recommend a detailed two-step anomaly scan including mid-gestation fetal echocardiography for all twins.

Second and third trimesters

In 1999, Quintero and colleagues proposed a method of TTTS staging, which did not include consideration of the fetal heart.[2] However, in the typical presentation of TTTS, differences in cardiac size are seen (Figure 12.2). Indeed, different functional cardiac anomalies have been observed as early as 18 weeks' gestation, strongly suggesting that cardiac malfunction is one of the first abnormalities of TTTS detectable by ultrasonography.

Other observations suggest that the earliest symptom of fetal hypervolemia in the recipient is pulmonary regurgitation (Figure 12.3), probably due to high pulmonary resistance at

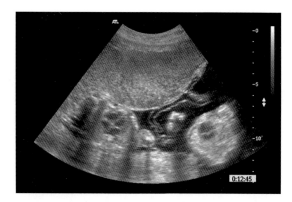

Figure 12.2 Discordant size fetal hearts suggestive of twin–twin transfusion syndrome

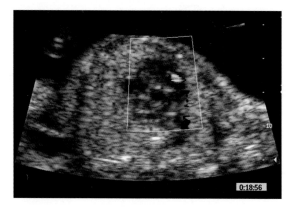

Figure 12.3 Pulmonary regurgitation with normal heart anatomy: this is suggested as the first functional sign of twin–twin transfusion syndrome due to blood volume overload in the recipient

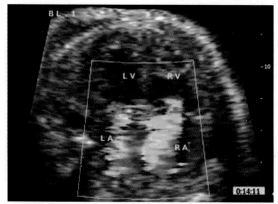

Figure 12.4 Tricuspid and mitral regurgitation due to volume overload in the recipient: LA, left atrium; LV, left ventricle; RA, right atrium; RV, right ventricle

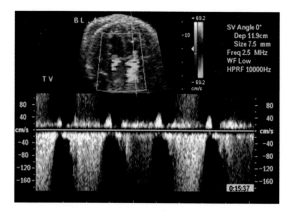

Figure 12.5 Tricuspid valve holosystolic regurgitation (spectral Doppler tracing)

this stage of pulmonary vascular bed development. This is followed by myocardial hypertrophy, an increase in size of the heart and leaking of the atrioventricular valve. Myocardial hypertrophy often mimics fetal cardiomyopathy, which usually affects the right heart, but rarely also the left. Hecher and associates[3] reported that tricuspid regurgitation was present during systole in 40% of TTTS recipients (Figure 12.4). In 6 out of 19 cases, the E and A waves of the tricuspid valve fused during diastole (this phenomenon was not noted in the donor), probably due to increased blood flow into the right ventricle (Figure 12.5).

The donor's heart is usually normal in echographic terms; however, blood flow velocity across the atrioventricular valves may be increased at the initial stage of hyperdynamic contractility. Lachapelle and colleagues[4] reported that the donor exhibits a hyperdynamic cardiac state, with significantly increased left ventricular shortening fractions and outputs. Hecher and associates,[3] on the other hand, reported significantly decreased mean values of atrioventricular flow velocities.

Fetal hydrops in the donor is very rare, and its cause is unclear. It might be due to myocardial dysfunction and ischemia or redirected blood flow from the recipient to the donor. In contrast, hydrops in the donor is not rare after invasive laser therapy, and is present in 25% of cases.[5] It was postulated that a sudden increase in volume load after the procedure affects the

131

donor, and that this clears a few days later in 90% of cases.[5]

FETAL ECHOCARDIOGRAPHY IN THE TWIN REVERSED ARTERIAL PERFUSION SEQUENCE

Chorioangiopagus parasiticus, the classic acardiac monster, is currently termed twin reversed arterial perfusion (TRAP) sequence (see Chapter 14). An acardiac twin is a rare complication that affects less than 1% of monochorionic multiple pregnancies or roughly one in 35 000 pregnancies. In this anomaly, as the name implies, the heart is absent or rudimentary, and the circulation is maintained by vascular communications with the co-twin (the 'pump' twin). The 'pump' twin is structurally normal, but is at risk for *in utero* cardiac failure and fetal or neonatal demise.

The final outcome and treatment modality are based on frequent echocardiographic assessments.[6] The main issue is to detect early signs of *in utero* congestive heart failure of the 'pump' twin,[7] because this complication may cause death in as many as 50% of these otherwise normal co-twins. The surviving 'pump' twin may present with heart failure and persistent myocardial hypertrophy after birth, which may mimic hypertrophic cardiomyopathy.

CONGENITAL HEART DEFECTS IN MULTIPLE PREGNANCIES

The prevalence of structural malformations is increased in twin compared with singleton pregnancies. This axiom indicates careful examination of the fetal anatomy as an integral part of perinatal care. Twins may be discordant for a given anomaly (e.g. one twin with normal heart anatomy and the other with hypoplastic left heart) or both twins may have an anomaly, but of a different nature (e.g. one twin with a cardiac anomaly and the other with a central nervous system anomaly). In the majority of cases, structural heart defects present in dizygotic twins (for instance hypoplastic left heart syndrome or atrioventricular septal

defect with normal heart anatomy in the co-twin) occur during heart embryogenesis. They should not be confused with 'acquired' structural defects in monozygotic, monochorionic twins, such as pulmonary stenosis which develops late during pregnancy. Needless to say, a cytogenetic work-up is often necessary when cardiac structural malformations are detected. Discordant heart disease in a monochorionic set may mimic TTTS. Koike and colleagues[8] reported hydrops fetalis due to Ebstein's anomaly at 22 weeks in one of monochorionic twins. The hydrops was treated with maternal digitalization and resolved by the 28th week of gestation. The twin with Ebstein's anomaly died 22 h after birth at 33 weeks; the non-affected twin survived, and was normal at 19 months of age.

Two recent articles focused on congenital heart disease (CHD) in multiple pregnancies. The first was by Paladini et al,[9] who assessed the diagnostic accuracy of fetal echocardiography and evaluated the type and the outcome of CHD detected in fetuses from multiple pregnancies. CHD was present in 45 of 711 fetuses from 282 twin, 45 triplet, and 3 quadruplet pregnancies. In the study population, the sensitivity of echocardiography was 88.8%, the specificity was 99.8%, the positive predictive value 97.6%, and the negative predictive value 99.2%. As for the 45 cases with CHD, the type of CHD was evenly distributed among the left and right heart, cono-truncal and septal defects, with 6/7 right heart lesions occurring in recipient fetuses of pregnancies complicated by TTTS. The aneuploidy rate was 7.0% (3/43). These authors concluded that the diagnostic performance of fetal echocardiography in twin gestations is comparable with that obtained in singletons. In another study, also from Naples, Italy, the authors focused on CHD in dizygotic twins.[10] They enrolled 1743 CHD patients with at least 1 sibling, and 66 pairs of dizygotic twins. Considering only the sibling nearest in age for each non-twin patient, the recurrence was 3.8% and half of the affected siblings had the same or similar CHD. Conversely, considering all 1886 siblings, recurrence of CHD in the non-twin group was 4%, half of which had a sibling with the same suspected pathogenic mechanism of CHD. Concordant CHD was found in 9/66 pairs of twins (13.6%), and in all (100%) the type of anomaly was also concordant (based on the suspected pathogenic mechanism).

FETAL ARRHYTHMIAS IN TWINS

The most common arrhythmias are premature atrial contractions, which are usually benign, require no pharmacologic treatment, and commonly resolve during pregnancy or during the first few days after delivery. However, the 'benign' nature of the arrhythmia should be carefully verified, because fetal premature atrial contractions can co-exist with congenital heart defects such as ventricular septal defect (VSD) or transposition of the great arteries (TGA). Some types of fetal arrhythmias, in particular bradyarrhythmias, may be the first sign of neonatal myocarditis. Supraventricular tachycardia in one twin requires special attention. Edwards and co-workers[11] reported good results with transplacental flecainide therapy in one such case, without evidence of maternal or fetal side-effects. However, such a situation may raise ethical and possible legal concerns regarding the best management option for this condition, which, at the same time, may cause complications in the co-twin and/or the mother.

FETAL ECHOCARDIOGRAPHY IN CONJOINED TWINS

The most common form (52.4%) of conjoined twins is thoracopagus (see Chapter 16). By definition, a conjoined heart is present, but the extent of sharing is variable. The hearts can be joined as a pericardial junction, minor venous/atrial connections or, more commonly (75%), an extensive conjunction with intermixing of chambers and valves. A typical example of conjoined hearts is shown in Figure 12.6. Figure 12.7 is the same thoraco-omphalopagus after delivery at 22 weeks of gestation.

Clearly, the presence and extent of the cardiac union is a major determinant of the

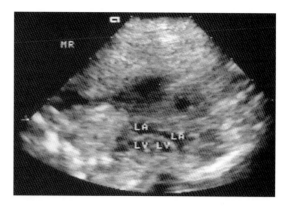

Figure 12.6   Conjoined hearts: LA, left atrium; LV, left ventricle

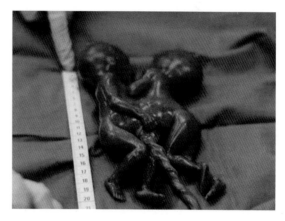

Figure 12.7   Thoraco-omphalopagus after delivery at 22 weeks of gestation

potential to separate the twins. According to Raffensperger,[12] sharing of atrioventricular valves and ventricles virtually precludes successful separation, even if one twin is sacrificed. Often a common atrium is present in conjoined twins, connecting with the inferior vena cava and the hepatic veins from each fetus. Anomalous pulmonary venous connection is also common. Two or three ventricles are usually present. Single ventricles, one from each twin, are often joined and have one or more defects in the common wall, allowing communication between the chambers. Common or straddling atrioventricular valves often attach into the ventricular components

Table 12.3   Treatment and outcome options in thoracopagi twins

Heart anatomy	Possible outcome
Two separated hearts, both with normal anatomy	separation and survival possible for both twins
Two separated hearts: one with congenital heart defect, one normal	separation and survival possible for the twin with normal heart anatomy

Conjoined hearts
  at level of atria
  at level of ventricles
	
	single survivor after cardiac surgery
	no survivors

Table 12.4   Etiology of fetal congestive heart failure

(1) Heart failure due to myocardial dysfunction (myocarditis, cardiomyopathy, volume overload)
(2) Disorders of cardiac rhythm (tachycardia: FHR > 220/min, or persistent bradycardia)
(3) High output failure due to anemia, arteriovenous fistula, Galen's malformation, sacrococcygeal teratoma, etc.
(4) Abnormal peripheral impedance with fetal growth failure
(5) Twin–twin transfusion syndrome or acardiac twin
(6) Congenital heart defect and progressive valvular regurgitation and/or 'acquired' *in utero* myocarditis

FHR, fetal heart rate

from both twins. The right ventricles are often hypoplastic or rudimentary. Abnormal ventriculo-arterial connections, including transposition or double-outlet right ventricle, are common in at least one twin. Abnormalities of the great arteries, including truncus arteriosus or interruption of the aortic arch, are also common.[13] Other reported defects include tricuspid atresia, mitral atresia, hypoplasia of ventricle, tetralogy of Fallot, and ventricular septal defect. Very rarely, an acardiac twin is involved in the conjoined set.[14]

For those patients who consider continuation of the conjoined twin pregnancy, further fetal echocardiographic assessment is crucial. After completion of fetal echocardiographic evaluation at around 20 weeks' gestation, counseling about the possible surgical procedures after birth can be offered. It should be remembered, however, that neonatal echocardiography is technically much more difficult and usually provides only screening information during the first examination.

When conjoined twins are diagnosed during the later stages of pregnancy, obstetric ultrasound as well as fetal echocardiography is much more difficult to perform, and sometimes three-dimensional and/or fast magnetic resonance imaging is necessary for better anatomic delineation of the twins. However, even if not all the anatomic details are clarified by fetal echocardiography, there is usually sufficient information to support a 'no resuscitation' decision after elective cesarean. Out of 11 cases of conjoined twins reported by Sanders,[13] there were 9 thoracopagi: 6 with conjoined hearts and 3 with shared pericardium. Survival is possible only in those with normal heart anatomy, as was the experience of Mackenzie and co-workers.[15] Recently, Andrews et al[16] determined the accuracy of prenatal and post-natal echocardiography in delineating the degree of cardiac fusion, intracardiac anatomy, and ventricular function of 23 sets of conjoined twins with thoracic level fusion. Twins were classified according to the degree of cardiac fusion: separate hearts and pericardium (group A, $n = 5$), separate hearts and common pericardium (group B, $n = 7$), fused atria and separate ventricles (group C, $n = 2$), and fused atria and ventricles (group D, $n = 9$). The degree of cardiac fusion was correctly diagnosed in all but one set. Intracardiac anatomy was correctly diagnosed in all cases, although the antenatal diagnosis was revised postnatally in three cases. Abnormal intracardiac anatomy was found in one twin only in two group A pairs, one group B pair, and both group C pairs. All group D twins had abnormal anatomy. Ventricular function was good in all twins scanned prenatally, and postnatally function correlated well with the clinical condition. These authors concluded that prenatal and postnatal echocardiography accurately delineates cardiac fusion, intracardiac anatomy, and

ventricular function in the majority of twins with thoracic level fusion.

Based on fetal echocardiographic findings in conjoined twins, one may construct a follow-up scheme to confirm or rule out an option for successful separation (Table 12.3).

FETAL CONGESTIVE HEART FAILURE

Fetal congestive heart failure (CHF) is defined as inadequate tissue perfusion, which results in a series of complex reflexes and adaptation to improve forward flow or redirect flow to vital organs. Several conditions may lead to fetal CHF (Table 12.4). Although fetal CHF is a serious condition, it can be successfully managed with extensive co-operation between the obstetrician and fetal cardiologist. Once the diagnosis is made and the fetuses have reached maturity, fetal CHF is an indication for elective cesarean section. Before this stage, fetal therapies can be considered, including maternal digoxin administration, and dexamethasone or other drugs administered to the mother or directly to the fetus.

REFERENCES

1. Maymon R, Weinraub Z, Herman A. Pregnancy outcome of euploid fetuses with increased nuchal translucency: how bad is the news? J Perinat Med 2005; 33: 191–8.

2. Quintero RA, Morales WJ, Allen MH et al. Staging in twin–twin transfusion syndrome. J Perinatol 1999; 19: 550–5.

3. Hecher K, Sullivan ID, Nicolaides KH. Temporary iatrogenic fetal tricuspid valve atresia in a case of the twin–twin transfusion syndrome. Br Heart J 1994; 72: 457–60.

4. Lachapelle MF, Leduc L, Cote JM, Grignon A, Fouron JC. Potential value of fetal echocardiography in the differential diagnosis of twin pregnancy with presence of polyhydramnios–oligohydramnios syndrome. Am J Obstet Gynecol 1997; 177: 388–94.

5. Gratacos E, Van Schoubroeck D, Carreras E et al. Impact of laser coagulation in severe twin–twin transfusion syndrome on fetal Doppler indices and venous blood flow volume. Ultrasound Obstet Gynecol 2002; 20: 125–30.

6. Osborn P, Gross TL, Shah JJ, Ma L. Prenatal diagnosis of fetal heart failure in twin reversed arterial perfusion. Prenat Diagn 2000; 20: 615–17.

7. Donnenfeld AE, van de Woestijne J, Craparo F, Smith CS, Ludomirski A, Weiner S. The normal fetus of an acardiac twin pregnancy: perinatal management based on echocardiographic and sonographic evaluation. Prenat Diagn 1991; 11: 235–44.

8. Koike T, Minakami H, Shirashi H et al. Digitalization of the mother in treating hydrops fetalis in monochorionic twin with Ebstein's anomaly. Case report. J Perinat Med 1997; 25: 295–7.

9. Paladini D, Vassallo M, Sglavo G, Russo MG, Martinelli P. Diagnosis and outcome of congenital heart disease in fetuses from multiple pregnancies. Prenat Diagn 2005; 25: 403–6.

10. Caputo S, Russo MG, Capozzi G et al. Congenital heart disease in a population of dizygotic twins: an echocardiographic study. Int J Cardiol 2005; 102: 293–6.

11. Edwards A, Peek MJ, Curren J. Transplacental flecainide therapy for fetal supraventricular tachycardia in a twin pregnancy. Aust NZ J Obstet Gynecol 1999; 39: 110–12.

12. Raffensperger J. A philosophical approach to conjoined twins. Pediatr Surg Int 1997; 12: 249–55.

13. Sanders SP. Conjoined twins. In: Allan L, Hornberger L, Sharland G, eds. Textbook of Fetal Cardiology. Greenwich: Medical Media Ltd, 2000: 366–76.

14. Sukcharaeon N, Wannakrairot P. Sonographic prenatal diagnosis of congenital heart defects in thoraco-omphalopagus. Asia Oceania J Obstet Gynecol 1992; 19: 43–9.

15. Mackenzie TC, Crombleholme TM, Johnson MP et al. The natural history of prenatally diagnosed conjoined twins. J Pediatr Surg 2002; 37: 303–9.

16. Andrews RE, McMahon CJ, Yates RW, et al. Echocardiographic assessment of conjoined twins. Heart 2006; 92: 382–7.

13

Sonographic diagnosis of twin-to-twin transfusion syndrome

INTRODUCTION

Although the diagnosis and treatment of twin-to-twin transfusion syndrome (TTTS) has improved greatly in recent decades, this condition remains one of the greatest challenges in modern fetal medicine for several reasons. First, two fetuses are involved. Second, the natural history of fetal loss or damage is extremely high compared with other fetal pathologies. Third, because the defect originates in the placenta, the affected fetuses are structurally normal and thus potentially completely salvageable. Finally, it is relatively common, occurring in 10–15% of monochorionic (MC) twins, and thus affecting about 1:3200 pregnancies or 1:1600 fetuses.[1] The two most significant barriers to developing rational treatments for this condition have been the lack of understanding of the underlying vascular pathophysiology, as well as the lack of an appropriate animal model.

CLINICAL FEATURES

For many years, the clinical diagnosis of TTTS was based on neonatal discordance in hemoglobin of ≥5 g/dl, which often was accompanied by marked differences in skin color. Such criteria are now regarded as obsolete, however. At present, the diagnosis is made antenatally by the simple criterion of ultrasonically observed discordance in amniotic fluid volume in MC twins, usually between 15 and 28 weeks' gestation, and in the presence of the oligopolyhydramnios sequence, in which the deepest vertical pool in the donor is ≤2 cm and in the recipient ≥8 cm.[2] Other features in the donor twin are a small or non-visible bladder, abnormal umbilical artery Doppler waveforms (absent or reverse end-diastolic frequencies) (AEDF/REDF), and growth restriction (Figure 13.1). Anhydramnios in the donor often leads to the appearance of a 'stuck' twin. Quintero and Chmait described the 'slung' appearance in 16% of cases where a non-'stuck' donor is cocooned in its amniotic membrane similar to a chrysalis.[3] In contrast, the recipient shows signs of hypervolemia including atrial natriuretic peptide-mediated polyuria, polyhydramnios, visceromegaly, abnormal venous Dopplers,[4,5] cardiac enlargement/failure and, in extreme cases, hydrops.

The differential diagnosis of TTTS includes discordant intrauterine growth restriction which complicates up to 40% of MC twins. This is distinguished by the absence of recipient phenotypic features in the co-twin, along with the absence of polyhydramnios. Controversy surrounds whether TTTS can occur in monoamniotic (MA) twins, presumably because MA twins are themselves rare and because the absence of an intervening membrane in MA twins would be expected to disguise some of the characteristics of TTTS. Indeed, mild TTTS features in MA twins occur only very rarely, and, therefore, monoamnionicity would appear to be largely protective against TTTS.

Ex vivo placental injection studies have shown that almost all MC placentas contain vascular anastomoses (Figures 13.2–13.4). Thus, the intertwin transfusion syndrome must be considered a normal event in MC

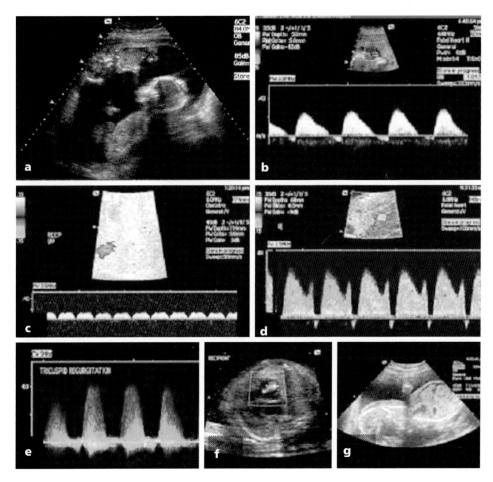

Figure 13.1 Ultrasound and Doppler findings in twin-to-twin transfusion syndrome (TTTS). Features of stage II TTTS include oligohydramnios–polyhydramnios sequence with growth discordance and non-visualization of donor bladder (a). Manifestations of hemodynamic compromise in stage III TTTS include reversed end-diastolic frequencies (REDF) in umbilical artery of donor twin (b), and pulsatile flow in umbilical vein (c), reversed flow in ductus venosus (d), and marked tricuspid regurgitation (e,f) in recipient. Worsening cardiovascular dynamics in recipient result in fetal hydrops, i.e. stage IV (g)

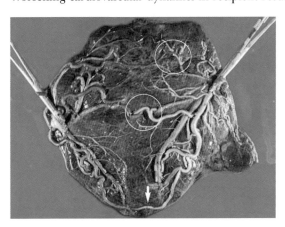

Figure 13.2 An injection study of a monochorionic placenta. Arteries from the left and right twins' placental cord insertions are shown in red and yellow with veins in blue and green, respectively. An arterio-arterial anastomosis is seen (arrow) along with multiple arterio-venous anastomoses (circles). Reproduced with permission from reference 6

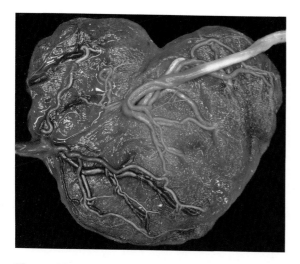

Figure 13.3 Typical placenta delivered at 26 weeks of monochorionic diamniotic twins, TTTS, and preterm rupture of membranes showing 1 AV-1VA anastomosis. Recipient's cord on the right. Image of courtesy of Liesbeth Lewi, Leuven, Belgium

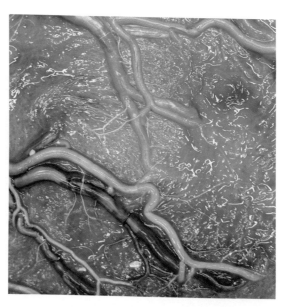

Figure 13.4 Detail of the AV anastomosis. Image courtesy of Liesbeth Lewi, Leuven, Belgium

twins. If, however, intertwin transfusion is a normal event in MC twins, it must be relatively balanced in order to avoid clinical manifestations. It follows that TTTS is a consequence of unbalanced intertwin transfusion, as suggested more than a century ago by the landmark pathologic studies of Schatz, and more recently supported by both computer modeling and *ex vivo* and *in vivo* studies of anastomotic configurations in TTTS.

Three types of interplacental anastomoses are identifiable on the chorionic surface or plate: arterio-arterial (AA), veno-venous (VV) and arterio-venous (AV). AA and VV anastomoses are superficial and permit bidirectional flow. In contrast, deep AV anastomoses characterize a cotyledon supplied by a chorionic artery from one twin, and drained by a chorionic vein of the co-twin. Strictly speaking, an AV anastomosis is not an anastomosis, as it does not bypass the normal capillary circulation, and more correctly represents a shared cotyledon. Whereas AA and AV anastomoses are found in the majority of MC placentas, VV anastomoses are present in fewer than 25% of them.

Initial *ex vivo* injection studies confirmed that TTTS placentas have more deep than superficial anastomoses compared with MC controls.[6] The largest study to date of placental angioarchitecture in TTTS compared 21 TTTS with 49 non-TTTS MC placentas and demonstrated that only the frequency of AA anastomoses was different, in contrast to the AV or VV anastomoses.[7] Not only were those affected by TTTS less likely to have AA anastomoses, present in only 24% compared with 84% of MC controls, but at least one AV anastomosis was always present in TTTS placentas in contrast to none in 16% of MC controls. Seventy-eight percent of twins connected to a placenta with ≥ 1 AV and no AA anastomoses developed TTTS. Under these circumstances, it appears that AA anastomoses have the potential for compensating any hemodynamic imbalance that derives from unidirectional AV anastomoses by virtue of their high pressure differential. Indeed, the protective role of AA anastomoses in MC twin pregnancies has been validated by imaging studies.[8,9] AA anastomoses can be identified antenatally by color

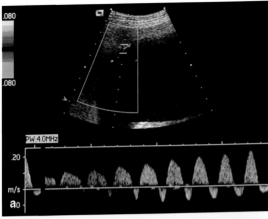

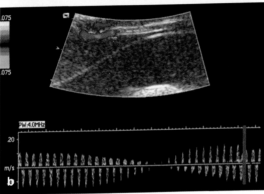

Figure 13.5 The characteristic interference pattern (a) seen with pulsed wave Doppler insonation of an arterio-arterial anastomosis. Superimposition of two umbilical artery waveforms results in the three characteristics: a bidirectional waveform, a speckled appearance when viewed by spectral Doppler, and a periodicity dependent upon the difference in twin heart rates. Reproduced with permission from *Human Reproduction*. The periodicity of the Doppler waveform is highlighted by using a slower sweep (b) (25 mm/s vs. 50 mm/s)

Doppler from as early as 11 weeks' gestation (Figure 13.5), and *in vivo* studies have validated the absence of AA anastomoses as being associated with an increased risk of TTTS (61% vs 15%, odds ratio 8.6).[8]

CARDIOVASCULAR PATHOPHYSIOLOGY

Unbalanced net intertwin transfusion accounts for much of the hemodynamic change present in TTTS. Doppler studies of recipients show venous waveform patterns consistent with increased central venous pressure. Typically, donor fetuses display little abnormality in cardiac function, whereas recipient fetuses frequently develop cardiomegaly, tricuspid regurgitation, and ventricular hypertrophy. Decreased glomerular filtration and renal perfusion in the donor may be responsible for a renal defect which may be more developmental rather than secondary to ischemia. High atrial natriuretic peptide, secreted in response to fluid overload, along with concomitant suppression of antidiuretic hormone, mediates the associated polyuria and polyhydramnios.[10] Hypervolemia also elevates cardiac preload. Findings of hypertension in the recipient[11] indicate that elevated afterload may also contribute to cardiovascular dysfunction. Cardiac hypertrophy secondary to increased afterload sometimes results in functional right ventricular outflow obstruction of sufficient severity to warrant valvotomy in infancy. Recipient kidneys are enlarged, congested, and show hemorrhagic infarction, with glomerular and arterial changes resembling those found in polycythemia and hypertension.

Several features of TTTS are not explained by fluid volume disturbances. In the recipient, these include systemic hypertension and hypertrophic outflow tract obstruction. In the donor, these include increased placental vascular resistance *in utero* and reduced arterial compliance in infancy. Further, little correlation exists between hemoglobin discordance and disease severity. Discordant long-term vascular programming in genetically 'identical' survivors, which appears preventable with timely intrauterine therapy, implicates deranged fetoplacental vascular function *in utero*.[12]

DIAGNOSIS OF TWIN-TO-TWIN TRANSFUSION SYNDROME

In the past, diagnosis of the syndrome was made only after delivery of the affected twin pair and careful examination of the placenta. The standard neonatal criteria comprised a difference in *cord hemoglobin* concentrations of

Table 13.1 Step-by-step diagnosis of twin-to-twin transfusion syndrome

Step 1	look for chorionicity (preferably between 11 and 14 weeks)
Step 2	look for discordance in amniotic fluid volume/bladder size
Step 3	look for discordance in size between twins (abdominal circumference)
Step 4	assess Doppler blood flow in fetal vessels (UA, DV, UV)/fetal heart (transtricuspid flow)
Step 5	look for signs of fetal hydrops (echocardiography)
Step 6	look for placental brightness or other ancillary signs

UA, umbilical artery; DV, ductus venosus; UV, umbilical vein

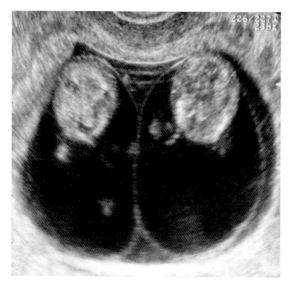

Figure 13.6 Example of a monochorionic twin pregnancy at 11 weeks of gestation, showing a thin dividing membrane without chorion between the amnion layers

5 g/dl or more and a difference in *birth weights* of 20% or more. Danskin and Neilson,[13] in 1989, revisited the neonatal criteria for diagnosis of TTTS, finding that an intertwin hemoglobin disparity of 5 g/dl or more and birth weight differences of more than 20% were present in both MC and DC twins in similar proportions. Wenstrom and colleagues[14] shortly thereafter also found that weight and hemoglobin level discordance were relatively common among MC twins. With the publication of these two reports, it became clear that making a diagnosis of TTTS based solely on neonatal criteria was totally insufficient. Fortunately for all concerned, sonographic criteria for antenatal diagnosis of TTTS were waiting in the wings. It is clearly a credit to countless obstetric sonographers in diverse locations, having at their disposal increasingly sophisticated technology, that not only did the diagnosis become ultrasonically based, but more recently a composite of ultrasonographic features has been proposed to identify TTTS correctly and minimize false-positive errors (Table 13.1). The following paragraphs elaborate the steps listed in the table.

Determination of monozygosity and monochorionicity

TTTS is a syndrome unique to MC pregnancies. As such, the first step towards diagnosis is the establishment of chorionicity (approximately 100% correct chorionic assignment is possible during the first trimester of pregnancy). The concomitant appearance of several sonographic criteria assists in the correct diagnosis of chorionicity, the most determinant factor in terms of perinatal prognosis:

(1) One placenta with a paper-thin, reflective hair-like septum without a chorion between the two amnions (T-sign) at 10–14 weeks of gestation (Figure 13.6);
(2) Very thin septum of < 2 mm in thickness;
(3) Same sex in the observed pair.

In contrast, TTTS can be ruled out if signs of dichorionicity are present, i.e. two separate placentas or two fetuses of unlike sex, and a lambda or twin-peak sign with chorion between each layer of amnion at 10–14 weeks of gestation.

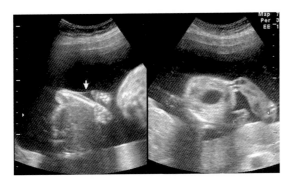

Figure 13.7 'Stuck twin'. The right image shows the recipient surrounded by severe polyhydramnios. The left image shows the donor entrapped in its membranes (arrow), surrounded by the severe polyhydramnios of the recipient. If the thin membrane is missed, the image could be erroneously diagnosed as monoamniotic twins. Image courtesy of B. Caspi, Kaplan Medical Center

Discordance in size

Discordant growth is a common complication of twin pregnancies and, as noted above, is no longer considered as a critical sign of TTTS, although many cases will exhibit size differences.[13,14]

Discordance in amniotic fluid volume (poly-oligohydramnios sequence)

In 1988, Chescheir and Seeds[15] described a powerful diagnostic clue for TTTS based on the fact that six out of seven twin pregnancies with monochorionic placentas and TTTS had concurrent polyhydramnios and oligohydramnios. This is not surprising when one considers that TTTS is a clinical manifestation of an intertwin hemodynamic imbalance as described above. Subsequently, more uniform criteria were proposed by Chamberlain et al for a quantitative definition of the oligohydramnios sequence: the deepest vertical pool in the donor sac should be < 2 cm and > 8 cm in the recipient sac.[16] Not infrequently, the oligohydramnios becomes anhydramnios within the donor sac and this circumstance results in the donor becoming 'stuck', that is, shrouded by the intertwin membrane. At the same time, however, the recipient sac becomes severely polyhydramniotic (Figure 13.7). The importance of using all the criteria listed in Table 13.1 lies in the observation that, in the presence of discordant anomalies in twins that cause differences in amniotic fluid volume such as esophageal atresia or renal agenesis, the olygohydramnios/anhydramnios sequence can also be present, albeit without the other diagnostic criteria. Other related confirmatory features include a small or non-visible bladder due to hypovolemia and renal hypoperfusion in the donor, along with a distended urinary bladder and resulting excessive micturition in the recipient. The poly-oligohydramnion sequence constitutes Quintero's stage I whereas the absent bladder in the donar constitutes stage II of severity of TTTS.

Abnormal Doppler findings

Alterations in cardiac hemodynamics are indirectly captured by alterations in venous blood flow waveforms. The abnormal pulsatile pattern consists of an increased velocity of blood flow away from the heart during atrial contraction, and this phenomenon has been reported in the fetus with a failing heart.

Studies concerning arterial Doppler velocimetry in TTTS are not in agreement. On the one hand, some authors[17,18] report no or little difference in the indices of the umbilical arteries in TTTS, whereas others find various changes in vascular resistance.[19,20] Ohno and colleagues suggested that Doppler velocimetry in the umbilical artery might detect TTTS before the appearance of fetal hydrops. This disagreement aside, Doppler was found useful in monitoring of the fetoplacental circulation and fetal condition, especially during treatment, but no benefit was shown regarding fetal outcome.[19]

A cross-sectional study investigating the circulatory profile of co-twins in TTTS in mid-pregnancy was reported by Hecher and co-workers.[20] These investigators found an increased resistance to flow in the umbilical arteries of both donor and recipient, but beyond 21 weeks of gestation, the resistance was increased only in the recipient. They suggested that this high resistance could be a consequence of compression of placental vessels due to two possible mechanisms. The first might be increased intra-amniotic pressure in polyhydramnios, and the second might be placental edema resulting from hypervolemia-related heart failure. The increased resistance to flow in the donor's umbilical artery may either reflect a primary maldevelopment of the donor's placenta or may be caused by compression of the cord due to polyhydramnios in the recipient's sac. The donor fetus could be expected to have severe utero-placental insufficiency with additional chronic hypovolemia. Currently, Doppler studies of the umbilical artery are an integral part of assigning the severity of TTTS.[21] Abnormal Dopller velocimetry constitutes Quintero's stage III of severity of TTTS.

Doppler studies of the middle cerebral artery (MCA) in TTTS show a decreased pulsatility index (PI) in the recipient, whereas PI values in the donor vary within the normal range, but are occasionally lower or higher.[20] Hecher and co-workers speculated that the changes in blood flow in the recipient's MCA might be the consequence of hypervolemia-related congestive heart failure, and might represent vasodilatation in response to heart failure-related hypoxemia.[20] The Doppler values in the donor's MCA suggested the absence of redistribution in the fetal circulation. The increased PI values in some cases could also be the result of head compression by polyhydramnios of the recipient's sac, or a result of reduction in the left ventricular output, suggesting decompensation of fetal cerebral circulation.[20] At present, the best explanation for the Doppler findings in the donor is hypovolemia rather than anemia and hypoxemia, and, in the recipient, hypervolemia and congestive heart failure might partly explain the observed changes. Suzuki and colleagues studied the MCA and the umbilical artery Doppler waveforms in growth-restricted fetuses with and without TTTS, and found that the MCA PI values in the TTTS group, especially in fetuses who subsequently developed periventricular leukomalacia, were significantly higher than normal values.[22] This finding suggests an absence of blood flow redistribution, as observed in hypoxemic and IUGR fetuses due to placental insufficiency.[22]

Senat et al[23] assessed the value of the fetal MCA-peak systolic velocity (PSV) in the prediction of anemia within 24 hours of the death of one MC twin in TTTS. Doppler examination of the MCA-PSV was performed in 20 MC survivors of pregnancies complicated by TTTS between 20 and 34 weeks' gestation. The sensitivity and specificity of MCA-PSV in the prediction of severe fetal anemia were 90%, with a false-negative rate of 10%. The correlation between PSV and hemoglobin concentration was strongly significant. The authors concluded that in fetuses at risk of acute anemia, the measurement of MCA-PSV is a reliable non-invasive diagnostic tool and may be helpful in counseling and planning invasive assessment and therapy. More recently, Robyr and co-workers[24] reported on the prevalence and management of late complications in TTTS treated by laser therapy when both twins remained alive 1 week after surgery. MCA-PSV Doppler measurements were useful in the follow-up of double survivors to detect recurrence of TTTS with (14%) and without (13%) polyhydramnios–oligohydramnios sequence, but manifesting as anemia and polycythemia that result from unidirectional feto-fetal blood transfusion, mainly from former recipients into former donors.

The umbilical artery PI values in the smaller twin were significantly higher in the TTTS group compared with the non-TTTS group; however, these values decreased after amnioreduction, and were associated with recovery of fetal circulation.[25] The variable umbilical artery Doppler findings for TTTS are probably a result of the complex pathophysiologic features of this condition, for which there is no predictable pattern of vascular anastomoses and no uniform pattern of umbilical artery blood flow abnormalities. The literature is without consensus whether fetuses presenting signs of increased placental resistance may be fetuses with TTTS or rather fetuses suffering from placental insufficiency.

The most striking feature in TTTS is reduced or reversed flow during atrial contraction in the ductus venosus (DV). This

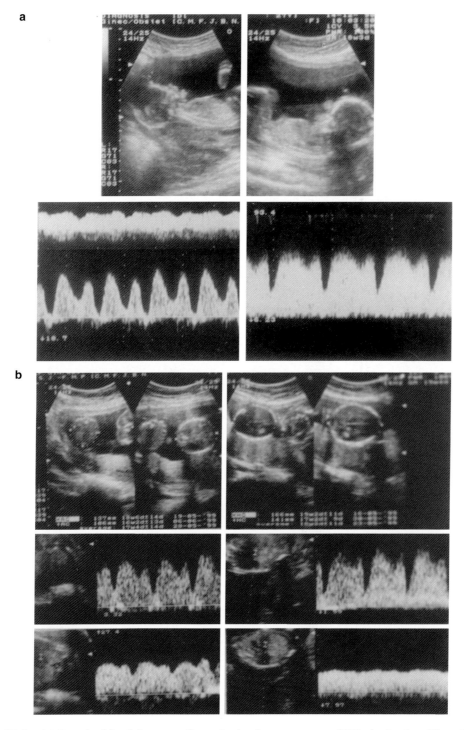

Figure 13.8 (a) Doppler blood flow waveforms in the ductus venosus (DV) obtained at 18 weeks of gestation, when twin-to-twin transfusion was detected. Abnormal flow in the DV (absent flow during atrial contraction) and umbilical vein (pulsatile flow) was recorded in the recipient. (b) Improvement in DV waveforms in the recipient 1 week after fetoscopic laser coagulation

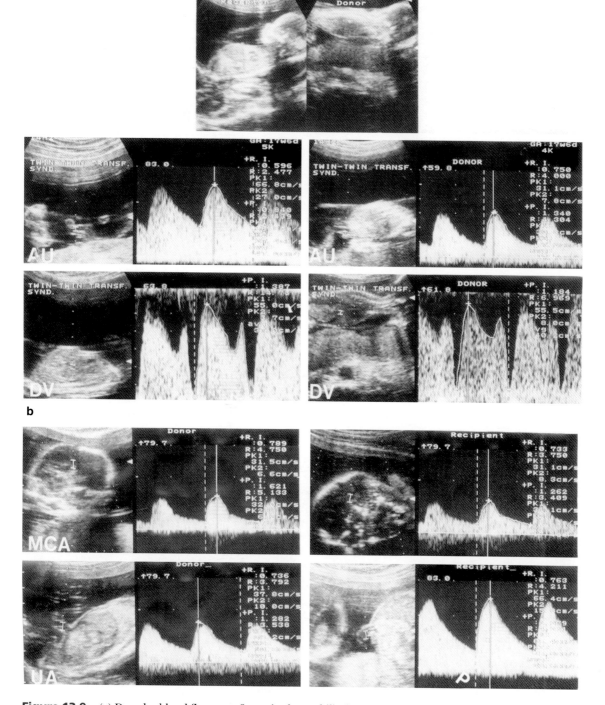

Figure 13.9 (a) Doppler blood flow waveforms in the umbilical artery (AU) and ductus venosus (DV) obtained at 17 weeks of gestation, when twin-to-twin transfusion was detected. In both fetuses, abnormal flow in the DV (decreased velocity during atrial contraction) was recorded. The umbilical artery showed

b *Continued*

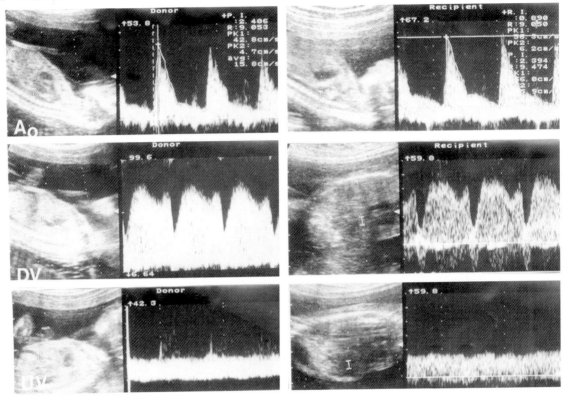

Figure 13.9 *Continued*
normal blood flow waveforms. Note the 'stuck twin' with oligohydramnios (donor) and the polyhydramnios around the recipient. (b) Normal Doppler blood flow profiles (arterial and venous) obtained in both fetuses 1 week after fetoscopic laser coagulation. MCA, middle cerebral artery; UA, umbilical artery; Ao, descending aorta; UV, umbilical vein. Reproduced with permission from reference 26

feature is commonly found in fetuses with congenital heart defects, growth restriction, and TTTS (Figures 13.8 and 13.9). In all these clinical situations, this particular hemodynamic alteration seems to reflect impaired cardiac performance and appears as a sign of dismal prognosis. Hecher and co-workers[27] described highly pulsatile venous waveforms in the recipient with fully established TTTS. Umbilical vein pulsations and absent or reversed flow during atrial contraction in the DV are signs of congestive heart failure due to hypervolemia and increased preload from placental vascular anastomotic transfusion.

Echocardiography

The advantages of fetal echocardiography in TTTS include an accurate assessment of the cardiovascular adaptation to intertwin transfusion, the early recognition of deterioration, and the possibility of an evaluation of antenatal management. Considering the hemodynamic imbalance between each of the circulations, a process that involves an excess of blood flowing from the donor to the recipient fetus, cardiac involvement is logically expected. Echocardiography is a well-established tool for antenatal assessment of both structural and functional heart disease.

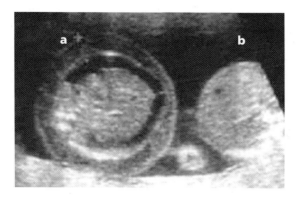

Figure 13.10 Severe hydrops of the recipient twin (a) is seen on the left, with skin edema and liver floating in massive ascites. On the right is the donor twin (b). Image courtesy of B. Caspi, Kaplan Medical Center

In one study, all recipient fetuses (17 pairs of MC twins with TTTS) showed cardiac hypertrophy and dilatation, well-known compensatory mechanisms for blood volume overload and high cardiac output (the so-called Frank–Starling mechanism).[28] The cardiac involvement in the recipient twins was of variable severity, however, ranging from biventricular hypertrophy and dilatation to impaired contraction, with massive signs of tricuspid regurgitation and hydrops fetalis. A larger study showed unquestionable functional changes but a lower prevalence (less than 80%) of hemodynamic abnormalities in recipients.[12] That the ultrasound changes are real and persistent is demonstrated by the observation that, after birth, about half of the recipients show biventricular hypertrophy, with prevalent left ventricular hypertrophic cardiomyopathy. Of equal importance, a smaller subgroup will develop right ventricular tract obstruction (functional pulmonary stenosis) and pulmonary hypertension in the neonatal period,[29] which may be aggravated by systolic right ventricular dysfunction. Diastolic abnormalities have also been described in the right ventricle, with abnormal filling patterns, prolonged isovolumic relaxation time, and abnormal flow patterns in the inferior vena cava and ductus venosus.

Finally, it is important to remember that the conflicting Doppler results in TTTS may be explained by different pathophysiologic mechanisms and different stages of severity of the disease at the time of examination. Further and additional assessments of fetal cardiac function and a better understanding of the pathophysiology of cardiac dysfunction in TTTS may help not only in determining the best therapeutic regimen but also in potentially improving the fetal outcome.

Other ultrasonographic findings

These include, among other things, *identification of the cord insertion*, specifically a velamentous insertion of the cord. Also, *funipuncture* may theoretically allow the antenatal assessment of the intertwin hemoglobin difference, the degree of fetal anemia in the donor twin, and the twins' zygosity through various genetic studies. However, the possible benefit of this procedure seems to be questionable purely on clinical grounds, and the risks of invasive procedures like funipuncture significantly outweigh the informative gain. Other ultrasonographic findings might include *signs of hydrops in the recipient twin*. In an advanced stage of TTTS, the recipient twin, affected by congestive heart failure, may present signs of serosal effusions, such as ascites, pleural effusion, or subcutaneous edema (Figure 13.10). Hydrops constitutes Quintero's stage IV of severity of TTTS.

Placental brightness

There may be a *difference in color of the placentas*. Owing to blood transfusion from one twin to the other, the placenta of the donor twin tends to be whitish ('pale'), and the placenta of the recipient a denser (darker) color (excess of blood) (Figure 13.11). This phenomenon can

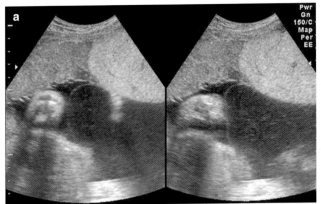
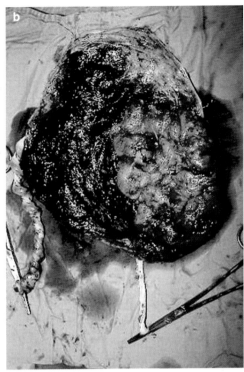

Figure 13.11 (a) This case was diagnosed as a monochorionic twin pregnancy. However, the twins exhibited many signs of twin-to-twin transfusion syndrome, but both sacs showed polyhydramnios. At 32 weeks, a clear difference in echogenicity between the two parts of the placenta could be seen. After birth, an H-type tracheo-esophageal fistula was found in the donor, explaining the dual polyhydramnios. (a) The maternal surface of the placenta seen in (b). The dark color was due to congestion and the pale part due to blood depletion. Images courtesy of B. Caspi and I. Blickstein, Kaplan Medical Center

sometimes be seen in the ultrasound scan as differences in the brightness of the placenta, and confirmed after birth by visual and necropsy examination.

PREDICTION OF TWIN-TO-TWIN TRANSFUSION SYNDROME

Based on the formidable complications that may be encountered in TTTS, targeted surveillance of MC twins at earlier stages of gestation could anticipate and provide timely management of the pregnancies at risk, and in particular of the TTTS. The potential to predict TTTS at an early gestational age comes mainly from the observation that increased NT in multiple pregnancy and abnormal blood flow in the DV seem to be related not only to chromosomal abnormalities or severe cardiac defects but also to specific complications of MC twins such as TTTS.

Nuchal translucency

Increased nuchal translucency thickness (NT) at 10–14 weeks of gestation is twice as common in MC twins compared with singleton pregnancies, and the likelihood ratio of developing TTTS in twins with increased NT is 3.51. Considering that MC pregnancies do not show a higher prevalence of chromosomal abnormalities, the higher prevalence of increased NT in twins could be ascribed to cardiac dysfunction. With advancing gestation, this transient heart failure eventually resolves, with increased diuresis and ventricular compliance.

Ductus venosus flowmetry

In recent studies of vascular hemodynamics in fetuses with increased NT at 10–14 weeks, the abnormal flow in the DV more frequently recorded in fetuses with chromosomopathies, with or without cardiac defects, was related to

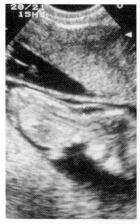
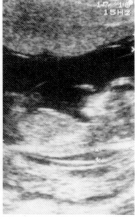
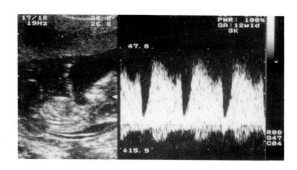

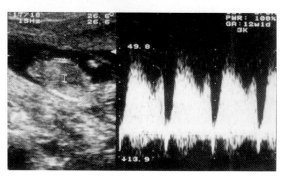

Figure 13.12 A monochorionic–diamniotic twin pregnancy was established at 12 weeks of gestation Doppler blood flow waveforms in both fetuses were obtained in the ductus venosus (DV). A discrete nuchal translucency (NT) discrepancy was noted (NT = 3.3/3.7 mm). The fetus with the highest NT showed an inverted A-wave in the DV and later developed signs of twin-to-twin transfusion syndrome at 18 weeks of gestation

heart strain. These findings are in general agreement with the overt hemodynamic alterations found in TTTS later in pregnancy. Therefore, accumulated evidence suggests that increased NT along with abnormal flow in the DV, even in the presence of a normal karyotype, may be early signs of cardiac impairment or defect. Matias et al reported that in all cases with both discrepant NT and abnormal blood flow in the DV, TTTS eventually developed (Figures 13.12 and 13.13). In contrast, whenever NT was abnormal but with normal flow in the DV, no cases of TTTS were found.[30,31]

Arterio-arterial anastomoses

Arterio-arterial anastomoses were recruited for an ultrasonographic survey of the chorionic plate using color Doppler energy, and were identified by their characteristic bidirectional interference pattern on spectral Doppler[32] (Figures 13.14 and 13.15). This

search for AA anastomoses in the placental plate was, until now, mainly used to exclude TTTS: only 5% of MC twins develop TTTS if AA anastomoses are present. In contrast, if AA anastomoses are absent, 58% develop TTTS. The studies of Taylor and co-workers[33] show a sensitivity and positive predictive value for absent AA anastomoses in predicting TTTS of 74% and 61%, respectively. The major limitation to the use of absent AA anastomoses in predicting TTTS, however, is the difficulty in being sure that an AA anastomosis is really absent or simply not yet seen, as frequently happens before 18 weeks. A recent Italian study[34] evaluated the reproducibility of Doppler antenatal detection of AA anastomoses in MC placentas, searched by color or power and spectral Doppler and confirmed postnatally by placental injection studies. Sensitivity and specificity of Doppler for detecting AA anastomoses were 75 and 100%,

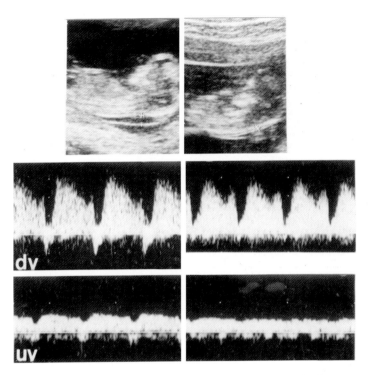

Figure 13.13 A monochorionic–diamniotic twin pregnancy was established at 12 weeks of gestation. Doppler blood flow waveforms in both fetuses were obtained in the umbilical vein (uv) and ductus venosus (dv) in the same scan. A nuchal translucency (NT) discrepancy was noted (NT = 3.7/1.0 mm). The fetus with increased NT showed an inverted A-wave in the ductus venosus and dicrotic pulsatility in the umbilical vein. Twin-to-twin transfusion syndrome developed at 17 weeks and the patient was referred for laser ablation of anastomosis. Reproduced with permission from reference 26

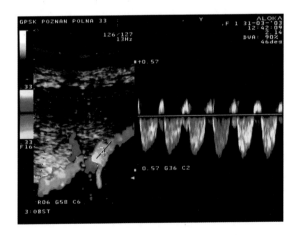

Figure 13.14 Color flow mapping of arterio-arterial (AA) anastomosis in twin-to-twin transfusion syndrome (left), and (right) pulsed Doppler waveforms obtained from superficial AA anastomosis indicating bidirectional blood flow

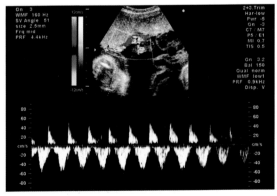

Figure 13.15 Color flow mapping of arterio-arterial anastomosis with signs of turbulent flow (top) and blood flow velocity waveforms (bottom)

respectively. Detection rates increased at advanced gestations and with an anterior/fundal placenta. As expected, the incidence of TTTS was higher in the group without AA anastomoses detected *in vivo* compared to the group with AA anastomoses found with Doppler (28.5 vs. 16.6%), but the difference was not statistically significant.

Superficial anastomoses have been implicated in the hemodynamic sequel of the death of a co-twin *in utero*, namely cerebral necrosis or intrauterine death. The visualization of superficial anastomoses by ultrasound may also have a role in monitoring therapy. Arterio-venous anastomoses have also been detected *in vivo* by color Doppler ultrasound.[35] This technique allows identification of pregnancies at risk of TTTS and may facilitate their treatment. Color Doppler ultrasound 'mapping' could make the endoscopic treatment of TTTS more selective and shorter, leading to less invasive techniques such as interstitial laser or focused ultrasound therapy.[36] In contrast, it is believed that color Doppler sonography is unlikely to play a major role in assisting endoscopic laser therapies in patients with acute polyhydramnios, as the communicating vessels cannot be identified in the majority of cases. However, further prospective studies are indicated to determine the utility of color Doppler energy for finding those anastomoses in establishing the prognosis in MC pregnancies.

REFERENCES

1. Fisk NM, Taylor MJO. The fetus(es) with twin twin transfusion syndrome. In: Harrison M, Evans M, Adzick S, Holzgreve W, eds. The Unborn Patient: The Art and Science of Fetal Therapy. Philadelphia: WB Saunders 2000: 341–55.

2. Danskin FH, Neilson JP. Twin-to-twin transfusion syndrome: what are appropriate diagnostic criteria? Am J Obstet Gynecol 1989; 161: 365–9.

3. Quintero RA, Chmait RH. The cocoon sign: a potential sonographic pitfall in the diagnosis of twin–twin transfusion syndrome. Ultrasound Obstet Gynecol 2004; 23: 38–41.

4. Wieacker P, Wilhelm C, Prompeler H et al. Pathophysiology of polyhydramnios in twin transfusion syndrome. Fetal Diagn Ther 1992; 7: 87–92.

5. Rosen DJ, Rabinowitz R, Beyth Y et al. Fetal urine production in normal twins and in twins with acute polyhydramnios. Fetal Diagn Ther 1990; 5: 57–60.

6. Bajoria R, Wigglesworth J, Fisk NM. Angioarchitecture of monochorionic placentas in relation to the twin–twin transfusion syndrome. Am J Obstet Gynecol 1995; 172: 856–63.

7. Denbow ML, Cox P, Taylor M et al. Placental angioarchitecture in monochorionic twin pregnancies: relationship to fetal growth, fetofetal transfusion syndrome, and pregnancy outcome. Am J Obstet Gynecol 2000; 182: 417–26.

8. Taylor MJ, Denbow ML, Tanawattanacharoen S et al. Doppler detection of arterio-arterial anastomoses in monochorionic twins: feasibility and clinical application. Hum Reprod 2000; 15: 1632–6.

9. Taylor MJ, Denbow ML, Duncan KR et al. Antenatal factors at diagnosis that predict outcome in twin–twin transfusion syndrome. Am J Obstet Gynecol 2000; 183: 1023–8.

10. Bajoria R, Ward RS, Sooranna SR. Atrial natriuretic peptide mediated polyuria: pathogenesis of polyhydramnios in the recipient to twin–twin transfusion syndrome. Placenta 2001; 22: 716–24.

11. Mahieu-Caputo D, Salomon LJ, Le Bidois J et al. Fetal hypertension: an insight into the pathogenesis of the twin–twin transfusion syndrome. Prenat Diagn 2003; 23: 640–5.

12. Gardiner HM, Taylor MJ, Karatza A et al. Twin–twin transfusion syndrome. The influence of intrauterine laser photocoagulation on arterial distensibility in childhood. Circulation 2003; 107: 1906–11.

13. Danskin FH, Neilson JP. Twin-to-twin transfusion syndrome: what are appropriate diagnostic criteria? Am J Obstet Gynecol 1989; 161: 365–9.

14. Wenstrom KD, Tessen JA, Zlatnik FJ, Sipes SL. Frequency, distribution and theoretical mechanisms of hematologic and weight discordance in MC twins. Obstet Gynecol 1992; 80: 257–61.

15. Chescheir NC, Seeds JW. Polyhydramnios and oligohydramnios in twin gestations. Obstet Gynecol 1988; 71: 882–4.

16. Chamberlain PF, Manning FA, Morrison I et al. Ultrasound evaluation of amniotic fluid volume. I. The relationship of marginal and decreased amniotic fluid volumes to perinatal outcome. Am J Obstet Gynecol 1984; 150: 245–50.

17. Giles WB, Trudinger BJ, Cook CM, Connelly AJ. Umbilical artery waveforms in triplet pregnancy. Obstet Gynecol 1990; 75: 813–16.

18. Rizzo G, Arduini D, Romanini C. Cardiac and extracardiac flows in discordant twins. Am J Obstet Gynecol 1994; 170: 1321–7.

19. Ohno Y, Ando H, Tanamura A et al. The value of Doppler ultrasound in the diagnosis and the management of twin-to-twin transfusion syndrome. Arch Gynecol Obstet 1994; 255: 37–42.

20. Hecher K, Ville Y, Nicolaides KH. Fetal arterial Doppler studies in twin–twin transfusion syndrome. J Ultrasound Med 1995; 14: 101–8.

21. Quintero RA, Dickinson JE, Morales WJ et al. Stage-based treatment of twin–twin transfusion syndrome. Am J Obstet Gynecol 2003; 188: 1333–40.

22. Suzuki S, Sawa R, Yoneyama Y et al. Fetal middle cerebral artery Doppler waveforms in twin–twin transfusion syndrome. Gynecol Obstet Invest 1999; 48: 237–40.

23. Senat MV, Loizeau S, Couderc S, Bernard JP, Ville Y. The value of middle cerebral artery peak systolic velocity in the diagnosis of fetal anemia after intrauterine death of one monochorionic twin. Am J Obstet Gynecol 2003; 189: 1320–4.

24. Robyr R, Lewi L, Salomon LJ et al. Prevalence and management of late fetal complications following successful selective laser coagulation of chorionic plate anastomoses in twin-to-twin transfusion syndrome. Am J Obstet Gynecol 2006; 194: 796–803.

25. Dickinson JE, Newnham JP, Phillips JM. The role of Doppler ultrasound prediction of therapeutic success in twin–twin transfusion syndrome. J Matern Fetal Invest 1995; 5: 39.

26. Matias A, Montenegro N, Areias JC. Anticipating twin–twin transfusion syndrome in monochorionic twin pregnancy. Is there a role for nuchal translucency and ductus venosus blood flow evaluation at 11–14 weeks? Twin Res 2000; 3: 65–70.

27. Hecher K, Ville Y, Snijders R, Nicolaides KH. Doppler studies of the fetal circulation in twin-to-twin transfusion syndrome. Ultrasound Obstet Gynecol 1995; 5: 318–24.

28. Fesslova V, Villa L, Nava S, Mosca F, Nicolini U. Fetal and neonatal echocardiographic findings in twin–twin transfusion syndrome. Am J Obstet Gynecol 1998; 179: 1056–62.

29. Zosmer N, Bajoria R, Weiner E, Rigby M, Vaughan J, Fisk N. Clinical and echographic features of in utero cardiac dysfunction in the recipient twin-to-twin transfusion syndrome. Br Heart J 1994; 72: 74–9.

30. Matias A, Montenegro N, Areias JC. Ductus venosus blood flow evaluation at 11–14 weeks in the anticipation of the twin–twin transfusion syndrome in monochorionic twin pregnancies. Ultrasound Rev Obstet Gynecol 2001; 1: 315.

31. Matias A, Ramalho C, Montenegro N. Search for hemodynamic compromise at 11–14 weeks in monochorionic twin pregnancy: is abnormal flow in the ductus venosus predictive of twin–twin transfusion syndrome? J Matern Fetal Neonatal Med 2005; 18: 79–86.

32. Denbow ML, Cox P, Talbert D, Fisk NM. Colour Doppler energy insonation of placental vasculature in monochorionic twins: absent arterio-arterial anastomoses in association with twin-to-twin transfusion syndrome. Br J Obstet Gynaecol 1998; 105: 760–5.

33. Taylor MJ, Denbow ML, Tanawattanacharoen S et al. Doppler detection of arterio-arterial anastomoses in monochorionic twins: feasibility and clinical application. Hum Reprod 2000; 15: 1632–6.

34. Fichera A, Mor E, Soregaroli M, Frusca TN. Antenatal detection of arterio-arterial anastomoses by Doppler placental assessment in monochorionic twin pregnancies. Fetal Diagn Ther 2005; 20: 519–23.

35. Taylor MJO, Farquharson D, Cox PM, Fisk NM. Identification of arterio-venous anastomoses in vivo in monochorionic twin pregnancies: preliminary report. Ultrasound Obstet Gynecol 2000; 16: 218–22.

36. Denbow ML, Rivens IH, Rowland IJ et al. Preclinical development of noninvasive vascular occlusion with focused ultrasonic surgery for fetal therapy. Am J Obstet Gynecol 2000; 182: 387–92.

14

Twin reversed arterial perfusion sequence

PATHOGENESIS

Abnormal placental vessels are common in monochorionic (MC) twinning. In the usual setting, blood from the placenta enters the fetal circulation through the umbilical veins and exits via the umbilical artery. Very rarely (1% of MC twins or 1:35 000 births), retrograde or reversed arterial perfusion takes place, from the placenta through the umbilical artery of one of the twins. In this setting, the twin with the reversed flow receives all of its blood supply from a normal co-twin who gains circulatory predominance – the so-called 'pump' twin. This vascular abnormality is currently termed the *twin reversed arterial perfusion* (TRAP) *sequence*. Often, the recipient twin demonstrates severe reduction anomalies of the upper part of the fetal body, and lacks a heart (*acardiac*, except for a few cases with a rudimentary – 'hemicardiac' – heart) and head (acephalic). Based on these observations, the TRAP sequence is also characterized as *chorioangiopagus parasiticus*, and as acardiac twinning.

The embryogenetic background of the TRAP sequence is still controversial. Opinions differ whether the underlying pathology is primary cardiac agenesis or cardiac dysmorphogenesis secondary to the reversed flow.[1] Some authors maintain that although TRAP might be a key diagnostic element for the acardiac condition, it need not necessarily be the primary cause, and a lethal heart malformation in early organogenesis – the so-called 'cardiac regression sequence' – seems more likely.[2] The theory holds further that the anomalous fetus is 'rescued' from an inevitable demise by the presence of a co-twin and the types of vascular connection that are required for TRAP, namely, close cord insertions and large arterio-arterial and veno-venous connections (Figure 14.1).

The alternative view holds that inadequate perfusion of the recipient twin is responsible for the development of the characteristic anomalies. In one recent report, the TRAP sequence was diagnosed several weeks after demonstrating independent embryonic heart rates by ultrasonography performed at 5–6 weeks.[1] The unique aspects of this case suggest that the pathogenesis of acardiac twining involves an arterio-arterial shunt with retrograde blood flow, and not a primary arrest in cardiac development.

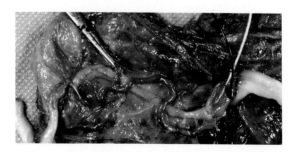

Figure 14.1 Twin reversed arterial perfusion. The cords are inserted very close together, with large arterio-arterial and veno-venous connections between their bases. The acardiac cord is to the left

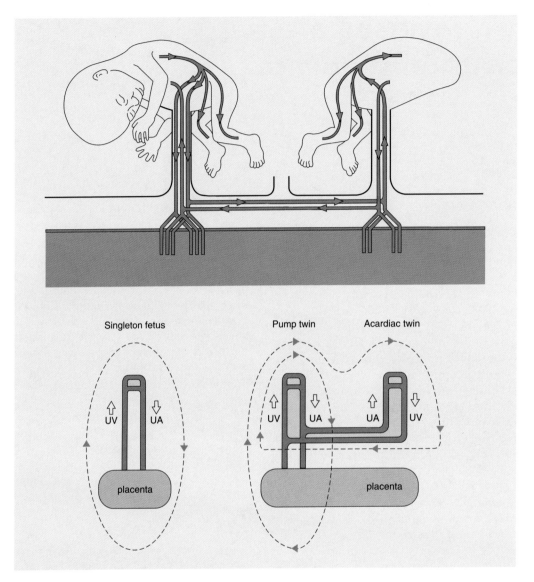

Figure 14.2 Twin reversed arterial perfusion (TRAP). Because the acardiac fetus has no active circulation, blood returns directly from its body to the pump twin without any passage through the placenta. This blood is therefore 'twice-used', hypoxic, possibly carrying thromboemboli from the veno-venous anastomosis and routed directly to the brain of the pump twin

Regardless, the pump twin perfuses the whole placenta and the acardiac twin represents a 'side-branch' of the pump twin's circulation (Figures 14.1 and 14.2). The venous blood returning from the acardiac to the pump twin via the veno-venous connection is 'twice-used', having perfused the bodies of both pump and acardiac twins without benefit of a cycle of placental purging. Furthermore, blood flow in the veno-venous connection is very slow, thrombosis frequently affects the vessel, and thromboembolism is a risk (Figure 14.3).

Although the TRAP sequence and the twin–twin transfusion syndrome (TTTS) share some similarities, they differ in several important aspects (Figure 14.4). First, whereas both

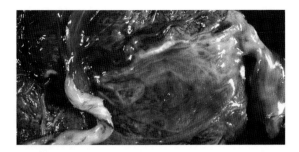

Figure 14.3 Thrombosis in the veno-venous return from the acardiac to the pump twin is caused by sluggish flow. Emboli from the veno-venous thrombosis would run immediately to the brain of the pump twin

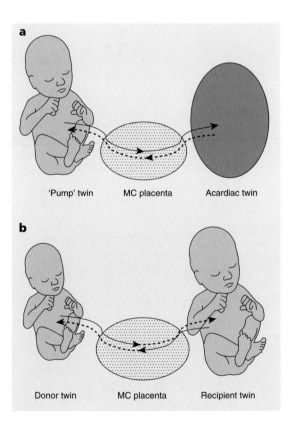

Figure 14.4 Schematic representation of vascular connections in twin reversed arterial perfusion (TRAP) and in twin–twin transfusion syndrome (TTTS). (a) In TRAP, the vascular connection is via a transplacental arterio-arterial anastomosis; (b) in TTTS, the vascular connection is via a transplacental arterio-venous anastomosis. MC, monochorionic

share a trans(MC)placental shunt from a donor to a recipient twin, in TTTS the shunt is via an arterio-venous anastomosis and in TRAP, on the other hand, the shunt is via an arterio-arterial connection. Second, the twins in TTTS are usually anatomically normal, whereas in TRAP, the recipient twin is grossly malformed. Finally, the strain on the fetal heart in TTTS is usually present in the recipient who suffers from cardiac overload, whereas the heart problem in TRAP is present in the donor, who needs to provide for both twins.

In 1981, Bieber and co-workers[3] identified two maternally derived chromosome sets and both maternal histocompatibility antigen haplotypes in the tissues of an acardiac twin. These findings were explained by proposing independent fertilizations, by two different spermatozoa, of a normal haploid ovum and its diploid first-meiotic-division polar body. More recently, however, Fisk and colleagues[4] performed polymerase chain reaction (PCR) on DNA extraction from nine twin sets with the TRAP sequence. Based on DNA fingerprinting patterns, Fisk and colleagues calculated that the chance that any of the acardiac twins resulted from fertilization of either the first or second polar body was < 4%, and the chance that they all resulted from polar body fertilization was < 1:100 000.[4]

NOMENCLATURE

The anomalies associated with TRAP are categorized according to the site of maldevelopment:

(1) Acardius anceps: a body and extremities are present, but the head and face are partially developed (Figure 14.5);

(2) Acardius acephalus: there are developed pelvis and lower limbs without a head, thorax, or arms;

(3) Acardius amorphus: this is an amorphous mass without recognizable organs, but with some form of axial structure (Figure 14.6); Figure 14.7 shows an X-ray image of an acardius amorphous twin;

(4) Acardius acormus: there is some cranial development.

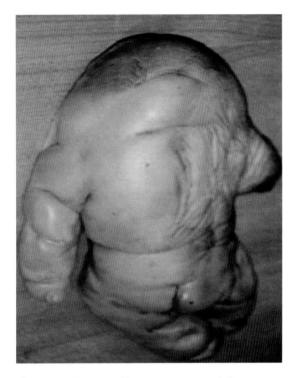

Figure 14.5 Acardiac monster post-delivery

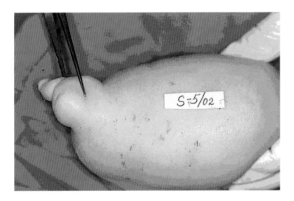

Figure 14.6 Acardius amorphus. This amorphous mass has no recognizable organs, but has some form of a limb

DIAGNOSIS

Sonographic imaging during the first trimester usually depicts MC twins, with absent or vague heartbeat in one. Sometimes, it is difficult to distinguish the fetal heart from

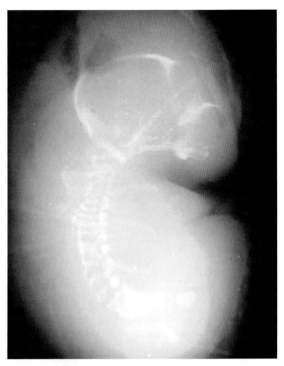

Figure 14.7 X-ray image of the acardiac twin shown in Figure 14.6. Note the underdeveloped skull, no facial contour and no limb bones

the large pulsating mediastinal vessels, which can be present in these fetuses, and this may lead to difficult diagnosis of embryonic death in an acardiac fetus in early pregnancy.[5,6]

Typically, the acardiac twin has a non-functioning heart, in addition to other characteristics, such as poorly developed or absent upper extremities or head[7] and severely malformed upper body with (variably) holoprosencephalus, anencephalus, or other brain malformations (Figure 14.8), facial cleaving and large cystic hygroma, abnormality of the thoracic viscera, severe abnormality of the thoracic bone structure, or severe abnormality or absence of the upper abdomen (liver, pancreas, and proximal intestine). Less frequently, the lower half of the body is affected, resulting in abnormalities of the external genitalia,[8] equinovarus and radial-ray deficiency, or

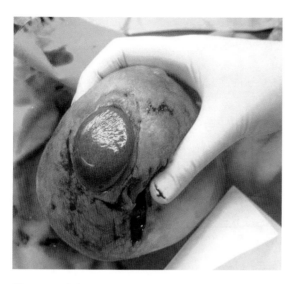

Figure 14.8 Cephalic end of the acardiac twin shown in Figure 14.6. Note the porencephalic cyst-like structure

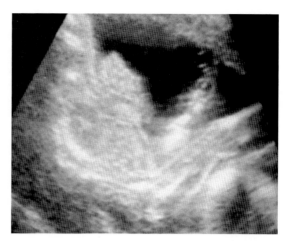

Figure 14.10 Acardiac twin at 22 weeks of gestation. Note the grotesque and malformed structure of the fetus

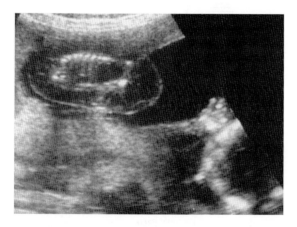

Figure 14.9 Acardiac twin: ultrasound image of the amorphic acardiac fetus. Note part of the fetal skeleton

abnormal or aberrant vasculature (single umbilical artery, persistent urachus, etc.).

Based on these structural malformations, the lumpy (Figure 14.9) or grotesque (Figure 14.10) phenotypic characteristics of the acardiac twin are easily recognized later in pregnancy. The sonographic diagnosis should be suspected on detection of a severe malformation, such as an unidentifiable head, trunk, or

extremities, in a monochorionic pair.[9] Other sonographic criteria include the absence of cardiac pulsations in one twin, generalized subcutaneous edema, polyhydramnios, and cystic masses in the upper fetal body. Among the complex constellation of malformations, omphalocele is particularly common (Figure 14.11a and b).[10] In one report of monoamnionic male twins, the acardiac twin demonstrated externalized intestines adherent to the placenta, absence of structures rostral to the thorax (except one poorly developed hand and arm), and the abdomen contained no organs. The entire intestine as well as two testes was located in a sac on the surface of the placenta.[10]

In rare instances, a heartbeat is noted in the acardiac twin, which may represent either a reflection of the pump twin's heartbeat or the presence of a rudimentary heart in the acardiac twin. Sometimes serial sonographic examinations are required to rule out single fetal death within the pair.

The diagnosis is confirmed by the characteristic reversed flow into the circulation of the acardiac twin by color Doppler studies of the umbilical vessels (Figure 14.12). In addition, the arterial umbilical systolic/diastolic (S/D) ratio is significantly high.[11–13]

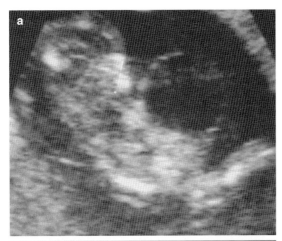

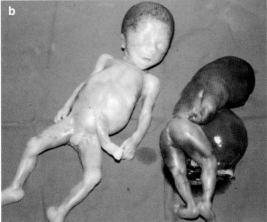

Figure 14.11 (a) Ultrasound image of another acardiac twin. Note the distended, fluid-filled abdomen. (b) Post-abortion image of the acardiac twin seen in (a). Note the malformed acardiac abortus in relation to the normal abortus

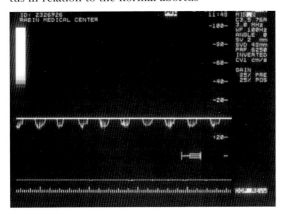

Figure 14.12 Doppler signals detected in the acardiac umbilical artery. Note shallow amplitude and absent end-diastolic flow

Table 14.1 Differential sonographic diagnosis of TRAP sequence

- Missed twin in an MC gestation
- Fetal teratoma
- Placental teratoma
- Conjoined twins
- Degenerating submucous fibroid

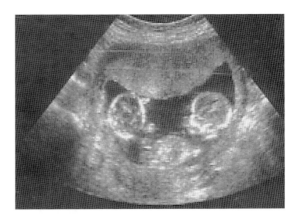

Figure 14.13 First-trimester sonography showing twins. One of the twins was diagnosed as a missed abortion, but was, in fact, an acardiac twin

Differential diagnosis (Table 14.1)

Regrettably, many cases are erroneously diagnosed during early ultrasound as a missed abortion of one twin (Figure 14.13). However, in a typical missed abortion, the size of the embryo/fetus decreases with time. In contrast, the size of the presumed acardiac twin *increases*. Since no dead embryo can increase in size, the diagnosis of TRAP sequence should be straightforward.

The sonographic differential diagnosis of an acardiac twin in the second trimester is a teratoma, wherein an amorphous trigerminal-layer mass is attached to a normal fetus. Teratoma can be differentiated by the completely disorganized nature of the tissue and the intrafunicular position.[11] In addition, the acardiac twin has a separate umbilical cord. Gillet et al[14] described an extremely rare case (less than 20 cases have been reported in the

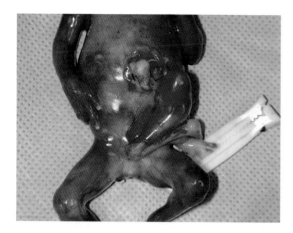

Figure 14.14 Completely formed fetus and an adjacent second body consisting of a pelvis with two lower extremities. Image courtesy of I. Timor, NY, USA

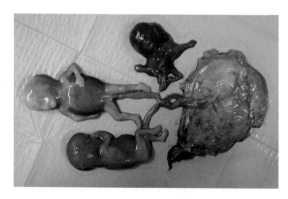

Figure 14.15 Monochorionic–monoamniotic triplet at 15 weeks gestational age with TRAP sequence and severe cord entanglement. Image courtesy of L. Lewi, Leuven, Belgium

literature since 1925) of placental teratoma erroneously mistaken for a TRAP sequence.

TRAP sequence and epigastric heteropagus conjoined twins may appear similar on antenatal sonography.[15] Differentiation between the two entities can be accomplished by three-dimensional (3D) ultrasound, which evaluates the relationship of a completely formed fetus and an adjacent second body consisting of a pelvis with two lower extremities (Figure 14.14). Indeed, 3D ultrasound may help to confirm uncertain cases of acardiac twins as depicted by regular 2D ultrasound.[16] Finally, an acardiac fetus can be misdiagnosed antenatally as a degenerated submucous fibroid.[17]

Diagnostic measures to help management decision

When the diagnosis is made sufficiently early, potential interception of the blood supply to the acardiac twin is possible. Later, the umbilical cord may be too large for simple procedures. Clinicians have two management options – conservative and interventional. The following information should be known, however, before any management decision is made:

(1) Amnionicity: TRAP occurs in the diamniotic as well as in monoamniotic variants of the MC gestation. Monoamniotic twinning has been reported in only 25% of cases of TRAP sequence.[18] When TRAP occurs in monoamniotic pregnancies, treatment of the TRAP alone does not reduce the risks associated with monoamnionicity. It follows that umbilical cord occlusion with transection of the cord is necessary in patients with monoamniotic or 'pseudomonoamniotic' TRAP to avoid subsequent entanglement and demise of the 'pump' twin.[19]

(2) TRAP sequence may occur in higher-order multiples, such as in dichorionic triplets.[20] In such circumstances, termination of the acardiac twin by severing its blood supply does not reduce the risk of twin–twin transfusion between the 'pump' twin and the third fetus of the triplet set that also shares the MC placenta (Figure 14.15). Because such a complication is extremely rare, no clear-cut management exists.

(3) Although 'pump' twins are in essence morphologically and chromosomally normal, anomalies are reported in these twins. It is therefore necessary to exclude malformations in order to avoid unnecessary invasive treatments. Van Allen and colleagues[9] reported that the incidence of chromosomal abnormality in the 'pump' twin might be as high as 9%.

Assessment of well-being in the 'pump' twin

Despite essentially being anatomically normal, heart failure of the 'pump' twin is the primary concern in the TRAP sequence. This is because of the excess demand from the abnormal circulation, whereby the 'pump' twin maintains its circulation as well as that of the acardiac co-twin. The imposed cardiac overload, which also leads to polyhydramnios and preterm birth, is a serious threat to the 'pump' twin and, if left untreated, may cause death in as many as 50–75% of cases.[1] In one large series of 49 cases, the overall prenatal mortality was 55%, primarily associated with prematurity.[21] In this series, gestational age at delivery was 29 ± 7.3 weeks, and the birth weights were 1378 ± 1047 and 651 ± 571 g for the normal twin and the acardiac twin, respectively.[21] It follows that frequent assessments of the cardiac function of the 'pump' twin are critical steps in the management of these pregnancies and should be established during pregnancy even if 'prophylactic' invasive procedures are not performed. Moreover, continuous follow-up may determine when cardiac function begins to deteriorate, necessitating intervention by either prompt delivery or by an invasive procedure to interrupt the blood supply to the acardiac twin.

Acardiac twin to 'pump' twin size ratio

Because polyhydramnios, the acardiac twin's weight, and the occurrence of preterm labor are all related to the cardiac function of the 'pump' twin, perinatal outcome is strongly related to the ratio between the acardiac and 'pump' twins' weights. Specifically, the higher the weight of the acardiac twin, the more likely is the development of cardiac insufficiency in the 'pump' twin, with the risk of congestive heart failure increasing to 94% when the acardiac twin's weight is more than half that of the 'pump' twin.[21] Conversely, if the estimated weight of the acardiac twin is less than one-quarter that of the 'pump' twin, the prognosis is excellent without further therapy. In the series described by Moore and associates, the mean

Table 14.2 Estimated weight of the acardiac twin calculated from the longest dimension of the acardiac mass

Longest dimension of the acardiac mass (cm)	Estimated weight of the acardiac twin (g)
10	103
12	152
14	211
16	280
18	358
20	446
22	543
24	650
26	767
28	893
30	1029
32	1174
34	1329
36	1494
38	1668
40	1852

overall ratio of the acardiac/normal twin weight was 0.52 ± 0.42; however, the ratio for patients delivered at < 34 weeks was 60 vs. 29% ($p < 0.04$).[21] In one-quarter of the cases, the twins' weight ratio was > 0.7, and the incidence of preterm births in these cases was 90%. It follows that when the acardiac/normal twin weight ratio is low, delivery at term or near term can be expected. In contrast, when the weight ratio is high due to massive edema of the acardiac twin, the cardiac dysfunction of the 'pump' twin may indicate early delivery. A publication concerning 10 cases managed expectantly by Sullivan and colleagues[22] reported nine women who delivered healthy 'pump' twins (one neonatal death), at a mean gestational age of 34.2 weeks, and mean weights of the 'pump' and acardiac twins of 2279 and 1372 g, respectively. This observation suggests that when the diagnosis of TRAP is made antenatally, neonatal mortality of the 'pump' twin may be considerably less than previously reported.

As the fetal indices used for sonographic estimations of fetal weight are not applicable to

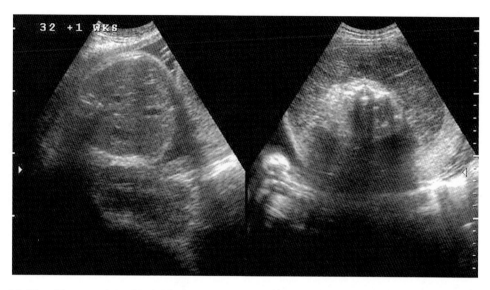

Figure 14.16 Characteristic third-trimester sonographic image of an acardiac twin (right). Note the vertebral column shown in this sonographic plane. Compare with the image of the 'pump' twin in the plane of the fetal liver (left)

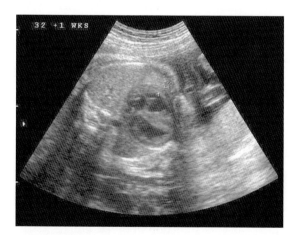

Figure 14.17 Measurement of cardiac wall hypertrophy of the 'pump' twin. Images 14. 16–17 courtesy of B. Caspi

acardiac twins, Moore et al[21] proposed the following equation:

$$\text{weight (g)} = 1.2L^2 - 1.7L$$

where L = longest dimension of the acardiac mass.[21] Table 14.2 shows the estimated weight of the acardiac twin by the length of the acardiac mass.

Alternatively, an approximate estimation of the weight of the acardiac twin can be made by comparing the abdominal circumferences of the twins (Figure 14.16), or by applying any formula that estimates the size of an ellipsoid.

Echocardiographic measures

As noted above, the final outcome and treatment modality are based on frequent echocardiographic assessments.[23] The main issue is to detect early signs of *in utero* congestive heart failure of the 'pump' twin.[24] Regardless, the surviving 'pump' twin may present with heart failure and persistent myocardial hypertrophy after birth (Figure 14.17), which may mimic hypertrophic cardiomyopathy. Chandra et al[25] described a twin pregnancy complicated by an acardiac, acephalic fetus diagnosed at 19 weeks' gestation. Serial amniocenteses were performed to decompress the hydramnios between 27 and 33 weeks. Ultrasonography indicated ventricular septal hypertrophy in the donor twin at 27 weeks, and cesarean delivery occurred at 33 weeks. The neonatal course was complicated by hypertrophic cardiomyopathy, which ultimately resolved without sequelae by 1 year of age.

Table 14.3   Fetal echocardiographic markers of congestive heart failure

Cardiomegaly: heart area/chest area ratio > 0.45
Heart circumference/chest circumference ratio > 0.55
Atrial enlargement
Holosystolic tricuspid valve regurgitation
Slow upstroke for tricuspid valve regurgitation (dP/dt)
Trivial and holosystolic mitral valve regurgitation
Pulmonary and aortic regurgitation
Decreased shortening fraction of right ventricle, left ventricle or both (normal values 28–40%)
Myocardial hypertrophy (wall thickness > 4 mm, sign of fetal hypertension)
Abnormal A/E ratio for mitral and/or tricuspid valve (in compromised fetus E = A, or E > A)
Dilatation of the inferior vena cava > 5 mm
Dilatation of the hepatic vein
Hepatomegaly
Reversal flow in ductus venosus
Abnormal pulsation in the inferior vena cava (A/S ratio > 0.15)
Pulsation in the umbilical vein
Ascites, pericardial effusion or hydrothorax
Polyhydramnios
Placentomegaly

P, pressure; t, time

The cardiac manifestations of the 'pump' twin may require intrauterine digoxin treatment, initiated after the sonographic diagnosis of fetal cardiac insufficiency. Simpson and co-workers reported more than two decades ago that the sonographic signs of cardiac insufficiency disappeared completely after treatment over 6 weeks, with survival of the 'pump' twin. It is not currently known how often this therapy is selected.[26]

Fetal echocardiographic markers of congestive heart failure are shown in Table 14.3.

Doppler assessment

Doppler blood flow velocimetry has a triple role in TRAP sequence cases. First, Doppler studies are able to confirm the presence of retrograde perfusion in the umbilical artery of the acardiac twin in early pregnancy.[27] Hence, they are a critical part of the diagnosis. Second, Doppler is used to support the pathogenesis of the TRAP sequence.[28] Finally, Doppler has an essential role in management strategy.

Shih and colleagues used Doppler velocimetry to analyze the blood flow pattern in the umbilical artery in the TRAP sequence and identified three patterns.[29] The first pattern, the so-called 'collision-summation', is characterized by two independent pulsation rates of bidirectional flow (abnormal pulsatile heart in the malformed twin) with cyclic alterations of blood flow. The second, reported as 'twin pulse', shows the flow away from the acardiac twin (with the presence of a primitive heart) with absent diastolic velocity, as well as the flow pumped into the acardiac twin with a prominent diastolic component. In other words, both flows are constantly pumping in opposite directions and at different rates. The third, a 'pump-in' pattern, demonstrates pulsatile flow towards the acardiac mass in the reverse direction. The authors suggested that the flow patterns of acardiac twins are determined by both the existence of a primitive heart and the nature of the vascular anastomoses.[29]

Dashe and co-workers[30] evaluated Doppler velocimetric findings in six pregnancies complicated by the TRAP sequence to determine the association of these findings with pregnancy outcome. Following confirmation of reversal of flow in all cases, the authors calculated the resistive index values and the difference in resistive index between the 'pump' and acardiac twin in each pair. Five of six 'pump' twins survived the immediate neonatal period. Although five of the acardiac twins had abnormally elevated Doppler index values, no ratio of systolic to diastolic velocity or resistive index value of the acardiac twin alone was associated with either a good or poor prognosis for the 'pump' twin. Larger differences in resistive index (> 0.20) were associated with improved outcome of the 'pump' twin, whereas smaller (and significantly different) resistive index differences were associated with poor outcome, including cardiac failure and central nervous system hypoperfusion.[30]

Brassard et al[31] identified and followed nine cases of TRAP sequence. Adverse outcome was defined as death, cardiac failure, or delivery before 30 weeks' gestation for reasons related to the presence of the acardiac twin. Four fetuses died, two *in utero* (22 weeks) and two after cesarean (26 and 31 weeks) for advanced cardiac failure. Outcome was favorable in the five other cases. The cardiothoracic ratio and presence of cysts or of a rudimentary heart did not correlate with outcome. A pulsatility index in the umbilical artery of the acardiac twin significantly lower than that of the normal twin (ratio of 0.71 compared with 1.04 for good outcome, $p < 0.05$), an elevated shortening fraction in the second trimester, and a rapid growth rate of the acardiac mass were all associated with a poor prognosis.

New types of reversed flow

Gembruch and colleagues presented a case of TTTS with death of a donor at 25 weeks of gestation and the development of the TRAP sequence,[32] observing reversed flow from the umbilical arteries through the aorta, left heart, right heart, inferior vena cava, ductus venosus, and back to the placenta through the umbilical vein. This finding suggests that if one fetus dies in an MC pair, the falling blood pressure in the dying fetus may lead to a shift in the pressure gradient and cause an acute transfusion of blood from the surviving twin to the dying one through the superficial arterio-arterial or veno-venous anastomoses. Moreover, *this reversed flow is one of the current explanations for the high prevalence of end organ damage in the survivor following single fetal demise in MC twins.*

The advent of modern therapy for TTTS by fetoscopic laser coagulation of the placental anastomoses led to the co-occurrence of anemic recipients and polycythemic donors following treatment. Lewi et al[33] used single-shot digital angiography as well as digital photography of the placental angioarchitecture to document residual vascular connections visible only on angiography that did not prevent the resolution of TTTS. These operation-elusive anastomoses may account for lesser degrees of feto-fetal transfusion, which sometime occurs in the reversed direction.

Diagnosis-based management

Table 14.4 shows the various options used to treat the TRAP sequence. The 'do nothing' policy – 'let Nature do its deed' – is not an applicable option in modern perinatal medicine. With the advent of sonography, echocardiography, and Doppler velocimetry, most clinicians

Table 14.4 Treatment options for the TRAP sequence

(1) Do nothing
(2) Observation
(3) Observation until deterioration (tailored intervention)
(4) Medical treatment of cardiac insufficiency (digoxin)
(5) Hysterotomy
(6) Interruption of blood supply to the acardiac twin (prophylactic or indicated)
   a. Embolization
   b. Cord ligation
   c. Diathermy (mono/bipolar)
   d. Intrafetal ablation
     • alcohol
     • monopolar diathermy
     • interstitial laser
     • radiofrequency

follow the pregnancy carefully, even if intervention is not considered. When an intervention is considered, this can be performed early in pregnancy – as a prophylactic measure – or later following the appearance of signs of cardiac decompensation of the 'pump' twin.

Although treatment with serial amniocenteses (to reduce the effect of polyhydramnios) and digoxin has been suggested, the main goal is interruption of the blood supply to the acardiac fetus.

In the past, treatment by selective delivery of the acardiac twin via sectio parvae (hysterotomy) was advocated. More recently, this aggressive and potentially complication-laden modality has been replaced by less invasive procedures, a logical approach in such circumstances. Because of the arterio-arterial shunt in TRAP, the artery must be interrupted, as simple thrombosis is quite difficult to achieve, and, if the vein is inadvertently thrombosed, the 'pump' twin may suffer from embolization related to the procedure.

Umbilical cord ligation was pioneered by Quintero and colleagues more than a decade ago.[34] Whereas this procedure is associated with a 70–80% success rate, it also entails risks of technical failure, premature rupture of the membranes, and bleeding. An alternative approach, first advocated in 1994 as well, is endoscopic coagulation of the umbilical cord vessels of the acardiac twin using a Nd:YAG (neodymium: yttrium–aluminum–garnet) laser.[35] Laser coagulation was successful in arresting blood flow to the acardiac fetus in cases treated at 17 and 20 weeks, but in pregnancies treated at 26 and 28 weeks, the umbilical cords were edematous and laser coagulation failed to arrest blood flow.[35] More recently, a tailored approach was proposed, whereby conservative treatment was offered to milder cases of the TRAP sequence with a low weights ratio, whereas larger acardiac twins had invasive intervention and cord occlusion.[36]

Recent attempts to further minimize the nature of the therapeutic intervention were reported by Tsao and colleagues.[37] Under direct real-time sonographic guidance, the operators percutaneously inserted a 3 mm (14 gauge) radiofrequency ablation needle through the maternal abdominal wall into the intrauterine fetal abdomen at the level of the cord insertion site of the acardiac twin. Energy was applied until termination of blood flow to the acardiac fetus was documented by Doppler ultrasound scanning. No major maternal complications were reported in 13 cases, and 12 out of 13 'pump' twins remained alive and well.

A review identified 32 reports involving 74 cases of acardiac twin treated by invasive techniques.[38] Seventy-one cases were included for analysis: 40 were treated by cord occlusion (5 embolizations, 15 cord ligations, 10 laser coagulations, 7 bipolar diathermy, and 3 monopolar diathermy) and 31 by intrafetal ablation (5 by alcohol, 9 by monopolar diathermy, 4 by interstitial laser, and 13 by radiofrequency). The overall median gestational ages at treatment and delivery were 21 and 36 weeks, respectively, with a median treatment–delivery interval of 13 weeks. The overall 'pump' twin survival rate was 76%. Intrafetal ablation was associated with increased gestational duration (37 vs. 32 weeks) and a longer median treatment–delivery interval (16 vs. 9.5 weeks) compared with cord occlusion techniques. It was also associated with a lower technical failure rate (13 vs. 35%), a lower rate of births or rupture of membranes.

SUMMARY

The diagnosis and management of the TRAP sequence has changed dramatically since the advent of sonography, echocardiography, Doppler flow analysis, and so-called 'minimally invasive' instrumentation. It is now possible to tailor the appropriate management to the individual case, based not only on inter-twin size ratio, but also on direct echocardiographic assessment of the cardiac function of the 'pump' twin. Expectant management, under close observation, is at present safer than ever before. Consequently, the chance of survival of the 'pump' twin has significantly improved with modern perinatal care.

REFERENCES

1. Coulam CB, Wright G. First trimester diagnosis of acardiac twins. Early Pregnancy 2000; 4: 261–70.

2. Ersch J, Stallmach T. Cardiac regression sequence: reversal of blood flow is diagnostic but not causative in an acardiac fetus. Early Hum Dev 1998; 52: 81–5.

3. Bieber FR, Nance WE, Morton CC et al. Genetic studies of an acardiac monster: evidence of polar body twinning in man. Science 1981; 213: 775–7.

4. Fisk NM, Ware M, Stanier P et al. Molecular genetic etiology of twin reversed arterial perfusion sequence. Am J Obstet Gynecol 1996; 174: 891–4.

5. Fusi L, Fisk N, Talbert D et al. When does death occur in an acardiac twin? Ultrasound diagnostic difficulties. J Perinat Med 1990; 18: 223–7.

6. Kamitomo M, Kouno S, Ibuka K et al. First-trimester findings associated with twin reversed arterial perfusion sequence. Fetal Diagn Ther 2004; 19: 187–90.

7. Al-Malt A, Ashmead G, Judge N et al. Color-flow and Doppler velocimetry in prenatal diagnosis of acardiac triplets. J Ultrasound Med 1991; 10: 341–5.

8. Izquierdo L, Smith J, Gilson G et al. Twin, acardiac, acephalus. Fetus 1992; 1: 1.

9. Van Allen MI, Smith SW, Shepard TH. Twin reversed arterial perfusion (TRAP) sequence: a study of 14 twin pregnancies with acardius. Semin Perinatol 1983; 7: 285–93.

10. Emery SC, Vaux KK, Pretorius D, Masliah E, Benirschke K. Acardiac twin with externalized intestine adherent to placenta: unusual manifestation of omphalocele. Pediatr Dev Pathol 2004; 7: 81–5.

11. Benson CB, Bieber FR, Genest DR et al. Doppler demonstration of reversed umbilical blood flow in the acardiac twin. J Clin Ultrasound 1989; 17: 291–5.

12. Pretorius DH, Leopold GR, Moore TR et al. Acardiac twin: report of Doppler sonography. J Ultrasound Med 1988; 7: 413–16.

13. Papa T, Dao A, Bruner JP. Pathognomonic sign of twin reversed arterial perfusion using color Doppler sonography. J Ultrasound Med 1997; 16: 501–3.

14. Gillet N, Hustin J, Magritte JP, Givron O, Longueville E. Placental teratoma: differential diagnosis with fetal acardia. J Gynecol Obstet Biol Reprod 2001; 30: 789–92.

15. MacKenzie AP, Stephenson CD, Funai EF, Lee MJ, Timor-Tritsch I. Three-dimensional ultrasound to differentiate epigastric heteropagus conjoined twins from a TRAP sequence. Am J Obstet Gynecol 2004; 191: 1736–9.

16. Bonilla-Musoles F, Machado LE, Raga F, Osborne NG. Fetus acardius: two- and three-dimensional ultrasonographic diagnoses. J Ultrasound Med 2001; 20: 1117–27.

17. Seckin NC, Turhan NO, Kopal S, Inegol I. Acardiac twin: a misdiagnosed, mismanaged case. Eur J Obstet Gynecol Reprod Biol 2003; 107: 212–13.

18. Petersen BL, Broholm H, Skibsted L, Graem N. Acardiac twin with preserved brain. Fetal Diagn Ther 2001; 16: 231–3.

19. Bermudez C, Tejada P, Gonzalez F et al. Umbilical cord transection in twin-reverse arterial perfusion syndrome with the use of a coaxial bipolar electrode (Versapoint). J Matern Fetal Neonatal Med 2003; 14: 277–8.

20. Malinowski W, Szwalski J. Monochorionic, diamniotic triplet pregnancy complicated by twin reversed arterial perfusion sequence. Postpartum autopsy of placenta and acardiac fetus. Ginekol Pol 2004; 75: 863–8.

21. Moore RT, Gale S, Benirschke K. Perinatal outcome of forty nine pregnancies complicated by acardiac twinning. Am J Obstet Gynecol 1990; 63: 907–12.

22. Sullivan AE, Varner MW, Ball RH et al. The management of acardiac twins: a conservative approach. Am J Obstet Gynecol 2003; 189: 1310–13.

23. Osborn P, Gross TL, Shah JJ, Ma L. Prenatal diagnosis of fetal heart failure in twin reversed arterial perfusion. Prenat Diagn 2000; 20: 615–17.

24. Donnenfeld AE, van de Woestijne J, Craparo F et al. The normal fetus of an acardiac twin pregnancy: perinatal management based on echocardiographic and sonographic evaluation. Prenat Diagn 1991; 11: 235–44.

25. Chandra S, Crane JM, Young DC, Shah S. Acardiac twin pregnancy with neonatal resolution of donor twin cardiomyopathy. Obstet Gynecol 2000; 96: 820–1.

26. Simpson PC, Trudinger BJ, Walker A, Baird PJ. The intrauterine treatment of fetal cardiac failure in a twin pregnancy with an acardiac, acephalic monster. Am J Obstet Gynecol 1983; 147: 842–4.

27. Schwarzler P, Ville Y, Moscoso G et al. Diagnosis of twin reversed arterial perfusion sequence in the first trimester by transvaginal color Doppler ultrasound. Ultrasound Obstet Gynecol 1999; 13: 143–6.

28. Fouron JC, Leduc L, Grigon A et al. Importance of meticulous ultrasonographic investigation of the acardiac twin. J Ultrasound Med 1994; 13: 1001–4.

29. Shih JC, Shyu MK, Hunag SF et al. Doppler waveform analysis of the intertwin blood flow in acardiac pregnancy: implications for pathogenesis. Ultrasound Obstet Gynecol 1999; 14: 375–9.

30. Dashe JS, Fernandez CO, Twickler DM. Utility of Doppler velocimetry in predicting outcome in twin reversed-arterial perfusion sequence. Am J Obstet Gynecol 2001; 185: 135–9.

31. Brassard M, Fouron JC, Leduc L, Grignon A, Proulx F. Prognostic markers in twin pregnancies with an acardiac fetus. Obstet Gynecol 1999; 94: 409–14.

32. Gembruch U, Viski S, Bagamery K et al. Twin reversed arterial perfusion sequence in twin-to-twin

transfusion syndrome after the death of the donor co-twin in the second trimester. Ultrasound Obstet Gynecol 2001; 17: 153–6.

33. Lewi L, Cannie M, Jani J et al. Placental angiography of double survivors and double fetal deaths after laser for twin twin transfusion syndrome (TTTS). Am J Obstet Gynecol 2004; S162.

34. Quintero RA, Reich H, Puder KS et al. Brief report: umbilical cord ligation of an acardiac twin by fetoscopy at 19 weeks of gestation. N Engl J Med 1994; 330: 469–71.

35. Ville Y, Hyett JA, Vandenbussche FP, Nicolaides KH. Endoscopic laser coagulation of umbilical cord vessels in twin reversed arterial perfusion sequence. Ultrasound Obstet Gynecol 1994; 4: 396–8.

36. Weisz B, Peltz R, Chayen B et al. Tailored management of twin reversed arterial perfusion (TRAP) sequence. Ultrasound Obstet Gynecol 2004; 23: 451–5.

37. Tsao K, Feldstein VA, Albanese CT et al. Selective reduction of acardiac twin by radiofrequency ablation. Am J Obstet Gynecol 2002; 187: 635–40.

38. Tan TY, Sepulveda W. Acardiac twin: a systematic review of minimally invasive treatment modalities. Ultrasound Obstet Gynecol 2003; 22: 409–19.

15

Monoamniotic twins

INTRODUCTION

Monoamniotic (MA) multiples are characterized by a single amniotic cavity, a single placenta, and two umbilical cords inserted close to each other (Figure 15.1). The first review to emphasize the significantly higher morbidity and mortality (40–70%) and the low prevalence of MA twin pregnancies (2–5% of all monochorionic (MC) twin pregnancies) appeared in 1935.[1] More recent reviews[2–5] reiterate the perinatal risk of monoamnionicity,[6] although it appears that intensive management and early delivery may reduce some of the antenatal mortality associated with these precarious pregnancies.[7,8] Modern technology, including high-resolution and three-dimensional (3D) ultrasound techniques, color Doppler, and fetal monitoring, provides the potential to anticipate the diagnosis of MA twins in the first trimester of pregnancy along with the possibility of closer surveillance and hopefully lower fetal loss.

PATHOPHYSIOLOGY OF MONOAMNIOTIC TWINS AND NATURAL HISTORY OF CORD ENTANGLEMENT

Monoamniotic placentation is the result of the process of amniogenesis and separation being delayed until day 12 or 13 post-fertilization. Current knowledge on the natural history of MA twins is mainly based on data derived from either prenatal sonographic reports in which the diagnosis was made after 18 weeks or postnatal studies. Recently, several groups reported observing cord entanglement in MA twins in the first trimester.[9–12] Although it is not currently known how early cord entanglements can occur, these observations support the conclusion that the umbilical cords are

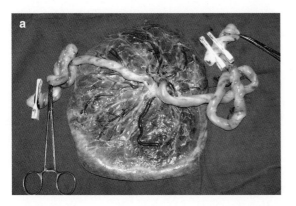
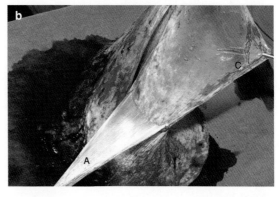

Figure 15.1 Monochorionic–monoamniotic twin placenta. (a) No septum or any amniotic folds between the umbilical cords inserted closely next to each other. (b) Examination of this pattern of placentation is similar to that of a singleton placenta. A, amnion; C, chorion

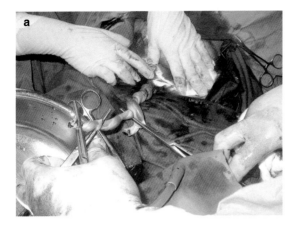

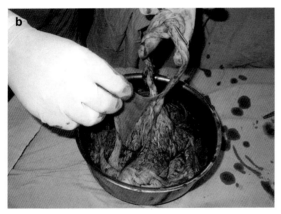

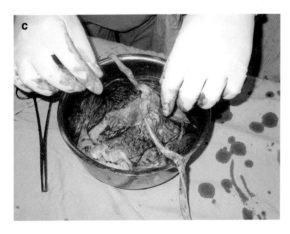

Figure 15.2 (a) Cord entanglement of a case believed to be monochorionic–diamniotic. (b) After the cords were untwisted, a thin, diamniotic membrane was found. (c) Membrane between the two juxtaposed cords: the proximity of the cords suggests a monoamniotic, rather than a diamniotic placenta

long enough and the twins are capable of sufficient movements to produce cord 'entanglement' as early as 10 weeks. It is possible that this phenomenon is facilitated when there is proportionately more amniotic fluid in relation to the small fetal body mass.[11]

The proximity of the cord insertions does not predict whether or not they become entangled. According to Benirshcke and Kaufmann,[13] a remnant of a bilaminar amniotic membrane can be noted in some MA placentas between closely adjacent cord insertions, suggesting that amniogenesis was in progress but was interrupted by the twinning process (Figure 15.2). In most instances, however, no such sign is visible between the cord insertion sites to suggest that twinning occurred and amniotic development was altered thereafter.[14] Female gender predominates in MA twins, and overall, the proportion of female like-sex pairs increases with proximity of the twins.[15] Whether the increased frequency of female sets reflects the effect of the mass of the X chromosome or some genetic factors on the inactivated X chromosome is unclear.

Aside from entanglement, the umbilical cord complications seen in MA twins are associated with abnormally long and single-artery cords. It remains unclear whether these abnormalities are coincidental or causally related to cord entanglement and perinatal death. The increased contact between the members of an MA twin pregnancy might to some degree explain why entanglement is facilitated, as neonates with long cords are relatively hyperkinetic compared with those with shorter cords. In cases with sudden intrauterine death and cord entanglement, it cannot be ascertained to what extent the cord entanglement, in combination with increased activity, caused hemodynamic interruption of blood supply, or whether previous changes of blood pressure might have facilitated a final obstruction of the entangled vessels.

DIAGNOSTIC APPROACH

Improvements in ultrasonographic resolution underlie the increasing numbers of prenatally

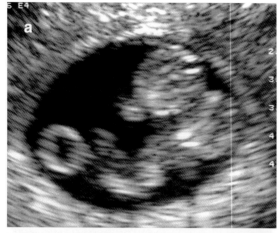

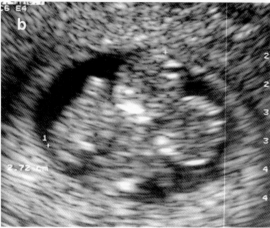

Figure 15.3 (a) Transvaginal sonogram of a pair of monoamniotic (MA) twins with one yolk sac. (b) Transvaginal sonogram of a pair of MA twins with close proximity

Table 15.1 Detection of chorionicity and amnionicity

(1) Absence of two separate chorionic sacs and absence of lambda sign: suspicion of MC multiple gestation
(2) Absence of the intertwin membrane and absence of a T sign: suspicion of MC–MA multiple gestation
(3) Further confirmation of MC–MA pregnancy is provided by
  • Single yolk sac (Figure 15.3a) with both allantoic vessels inserting into a single sac
  • Single placenta with close insertion of the two umbilical cords
  • Unusual intrauterine positioning of the two fetuses in close proximity to each other (Figure 15.3b)

detected MA twins. Moreover, new diagnostic tools such as color-flow mapping combined with Doppler velocimetry and, more recently, 3D ultrasound techniques have revolutionized the frequency as well as the accuracy of the diagnosis of cord entanglement in MA twins at any point in gestation.

First trimester

When early transvaginal or transabdominal sonography (TVS/TAS) reveals two separate fetuses and no clear evidence of a dividing membrane, MA twin pregnancy should definitely be suspected, especially if there is only one yolk sac (Figure 15.3).[9–11,16–18] The yolk sac is located in the chorioamniotic space, which disappears by the end of the first trimester. Whether MA twins have a single fused or two separate yolk sacs depends on the time of splitting of the germinal disk.[16–18] Therefore, visualization of two yolk sacs does not necessarily exclude an MA multiple pregnancy. This view is supported by a recent study of 22 cases of monochorionic multiple pregnancies scanned before 11 weeks of gestation in which the number of yolk sacs was recorded and compared with the presence or absence of a dividing membrane for all fetuses.[19] In 17/20 (85%) cases of monochorionic–diamniotic twins, two yolk sacs were seen. In one case of monoamniotic twins, a single yolk sac was observed. The authors of this study concluded that the presence of two yolk sacs in a monochorionic pregnancy predicts diamnionicity in 85% of the cases. The monoamnionicity diagnosis can be made only following a careful search for a dividing amniotic membrane since a single yolk sac was found in 3/20 (15%) cases of monochorionic–diamniotic twins as well as in MA twins.

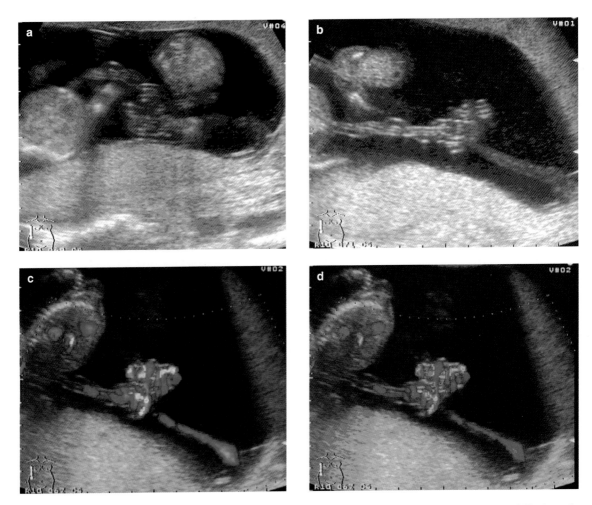

Figure 15.4 (a) Monoamniotic twins. A single amniotic cavity, a single placenta, and two umbilical cords closely inserted are criteria for diagnosis of monoamnionicity. (b) 2D image of cord entanglement in monoamniotic twins. 2D sonography is unable to distinguish between adjacent and entangled umbilical cords. (c) 2D color Doppler imaging of umbilical cord entanglement. (d) 2D power Doppler reconstruction of umbilical cord entanglement

If two yolk sacs and no dividing membrane are visualized before 9 gestational weeks, transabdominal (improved orientation) and transvaginal (improved resolution) scans should be repeated at a later stage (after 9 gestational weeks) when the dividing membrane should be clearly visible.[18] Using the 3D technique, it is possible to differentiate between monochorionic–diamniotic (MC–DA) and monochorionic–monoamniotic (MC–MA)

gestations as early as 6 weeks[20,21] (Figure 15.4). If MA twins are suspected, a systematic diagnostic protocol should be followed, as outlined in Table 15.1. One should remember, however, that the intertwin membrane in early pregnancy may be very thin and thus elusive to sonographic detection. Because of this, the role of the sonographer must exclude the presence of MA twins by subsequent meticulous searches for the dividing membrane.

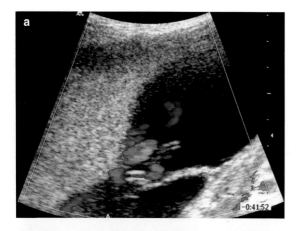

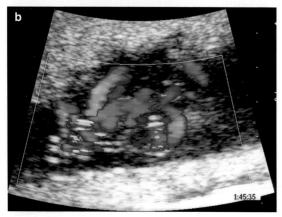

Figure 15.5 (a) Transabdominal color ultrasound in a dichorionic–diamniotic triplet pregnancy at 14 weeks. Note the simple loop of cord entanglement close to the placental insertion of the two cords of the monoamniotic triplets and Doppler velocimetry of the same segment, confirming cord entanglement by two different heart rates of the involved umbilical arteries. (b) Transabdominal color ultrasound of the same case at 18 weeks. Note the increased braiding with overlapping vessels of the two crossing cords, suggestive of 'branching'

Detection or exclusion of cord entanglement

Using 2D ultrasound, the detection or exclusion of cord entanglement is possible by noting the quality and number of loops. This procedure should be repeated at each new scan.

If, on the other hand, color Doppler is available, cord entanglement can be diagnosed or

excluded with greater certainty and at an earlier stage (Figure 15.5a), the earliest diagnosis having been made at 10 gestational weeks. Even in instances when cord entanglement is diagnosed, it is advisable to repeat the scan, as cord entanglement may worsen in the sense that either more loops may become involved (Figure 15.5a and b), or alteration of the normal Doppler profile suggests that partial compression may become detectable at a later stage in pregnancy.[22–24] Whether such a finding might have implications for further management is not yet clear, but nonetheless the finding is important.[25]

If Doppler velocimetry is available, the diagnosis can be further confirmed by demonstrating different fetal heart rate patterns in the same direction on umbilical artery Doppler analysis of a common mass of cord vessels visible by ultrasound between the ventral surfaces of the two fetuses (Figure 15.6a and b).

Detection or exclusion of gross structural anomalies

When the diagnosis of MA twin pregnancy is certain, detailed anatomic examination of both twins is important, as structural anomalies occurring in only one of the twins, or rarely in both, are very common.[11] Major anomalies can be diagnosed at an early stage of pregnancy (anencephaly, body-stalk anomaly, severe spina bifida, kyphoscoliosis, and, last but not least, conjoined twins). Sebire and colleagues[11] reported on a subset of 12 cases (3.8%) of MC–MA pregnancies detected by ultrasound scan at 11–14 weeks' gestation. Four of these were conjoined twins, and 4 out of the remaining 8 MA twin pregnancies showed structural anomalies confined to only one of the twins (anencephaly, body-stalk anomaly, diaphragmatic hernia, kyphoscoliosis).[11] The four normal twins had no signs of increased nuchal translucency (NT), but cord entanglement was demonstrated from the first trimester onwards, in agreement with the experience of others.[10] Other anomalies described in MA twins involve the central nervous system, urogenital tract, and cardiac systems.

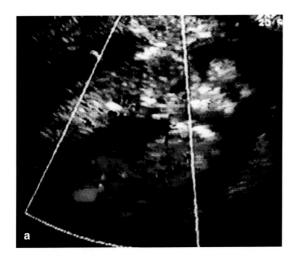

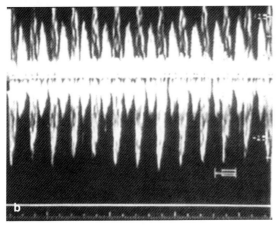

Figure 15.6 (a) Transabdominal color ultrasound of a monochorionic–monoamniotic twin pregnancy at 14 weeks. Note the cord entanglement of the two cords close to the umbilical insertion. (b) Doppler velocimetry of the same segment showing the flow velocity waveforms of four different arteries with two different heart rates

Measurement of NT and ductus venosus (DV) flow patterns may play a role in identifying or ruling out those multiples with increased risk of chromosomal or congenital anomalies. However, owing to the rarity of MA pregnancy it has not been possible to clarify whether also NT and DV measurements also may be predictive of chromosomal anomalies or adverse fetal outcome in these pregnancies.[26]

Second and third trimesters

When ultrasound examinations were not widely available, cord entanglement was only incidentally observed in the second or early third trimester and not uncommonly only at birth. Suspicion of an MA twin pregnancy was confirmed by amniography and intra-amniotic injection of indigo carmine dye,[27,28] injection of air bubbles to delineate the dividing membrane, and computed tomographic amniography.[29] It was even suggested early on that in the second and third trimesters, computed tomographic amniography might be more accurate than ultrasound in detecting MA twins. However, techniques other than sonography are rarely necessary and transabdominal and transvaginal ultrasonography are clearly highly reliable tools to diagnose or exclude MA twin pregnancy.

The observation of a large and common mass containing umbilical cord vessels clearly demonstrates entanglement (see Figure 15.5a and b). Color-flow Doppler may confirm the vascular nature of the mass, whereas pulsed Doppler analysis may show apparent 'branching' of the umbilical artery with evidence of two different heart rates in the two segments of the branches, another clear sign of cord entanglement.

Diagnosis of cord entanglement and cord compression

The mass of entangled umbilical cords is usually interposed between the ventral surfaces of the two fetuses (Figure 15.6a) or at the placental insertion (Figure 15.5a). However, the umbilical cord can also wrap itself around other parts of the body of one of the multiples. For example, color Doppler has shown that the cord of one twin was tightly wrapped around the neck of its dead co-twin.[30] The diagnosis of cord entanglement with 2D real-time sonography may require a relatively long examination period, and due to limited sectional imaging, the examination may be informative only in terms of quality and number of loops (Figure 15.4).

Cord entanglement may sometimes be confused with the clustering of segments of a single umbilical cord, sometimes referred to as a 'stack of coins' appearance.[31] Invariably, however, true cord entanglement shows each of the two cords lying in an orderly spiral fashion.[32–34] The distinction between adjacent and entangled cords may also be made by 3D power Doppler examination, outlining the specific curvatures of the umbilical cord. Moreover, the number of loops involved in the entanglement can be determined easily and used for longitudinal assessment of the effects of entanglement, i.e. tightening compression and subsequent fetal compromise.

Doppler analysis of the umbilical artery flow patterns can reveal the presence of a notch indicative of a true knot, or abnormally elevated systolic/diastolic ratios up to absent end-diastolic flow. The presence of a notch in the umbilical artery velocity waveform may reflect hemodynamic alterations in the fetal–placental circulation secondary to narrowing of the arterial lumen, with an increase in downstream resistance in the umbilical vessels involved in cord entanglement. High blood flow velocities in the umbilical vein detected by velocimetry and/or pulsation in the umbilical vein flow pattern are also indicative of tight entanglement.[32] The presence of pulsations in the umbilical venous flow profile is a poor prognostic sign, as they suggest tight entanglement, consequential increased placental resistance, and cardiac overload due to increased pressure in the constricted cord.[35,36]

The diagnostic criteria for MA pregnancies are reported in Table 15.2.

Twin-to-twin transfusion syndrome (TTTS)

No consensus exists as to whether TTTS occurs in MA multiple pregnancies. In MA multiple pregnancy, the common amniotic cavity may function as a buffer for intertwin differences leading to blood shunting.[13] Nevertheless, when extensive polyhydramnios is observed in MA pregnancies, it is likely due to unbalanced perfusion, whereby the direction and passage

Table 15.2 Diagnostic criteria for monoamniotic twin pregnancies

No observed dividing intertwin membrane
Single placenta
Single yolk sac
Same sex
Amniotic fluid surrounding each fetus
Unrestricted movement of both fetuses
Cord entanglement present (Doppler documentation of branching of double umbilical vessel signals)

of blood volume shifts remain unclear and may even occur in both directions.[11] Sebire and colleagues suggest that acute TTTS more than cord entanglement may be responsible for sudden fetal demise in MA twins, because the close insertion of the two umbilical cords may be associated with large-caliber anastomoses between the two fetal circulations.[11] Consequently, an imbalance between the two circulations cannot be sustained for a prolonged period of time, as is the case in the classic TTTS, but rather results in major and sudden hemodynamic effects causing fetal death.[11] Although pathologic analysis of the twins and their placenta might be helpful, at this point it remains difficult if not impossible to detect the 'true' cause of early fetal demise from retrospective analysis alone. It follows that collection of more data from MA placentas is mandatory to determine the frequency and impact of unbalanced transfusion in MA twins. Prenatal Doppler velocimetry of arterio-venous anastomoses and postnatal angiography of the placenta might help to evaluate this issue in the future.

PSEUDOMONOAMNIOTIC TWINS (PMA)

The term pseudomonoamniotic refers to the situation whereby the dividing membrane ruptures before birth. Although this was described as early as the 12th century, it is an extremely unusual event.[37]

Iatrogenic PMA refers to inadvertent or intentional creation of a hole in the intertwin septum. Megory and colleagues[38] reported PMA twins with cord entanglement following genetic funipuncture (cordocentesis) in 1991. In that case, cell growth failed twice following amniocentesis and the authors opted for a funipuncture at 24 weeks. The spatial anatomy of the uterine content dictated needle entry into the cord of one fetus through the sac of the other fetus. This procedure produced PMA with cord entanglement, which was noticed only at birth.[38] In 1998, Feldman and associates[39] reported inadvertent membrane puncture and creation of a PMA gestation following amnioreduction for TTTS, and cautioned against the adverse outcome. Interestingly enough, in the same year, Saade and co-workers[40] published the first series of intentional septostomy to alleviate severe TTTS.

Iatrogenic PMA twins should be suspected whenever significantly different amounts of amniotic fluid, such as would be the case in the polyoligohydramnios sequence, equalize abruptly following amniocentesis. When the diagnosis of a PMA gestation is made, the pregnancy should be followed as any other pregnancy with a monoamniotic placenta.

The frequency of spontaneous PMA is unknown and few descriptions of this occurrence exist. Recently, a thin intertwin-dividing membrane of an MC–DA twin gestation was confirmed at 32 weeks by ultrasound, but disappeared at 36 weeks.[41] This pregnancy ended a few days later with a combined vaginal-cesarean delivery, due to severe fetal heart rate deceleration of the second twin. Cord entanglement was noted at the time of delivery, which was assumed to occur due to antepartum rupture of the dividing membrane between 32 and 36 weeks.[41] Another case[42] described sonographic documentation of MC–DA twins at 26 weeks' gestation with concordant fetal growth and findings suggestive of a true knot of the umbilical cord. At cesarean delivery at 34 weeks' gestation, spontaneous antepartum septostomy with entanglement of the two separate umbilical cords was noted.[42]

Caution should be exercised before concluding that spontaneous PMA does exist. Figure 15.2a shows cord entanglement found at 33 weeks during cesarean section. After untwisting the cords, a diamniotic membrane was evident, pushed down by the entangled cords (Figure 15.2b). The proximity of the cords, however, so characteristic of monoamniotic twins (Figure 15.2c), cast serious doubt on the possibility of spontaneous PMA in this case. Rather, it is possible that this represents a monoamniotic placenta with a remnant of an intertwin membrane, suggesting that amniogenesis was in progress but was interrupted by the twinning process.[43]

NOTES ON CLINICAL MANAGEMENT

Traditionally, 95% of cases of reported fetal demise are attributed to fatal umbilical cord complications. Such cases increase by 2–5% every week after 15 weeks' gestation and total 30–40% by 30 weeks. In the case of survival, perinatal morbidity is high.

Many clinical reports of MA twins focus on cord entanglement and the resultant risks. However, as MA twins are rare, a management consensus has not yet been achieved independent of whether or not cord entanglement is identified prenatally. Statistical validity of any findings is limited by the small sample sizes and the variety in management protocols, such as early admission versus outpatient control,[44] or elective versus emergency cesarean section. Vaginal delivery of MA twins has been reported in cases of cephalic presentation of both twins, but should not represent the standard practice.

Timing of delivery is also controversial. Some authors recommend delivery at 32 weeks of gestation, while others state that the risk of cord accidents declines with advancing gestation, thus questioning the usefulness of routine delivery at 32 weeks. A retrospective review of the most comprehensive articles finds conflicting opinions on whether the risks of early delivery outweigh the risks of fetal death. In fact, looking carefully at the cases where cord entanglement was diagnosed prenatally, the decision for surveillance and timing of delivery varied according to what the obstetrician thought about continuation of pregnancy.

Specific interventions, such as attempts to untie the entanglement, have not yet been reported. Regardless, current monitoring techniques for multiple pregnancies should be applied in MA twin pregnancies. Finally, selective termination of a malformed twin by cord occlusion technique should be followed by cutting the occluded cord in order to avoid entanglement.

REFERENCES

1. Quingley JK. Monoamniotic twin pregnancy. Am J Obstet Gynecol 1935; 29: 354–62.
2. Bilardo CM, Arabin B. Prenatal diagnosis of cord entanglement in monoamniotic multiple pregnancies. Ultrasound Rev Obstet Gynecol 2001; 1: 365–71.
3. Allen VM, Windrin R, Barret J, Ohlsson A. Management of monoamniotic twin pregnancies: a case series and systematic reviews of the literature. Br J Obstet Gynaecol 2001; 108: 931–6.
4. Su LL. Monoamniotic twins: diagnosis and management. Acta Obstet Gynecol Scand 2002; 81: 995–1000.
5. Shveiky D, Ezra Y, Schenker JG, Rojansky N. Monoamniotic twins: an update on antenatal diagnosis and treatment. J Matern Fetal Neonatal Med 2004; 16: 180–6.
6. Demaria F, Goffinet F, Keyem G et al. Monoamniotic twin pregnancies: antenatal management and perinatal results of 19 consecutive cases. BJOG 2004; 111: 22–6.
7. Ezra Y, Shveiky D, Ophir E et al. Intensive management and early delivery reduce antenatal mortality in monoamniotic twin pregnancies. Acta Obstet Gynecol Scand 2005; 84: 432–5.
8. Heyborne KD, Porreco RP, Garite TJ, Phair K, Obstetrix/Pediatrix Research Study Group. Improved perinatal survival of monoamniotic twins with intensive inpatient monitoring. Am J Obstet Gynecol 2005; 192: 96–101.
9. Arabin B, Laurini RN, van Eyck J. Early prenatal diagnosis of cord entanglement in monoamniotic multiple pregnancies. Ultrasound Obstet Gynecol 1999; 13: 181–6.
10. Overton TG, Denbow ML, Duncan KR et al. First-trimester cord entanglement in monoamniotic twins. Ultrasound Obstet Gynecol 1999; 13: 140–2.
11. Sebire NJ, Souka A, Skentou H et al. First trimester diagnosis of monoamniotic twin pregnancies. Ultrasound Obstet Gynecol 2000; 16: 223–5.
12. Sherer DM, Sokolovski M, Hartas-Rubinstein N. Diagnosis of cord entanglement of monoamniotic twins by first-trimester color Doppler imaging. J Ultrasound Med 2002; 21: 137–9.
13. Benirschke K, Kaufmann P. Pathology of the Human Placenta, 2nd edn. New York: Springer, 1990.
14. Baldwin VJ. The pathology of monochorionic zygosity. In: Baldwin VJ, ed. Pathology of Multiple Pregnancy. New York: Springer, 1994: 215–75.
15. Derom C, Vlietinick R, Derom R et al. Population-based study on sex proportion in monoamniotic twins. N Engl J Med 1988; 319: 119–20.
16. Hill LM, Chenevey P, Hecker J et al. Sonographic determination of first trimester twin chorionicity and amnionicity. J Clin Ultrasound 1996; 24: 305–8.
17. Babinszki A, Mukherjee T, Kerenyi T et al. Diagnosing amnionicity at 6 weeks of pregnancy with transvaginal three-dimensional ultrasonography: case report. Fertil Steril 1999; 71: 1161–4.
18. Levi CS, Lyons EA, Dashefsky SM et al. Yolk sac number, size and morphologic features in monochorionic monoamniotic twin pregnancy. Can Assoc Radiol J 1996; 47: 98–1003.
19. Shen O, Samueloff A, Beller U, Rabinowitz R. Number of yolk sacs does not predict amnionicity in early first-trimester monochorionic multiple gestations. Ultrasound Obstet Gynecol 2006; 27: 53–5.
20. Bromley B, Benacerraf B. Using the number of yolk sacs to determine amnionicity in early first trimester monochorionic twins. J Ultrasound Med 1995; 14: 415–19.
21. Pedersen MH, Larsen T. Three-dimensional ultrasonography of monoamniotic twins. Ugeskr Laeger 2001; 163: 619.
22. Suzuki S, Ishikawa G, Sawa R et al. Umbilical venous pulsation indicating tight cord entanglement in monoamniotic twin pregnancy. J Ultrasound Med 1999; 18: 425–9.
23. Kofinas AD, Penry M, Hatijs CG. Umbilical vessel flow velocimetry in cord entanglement in a monoamniotic twin pregnancy. J Reprod Med 1991; 36: 314–16.
24. Entezami M, Ragosch V, Hopp H et al. Notch in the umbilical artery Doppler profile in umbilical cord compression in a twin. Ultraschall Med 1997; 18: 277–9.
25. Vayssiere C, Plumere C, Gasser B, Neumann M, Favre R, Nisand I. Diagnosing umbilical cord entanglement in monoamniotic twins: becoming easier and probably essential. Ultrasound Obstet Gynecol 2004; 24: 587–9.
26. Bilardo CM, Muller MA, Zikulnig L et al. Ductus venosus studies in high-risk fetuses: relationship with

nuchal translucency measurement and fetal outcome. Ultrasound Obstet Gynecol 2001; 17: 288–94.

27. Lavery JP, Gadwood KA. Amniography for confirming the diagnosis of monoamniotic twinning. A case report. J Reprod Med 1990; 35: 911–14.

28. Tabsch K. Genetic amniocentesis in multiple pregnancies: a new technique to diagnose monoamniotic twins. Obstet Gynecol 1990; 75: 296–8.

29. Strohbehn K, Dattel BJ. Pitfalls in the diagnosis of non-conjoined monoamniotic twins. J Perinatol 1995; 15: 484–93.

30. Westover T, Guzman ER, Shen-Schwarz S. Prenatal diagnosis of an unusual nuchal cord complication in monoamniotic twins. Obstet Gynecol 1994; 84: 689–91.

31. Tongsong T, Chanprapaph P. Evolution of umbilical cord entanglement in monoamniotic twins. Ultrasound Obstet Gynecol 1999; 14: 75–7.

32. Westover T, Guzman ER, Shen-Schwarz S. Prenatal diagnosis of an unusual nuchal cord complication in monoamniotic twins. Obstet Gynecol 1994; 84: 689–91.

33. Tongsong T, Chanprapaph P. Evolution of umbilical cord entanglement in monoamniotic twins. Ultrasound Obstet Gynecol 1999; 14: 75–7.

34. Aisenbrey GA, Catanzarite VA, Hurley TJ et al. Monoamniotic and pseudomonoamniotic twins: sonographic diagnosis, detection of cord entanglement, and obstetric management. Obstet Gynecol 1995; 86: 218–22.

35. Abuhamad AZ, Mari G, Copel JA et al. Umbilical artery flow velocity waveforms in monoamniotic twins with cord entanglement. Obstet Gynecol 1995; 86: 674–7.

36. Rosemond RL, Hinds NE. Persistent abnormal umbilical cord Doppler velocimetry in a monoamniotic twin with cord entanglement. J Ultrasound Med 1998; 17: 337–8.

37. Preuss J. Biblical–Talmudic Medicine, 2nd edn. New York: Hebrew Publishing Company, 1983: 428–30.

38. Megory E, Weiner E, Shalev E, Ohel G. Pseudomonoamniotic twins with cord entanglement following genetic funipuncture. Obstet Gynecol 1991; 78: 915–17.

39. Feldman DM, Odibo A, Campbell WA, Rodis JF. Iatrogenic monoamniotic twins as a complication of therapeutic amniocentesis. Obstet Gynecol 1998; 91: 815–16.

40. Saade GR, Belfort MA, Berry DL et al. Amniotic septostomy for the treatment of twin oligohydramnios–polyhydramnios sequence. Fetal Diagn Ther 1998; 13: 86–93.

41. Nasrallah FK, Faden YA. Antepartum rupture of the intertwin-dividing membrane in monochorionic diamniotic twins: a case report and review of the literature. Prenat Diagn 2005; 25: 856–60.

42. Sherer DM, Bitton C, Stimphil R et al. Cord entanglement of monochorionic diamniotic twins following spontaneous antepartum septostomy sonographically simulating a true knot of the umbilical cord. Ultrasound Obstet Gynecol 2005; 26: 676–8.

43. Baldwin VJ. Pathology of Multiple Pregnancy. New York: Springer-Verlag, 1994: 201.

44. DeFalco LM, Sciscione AC, Megerian G et al. Inpatient versus outpatient management of monoamniotic twins and outcomes. Am J Perinatol 2006; 23: 205–11.

Conjoined twins

16

EPIDEMIOLOGY

The true incidence of conjoined twinning is difficult to estimate because of several confounding factors. The reported incidence of births with conjoined twinning is somewhere between 1 in 50 000 and 1 in 100 000 births (or 1 in 500–600 twin births). It varies among countries, most probably due to racial differences in overall twinning rates as well as ascertainment biases. However, it is likely that the actual incidence of the phenomenon is greater, but underestimation is common because of spontaneous or induced abortions or births before 22 weeks' gestation (and the lack of reporting of these in national statistics). Interestingly, although monozygotic twinning is exceedingly rare in mammals (except for the human and the nine-banded armadillo), the veterinary literature contains numerous reports of conjoined twins among such diverse species as the hamster, guinea-pig, fish, goat, cow, mouse, chicken, and buffalo.

EMBRYOLOGY

Perhaps the most debated aspect of conjoined twinning is its embryologic origin. Two contradicting theories exist – fusion or fission – and neither is likely to be definitively proved or disproved due to the ethical limitations associated with human embryonic research. The most comprehensive review of the controversies surrounding both theories is provided by Spencer in her recent book on conjoined twins.[1] The fission theory, generally accepted for the past 20 years, proposes that conjoined twins are a variation of monozygotic twins, but the division of the fertilized ovum is only partial. In other words, during the normal course of monozygotic twinning, an unknown stimulus causes division to occur at around 13 days post-fertilization – a time at which the developing embryo is too large (or too old) to separate fully. Thus, the embryonic mass divides in its main bulk, but remains united at one pole or the other, or at a point between the two poles.[2]

Proponents of the less accepted fusion theory argue, on the other hand, that the inner cell mass divides fully but the two monozygotic embryos stay close enough together to share either the amnion alone or both the amnion and the yolk sac. Then, as the embryos continue their rapid growth, they might come in contact with one another (always homologously) and become reunited ('fused') to result in either ventrally or dorsally conjoined twins. It is equally important to note, however, that no matter which theory one accepts, the clinical manifestation of conjoined twins as well as their overall management remains the same and is equally challenging.

CLASSIFICATION

The various types of conjoined twins may be broadly classified as either equal or unequal. The equal forms (duplicatas completa) show equal or nearly equal duplication of structures. In the unequal forms, there is unequal duplication of structures, and these belong to the category duplicatas incompleta. In these cases, only part of the anatomic structure of the fetus is

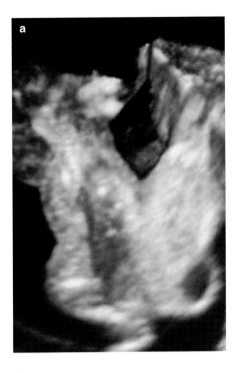

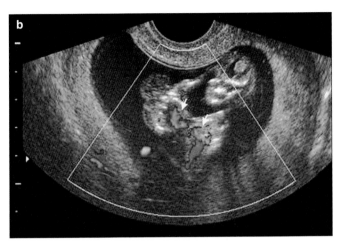

Figure 16.1 (a) Three-dimensional ultrasound image showing thoracopagus twins. (b) Doppler ultrasound image showing thoracopagus twins. Two hearts are depicted by the Doppler scan (arrows). Images courtesy of Y. Hazan, Kaplan Medical Center, Israel

duplicated. Classification of conjoined twins is typically based on the description of the fused anatomic region followed by the Greek suffix, 'pagus', to indicate fastened. The following classification of equal and unequal types of conjoined twinning was proposed by Potter and Craig[3] over 30 years ago and is still widely used.

Diplopagus

These are conjoined twins in whom the components, or components' parts, are equal and symmetrical.

Each component is complete, or nearly so

(1) Thoracopagus, sternopagus, xiphopagus, and sternoxiphopagus: connection in or near the sternal region, usually median, and the components are face to face (Figure 16.1);

(2) Pygopagus: connection at the sacrum and the components are back to back (Figure 16.2);

(3) Craniopagus: connection by the heads, usually median (Figure 16.3);

(4) Ischiopagus: connection in the lower pelvic region with the axes of the bodies

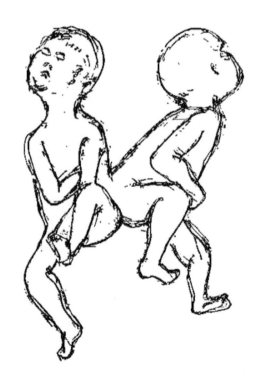

Figure 16.2 Pygopagus twins. Illustration courtesy of Raya Gabay, RN, Kaplan Medical Center, Israel

extending in a straight line in opposite directions (Figure 16.4).

The two components equal each other but each is less than an entire individual

(1) Duplication beginning in the cranial region:
  (a) Monocephalus diprosopus (single head):
    (i) Partial duplication of frontal region and nose;
    (ii) Partial duplication of frontal region, nose and mouth;
    (iii) Complete duplication of the face or with one eye of each face fused into a common median orbit;
  (b) Dicephalus (two heads, one body):
    (i) Dicephalus dipus dibrachius: two arms and legs with partial duplication of the spine and varying degrees of duplication of the median shoulder (Figure 16.5);

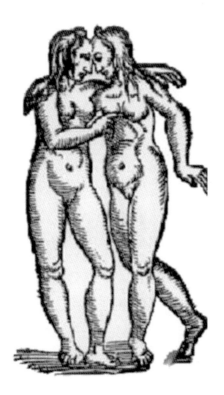

Figure 16.3 Craniopagus twins. Illustration by Ambroise Paré, a famous 16th century surgeon

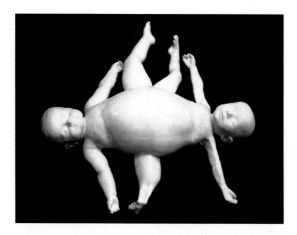

Figure 16.4 Ischiopagus tripus (three legs). Plaster cast of twins born in Warren county, Ohio, October 12, 1870. Image and text © 2004 Mütter Museum of the College of Physicians of Philadelphia

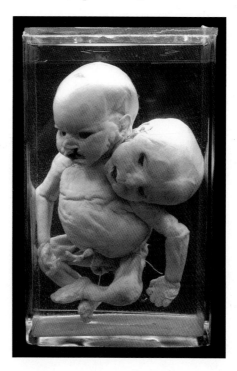

Figure 16.5 Full-term dicephalic twins, delivered in 1929. One head (left) shows also a cleft lip and palate. © 2004 Mütter Museum of the College of Physicians of Philadelphia

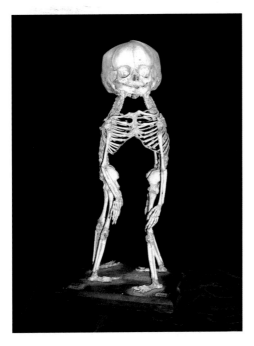

Figure 16.6 Skeleton of cephalothoracopagus twins. Image and text © 2004 Mütter Museum of the College of Physicians of Philadelphia

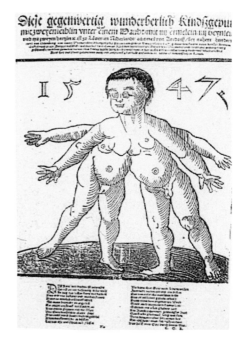

Figure 16.7 Cephalothoracopagus, syncephalus type. After a 1547 etching by an anonymous artist. These are the famous conjoined twins of Lowen[4]; of interest, both male and female genitalia are depicted by the artist

    (ii) Dicephalus dipus tribrachius: similar to dibrachius but with a median third arm or arm rudiment;

   (iii) Dicephalus dipus tetrabrachius: components united at the pelvis with varying degrees of fusion of the upper parts of the trunk but each component having a head and a pair of arms. The pelvis is partially duplicated but two legs are present;

(2) Duplication originating in the caudal region (dipygus):

  (a) Monocephalus tripus dibrachius: partial duplication of the pelvis with a third median leg that may be rudimentary or complete;

  (b) Monocephalus tetrapus dibrachius: partial or complete duplication of the pelvis with four legs, the pair belonging to one member often being fused in a sirenomelic limb;

(c) Cephalothoracopagus: two nearly complete components joined front to front over more or less the trunk region, but with a single neck and with heads more or less completely fused into a single compound mass (Figure 16.6):

    (i) Deradelphus: one face with two ears and a single normally formed cerebrum;

   (ii) Syncephalus: one face with four ears, two on the back of the head. The cerebrum is single or partially duplicated (Figure 16.7);

  (iii) Janiceps: two faces on opposite sides of the head with half of each belonging to each component (Figures 16.8 and 16.9);

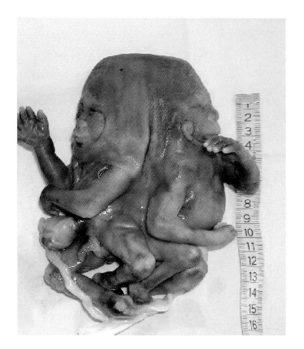

Figure 16.8 Cephalothoracopagus janiceps. Conjoined twins with two faces on opposite sides of the head. Figure courtesy of Dr Ido Solt, Rambam Medical Center, Haifa, Israel

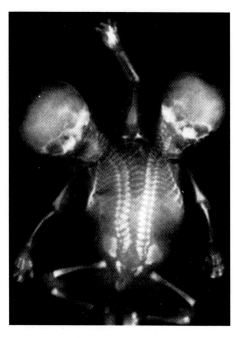

Figure 16.10 Dicephalus dipus tribrachius. X-ray of skeleton showing common arm with fused humerus and three bones in the forearm. Reproduced with permission from reference 3

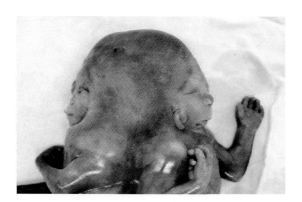

Figure 16.9 Close-up of cephalothoracopagus janiceps. Conjoined twins with two faces on opposite sides of the head. Figure courtesy of Dr Ido Solt, Rambam Medical Center, Haifa, Israel

(3) Duplication of both cranial and caudal regions (dicephalus dipygus):
  (a) Dicephalus tripus tribrachius: two members with a common trunk but two heads, two or three arms and three legs (Figure 16.10);

  (b) Similar to tripus tribrachius but with either upper or lower extremities or both completely duplicated;
  (c) Complete duplication of head, arms, and legs with anterior or lateral fusion of the trunk area.

Heteropagus

Unequal and symmetrical conjoined twins also exist in which one component is smaller and dependent on the other. The two members have very unequal degrees of development, one (autosite) being normal or nearly so, and the other (parasite) being incomplete and attached to the first as a dependent growth, usually at some point on the ventral surface.

Parasite attached to the visible surface of the autosite

(1) Parasite having arms, or a head and arms, usually attached to the autosite at or near the epigastrium;

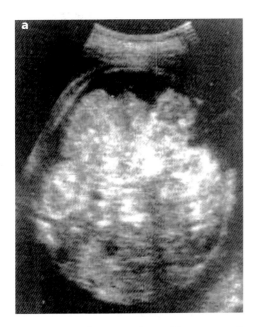 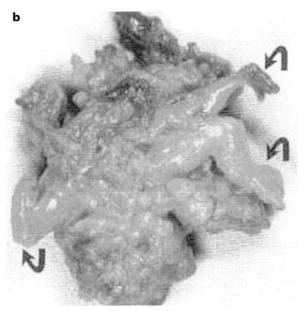

Figure 16.11 Fetus-*in-fetu*. This case was found in a miscarriage of 24 weeks. The sonographic scan (a) shows a large-for-dates fetal head (biparietal diameter 12.4 cm, head circumference 42 cm), with a large intracranial hyperechogenic and amorphic mass. The pathologic examination (b) revealed an immature teratoma, including well-defined fetal limbs. Images courtesy of I Solt MD and I Goldstein MD. Reprinted from Am J Obstet Gynecol Vol. 175. Goldstein I, Jakobi P, Groisman G, Itskovitz-Eldor J. Intracranial fetus-*in-fetu*, 1389–90 (1996), with permission from Elsevier

(2) Parasite having legs and varying portions of abdomen usually attached at or near the epigastrium;

(3) Parasite having arms and legs with or without a head with attachment at or near the epigastrium;

(4) Parasite attached to the head of the autosite;

(5) Parasite attached to the palate of the autosite;

(6) Parasite attached to the back, sacrum, or pelvis of the autosite.

Parasite developed in the autosite, usually in the thoracic or abdominal cavity, but occasionally in other regions (usually classified as tumors)

(1) Fetus-*in-fetu*: well-differentiated parasitic growth showing some degree of internal symmetry and cranial caudal differentiation (Figure 16.11);

(2) Teratoma: amorphous growth derived from the germ layers and lacking differentiation.

Other attempts have been made to standardize the terminology of conjoined twins and the more simplified classification proposed by Guttmacher and Nichols is also used by some authors (Table 16.1).[5]

The most common type of conjoined twinning, constituting approximately 60% of cases, involves conjunction in the mid-body (thoracophagus, xiphopagus, omphalopagus, or some combination thereof). In contrast, unequal conjoined twins are rare, accounting for less than 10% of cases.

CONJOINED TWINS COMPLICATING TRIPLET PREGNANCIES

Sepulveda and colleagues[6] reported two cases of conjoined twins complicating a triplet

Table 16.1 Types of conjoined twins (modified from reference 5)

Inferior conjunction
Diprosopus: 2 faces, 1 head, 1 body
Dicephalus: 2 heads, 1 body
Ischiopagus: inferior sacrococcygeal fusion
Pygopagus: posterolateral sacrococcygeal
  fusion

Superior conjunction
Dipygus: 2 pelves, and 4 legs
Syncephalus: facial + thoracic fusion
Craniopagus: cranial fusion

Middle conjunction
Thoracopagus: thoracic fusion
Omphalopagus: fusion from the umbilicus
  to the xyphoid cartilage
Rachipagus: vertebral fusion above the
  sacrum

pregnancy diagnosed by two-dimensional (2D) ultrasound in the first trimester and evaluated further by three-dimensional (3D) ultrasound. A review of the literature over the past 30 years reveals 11 other cases diagnosed prenatally by ultrasound. Overall, 3 (23%) of these 13 pregnancies followed assisted reproductive technologies, and 10 (77%) were diagnosed before 18 weeks. Four women opted for termination of the entire pregnancy and three were managed expectantly, with two delivering before 32 weeks. Two monochorionic pregnancies underwent selective feticide, with intrauterine demise of the non-conjoined fetus in both cases. All four dichorionic pregnancies undergoing selective termination or spontaneous embryo reduction to a singleton in the first trimester resulted in term delivery of the non-conjoined fetus. The rare condition of conjoined twins in a triplet pregnancy poses a significant obstetric diagnostic and management challenge. Accurate determination of chorionicity in these cases plays a critical role in determining management and outcome (see Chapter 5).

PRENATAL DIAGNOSIS

Conjoined twins can be diagnosed during routine antenatal ultrasonography. In the absence of clear-cut signs of fusion, additional sonographic findings summarized by Koontz and colleagues include:[7]

(1) The lack of a separating membrane;
(2) Inability to separate the fetal bodies;
(3) Detection of other anomalies in a twin gestation;
(4) More than three vessels present in the umbilical cord;
(5) Both fetal heads persistently at the same level;
(6) Backward flexion of the cervical and upper thoracic spine;
(7) No change in the relative positions of the fetuses despite attempts at manual manipulation of the twins.

Serial examinations are indicated to monitor fetal growth, nature of the fusion, and the development of hydrops, and to detect fetal demise.

The use of Doppler umbilical arterial velocity waveform analysis can reveal a characteristic 'double layer' spectral velocity waveform from the umbilical arteries. This is the result of signals originating from two separate arterial supplies adjacent to each other in a single umbilical cord. Such a characteristic feature provides an additional sonographic sign in the diagnosis of conjoined twins.[8]

Although first-trimester diagnosis of conjoined twins is possible, false-positive cases may occur before 10 weeks because fetal movements are limited earlier in gestation, and monoamniotic twins may appear conjoined.[9] A recent detailed analysis of case reports in which 3D imaging was used suggests that, at present, this modality does not improve the diagnosis made by 2D ultrasound. Overall, very early prenatal diagnosis and first-trimester 3D imaging provide very little additional practical medical information compared to the 11–14 weeks' ultrasound examination.[9] However, at times, twin reversed arterial perfusion sequence and epigastric heteropagus conjoined twins may appear similar antenatally and can be differentiated by 3D ultrasound by demonstrating the relationship of a completely formed fetus and an adjacent second body consisting of a pelvis with two lower extremities.[10]

Andrews et al[11] recently determined the accuracy of pre- and postnatal echocardiography in delineating the degree of cardiac fusion, intracardiac anatomy, and ventricular function of 13 thoracopagus, 5 thoraco-omphalopagus, and 5 parapagus pairs with thoracic-level fusion presenting to a single center over a 20-year period. These twins were classified according to the degree of cardiac fusion. The data indicate that the degree of cardiac fusion was correctly diagnosed in all but one set. Intracardiac anatomy was correctly diagnosed in all instances, although the antenatal diagnosis was revised postnatally in three cases. Ventricular function was good in all twins scanned prenatally, and postnatal function correlated well with clinical condition. Thirteen sets of twins with separate hearts and pericardia, separate hearts and common pericardia, or fused atria and separate ventricles underwent surgical separation, but only 16/26 survived. There were no survivors from sets with fused atria and separate ventricles or fused atria and ventricles. This study suggests that pre- and postnatal echocardiography accurately delineates cardiac fusion, intracardiac anatomy, and ventricular function in the majority of twins with thoracic-level fusion and, therefore, should be an integral part of assessing feasibility of separation.[11]

Magnetic resonance imaging can also be used prenatally to more precisely determine the extent of fusion and to begin planning for immediate postnatal management (i.e. survivability within a few hours after delivery). No prenatal imaging technique is sufficiently precise to aid the surgeon in determining the approach to surgical separation and probability of success. However, such decisions and conclusions can only be reached after careful postnatal considerations.

POSTNATAL IMAGING

Conjoined twins present a unique challenge to pediatric surgeons and radiologists. Planning of surgical separation is aided by accurate preoperative imaging. The area of fusion largely determines the imaging modalities used. Thoracic conjunction is most common and requires cardiac assessment, preferably by echocardiography, but contrast studies can enhance the finer details.[6,12] Magnetic resonance imaging and computed tomography provide excellent anatomic and bone detail, demonstrating organ position, shared viscera, and limited vascular anatomy. Contrast-material radiography allows evaluation of the gastrointestinal and urogenital tracts, and a shared liver requires assessment of anatomy, vascularization, and biliary drainage. Angiography helps to define specific vascular supply, which is useful in determining the distribution of shared structures between the twins at surgery.

Functional magnetic resonance (fMR) imaging was used in adult craniopagus (temporoparietooccipital fusion) to evaluate hemispheric language dominance and the eloquent language areas in the preoperative planning stages of a recent operation.[13] Significant blood oxygen level-dependent activations were detected in the main language regions in each twin. Overall, the right-handed twin was strongly left lateralized for language, whereas the left-handed twin showed more bilateral activation during language tasks. Non-invasive language mapping with the aid of fMR imaging has been demonstrated for the first time in total craniopagus.[13]

It is axiomatic that each set of conjoined twins is unique. A complex imaging strategy to accurately define anatomic fusion, vascular anomalies, and other associated abnormalities is important for surgical planning and prognostic information.[11] A very useful diagnostic 'cheatsheet' has been provided by Sepulveda and colleagues,[6] which clearly shows the preferred imaging modalities used in different types of conjoined twinning (Table 16.2).

Table 16.2 Imaging modalities used in diagnosing the anatomy of conjoined twins[6]

Twin type	Overview	Cardiovascular	System evaluated*							
			Hepatobiliary	Pulmonary	Upper GI	Lower GI	Urologic	Genital	Neurologic	Vascular
Thoracopagus	plain radiography, MR imaging	echocardiography, cardiac catheterization	yes	yes	yes	no	no	no	no	yes
Omphalopagus	plain radiography, MR imaging	echocardiography	yes	yes	yes	maybe	no	no	no	yes
Pygopagus	plain radiography, MR imaging, CT of spine	echocardiography	no	no	no	yes	yes	yes	maybe	maybe
Ischiopagus	plain radiography, MR imaging, CT of pelvis	echocardiography, cardiac catheterization	maybe	maybe	maybe	yes	yes	yes	no	yes
Craniopagus	plain radiography, MR imaging, CT of skull	echocardiography	no	no	no	no	no	no	yes	maybe
Parapagus	plain radiography, MR imaging, CT of pelvis	echocardiography, cardiac catheterization	maybe	maybe	yes	yes	yes	yes	no	yes
Cephalopagus	plain radiography, MR imaging, CT of skull	echocardiography, cardiac catheterization	maybe	maybe	no	no	no	no	yes	yes
Rachipagus	plain radiography, MR imaging, CT of spine	echocardiography	no	no	no	no	no	no	maybe	no

MR, magnetic resonance; CT, computed tomography; GI, gastrointestinal

REFERENCES

1. Spencer R. Conjoined Twins: Developmental Malformations and Clinical Implications. Baltimore: Johns Hopkins University Press, 2003.

2. Machin GA, Sperber GH. Lessons from conjoined twins. Am J Med Genet 1987; 28: 89–97.

3. Potter EL, Craig JM. Pathology of the Fetus and the Infant. Chicago: Year Book Medical Publishers, 1975.

4. Blickstein I. The conjoined twins of Lowen. Twin Res 2000; 3: 185–8.

5. Guttmacher AF, Nichols BL. Teratology of conjoined twins. In: Bergsma D, ed. Birth Defects Original Article Series: Conjoined Twins. New York: The National Foundation–March of Dimes, 1967: 3–9.

6. Sepulveda W, Munoz H, Alcalde JL. Conjoined twins in a triplet pregnancy: early prenatal diagnosis with three dimensional ultrasound and review of the literature. Ultrasound Obstet Gynecol 2003; 22: 199–204.

7. Koontz WL, Herbert WN, Seeds JW, Cefalo RC. Ultrasonography in the antepartum diagnosis of conjoined twins: a report of two cases. J Reprod Med 1983; 28: 627–30.

8. Woo JS, Liang ST, Lo R. Characteristic pattern of Doppler umbilical arterial velocity waveform in conjoined twins. Gynecol Obstet Invest 1987; 23: 70–2.

9. Pajkrt E, Jauniaux E. First-trimester diagnosis of conjoined twins. Prenat Diagn 2005; 25: 820–6.

10. MacKenzie AP, Stephenson CD, Funai EF, Lee MJ, Timor-Tritsch I. Three-dimensional ultrasound to differentiate epigastric heteropagus conjoined twins from a TRAP sequence. Am J Obstet Gynecol 2004; 191: 1736–9.

11. Andrews RE, McMahon CJ, Yates RW et al. Echocardiographic assessment of conjoined twins. Heart 2005; 92: 382–7.

12. Kingston CA, McHugh K, Kumaradevan J et al. Imaging in the preoperative assessment of conjoined twins. Radiographics 2001; 21: 1187–208.

13. Ho YC, Goh KY, Golay X et al. Functional magnetic resonance imaging in adult craniopagus for presurgical evaluation. J Neurosurg 2005; 103: 910–16.

17

Complete hydatidiform mole with coexistent twin

INTRODUCTION

A hydatidiform mole coexisting with a live fetus is uncommon. Suspicion that this condition may exist arises when an ultrasound scan identifies a fetal pole alongside an abnormal placenta. The main issue clearly is to differentiate between two possible diagnoses: a singleton pregnancy consisting of a partial hydatidiform mole with an abnormal triploid fetus that usually dies *in utero* during the first half of pregnancy versus a twin gestation consisting of a complete hydatidiform mole along with a coexisting live fetus (CMCF). The latter is extremely rare,[1–4] however, and management is challenging because the fetus may be viable. Information about this entity is scant. Moreover, only a few case reports of a twin gestation with a coexisting hydatidiform mole have accurately distinguished between a partial mole with a live fetus and CMCF. Although CMCF is associated with fetal survival, it carries a significant risk of severe complications including pre-eclampsia, preterm delivery, and development of persistent gestational trophoblastic tumor (GTT).

This chapter discusses the diagnosis of complete hydatidiform mole with a coexisting fetus (Figure 17.1).

CYTOGENETICS AND MOLECULAR BASIS OF PARTIAL AND COMPLETE HYDATIDIFORM MOLE

Gestational trophoblastic diseases are heterogeneous conditions derived from the products of pregnancy. These conditions, including hydatidiform mole, invasive mole, choriocarci-

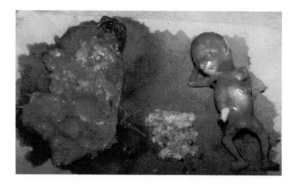

Figure 17.1 Complete hydatidiform mole (left) with a male co-twin (right) and a normal placenta (center). Pregnancy was terminated at 18 weeks because of severe pre-eclampsia and life-threatening thyrotoxicosis

noma, and placental-site trophoblastic tumors, are characterized by abnormal growth of the chorionic tissue with varying propensities for local invasion and metastasis. In all these conditions the presence of paternal genes is a prerequisite, as well as a distinguishing feature that separates it from other non-gestational tumors.

Hydatidiform mole is associated with an abnormal placenta with enlarged and edematous chorionic villi, accompanied by hyperplasia of the trophoblast. In the late 1970s, Vassilakos and colleagues[5] first described two distinct pathologic entities: partial and complete hydatidiform mole (CHM) with different mechanisms of origin based on cytogenetic analysis. Partial moles derive from dispermic fertilization of a haploid normal oocyte, and produce a triploid set of chromosomes. In the majority of instances, the extra set is of paternal origin, and fetal parts can be recognized. The incidence of persistent GTT following partial moles may be as low as 4%.[3] In contrast, a CHM contains a diploid set of 46 chromosomes, all of paternal origin (androgenic). Sex chromosomes are almost always XX, and most probably are derived from the fertilization of an anuclear ovum by a haploid (23X) spermatozoon, and subsequent duplication of its own chromosomes. No fetal parts can be identified, and the risk of developing persistent GTT is higher (12–20%) than in partial mole.[3,6] It is believed that the higher the ratio of paternal/maternal chromosomes, the greater is the molar change, as is the case with CHM (2:0 paternal/maternal ratio) compared with partial mole (2:1).

Golubovsky[7] questioned the two proposed mechanisms that are usually envisaged for this kind of diandric diploidy:

(1) Penetration by a haploid sperm of a nanuclear ('empty') oocyte with subsequent endoreduplication of the male pronucleus. Only 46,XX conceptions survive, and 46,YY are non-viable;
(2) Fertilization of an anuclear oocyte by two haploid sperms, resulting in the so-called heterozygous mole.

Clearly, both proposed mechanisms implicate the presence of some regular 'reservoir' of empty or anuclear oocytes – an implication that is unfounded by evidence. Enucleated oocytes are produced under experimental circumstances. However, they have not been described as a regular feature of oogenesis and as being potentially fertilized under natural conditions.[7] A detailed alternative theory has been proposed by Golubovsky but is beyond the scope of this chapter.

Differential diagnosis of the combination of a live fetus and a molar-appearing placenta includes three possibilities. The first is a singleton pregnancy consisting of a partial hydatidiform mole and a live fetus. The second consists of a twin pregnancy with one placenta exhibiting a complete mole (no fetus) and the other placenta (sometimes in close approximation with the first) sustaining a normal twin. The third possibility is a combination of partial mole and a twin in one sac and a normal twin in the other. In the last possibility, the option of CHM is easily excluded by the presence of two fetuses. The real challenge is to distinguish between the first two possibilities, because of the chance of survival in the instances which include a CMCF. Another very rare possibility is a diploid mole of biparental origin (a partial mole) and a coexistent fetus.[8] The prognosis and risk of persistent GTT of this obscure entity are currently unknown.

Complete and partial moles are associated with distinct fetal and maternal complications. In the combination of a partial hydatidiform mole, the fetus is almost always triploid, and the indication for a pregnancy termination is clear. In contrast, although the fetus may be normal in a twin pregnancy with a CMCF, continuation of the pregnancy is frequently associated with severe maternal complications, giving rise to a clear mother versus fetus clinical dilemma. The management of such pregnancies can be either immediate termination to avoid the potential maternal complications, or expectant management to save the fetus but endangering the mother with pregnancy complications or with a potentially persistent trophoblastic tumor.

INCIDENCE

The incidence of hydatidiform moles varies in different populations, and is much higher in Japan than in Europe or America.[9] The incidence of complete and partial hydatidiform moles varies between 1 and 3 per 1000 pregnancies.[10] The coexistence of a hydatidiform mole and a live fetus is much more uncommon, with a quoted range of incidence from 1 in 10 000 to 1 in 100 000 pregnancies. This estimate is based on old series reported before the era of distinguishing between partial and complete mole, and most of these cases were either aborted or resulted in *in utero* fetal death. Cases of molar pregnancy with a coexisting viable fetus are exceedingly rare, with only 16 cases with a living newborn reported before 1980.[11] In all instances except one, the diagnosis was made after delivery, and without differentiation between the partial and complete molar entities. More recently, accurately diagnosed complete hydatidiform moles were reported with a coexisting fetus,[10,12] but only a few with a living newborn. The true incidence of this rare entity is difficult to establish, and some authors suggest that the increased incidence of iatrogenic multiple gestations will result in a higher incidence of CMCF.[12] A final interesting observation, albeit without subsequent confirmation, is that of De George, who reported in 1970 a significantly increased frequency (1:225) of molar pregnancies before or after a twin pregnancy.[13]

DIAGNOSTIC TOOLS

As discussed above, the diagnosis of the different associations of a fetus with a mole has important clinical implications. High-resolution ultrasonography, the diagnostic tool of choice, is useful in such circumstances and allows determination of the number of gestational sacs as well as assessment of normal fetal development.

Most cases of molar pregnancies are diagnosed during the first trimester by the typical ultrasonographic visualization of the entire uterine cavity filled by a uniformly hyperechoic soft tissue comprising sharply defined echofree cysts of various sizes and shapes, the so-called 'snowstorm' pattern (Figure 17.2).

Twin pregnancies, consisting of CHM with a coexisting fetus, are usually diagnosed later in pregnancy. In these circumstances, the initial scan is not easy to interpret, and many cases present in the second trimester with the classical signs and symptoms of gestational trophoblastic disease. In CHM, the sonographic image typically shows a vesicular mass separate from a normal placenta, exhibiting a characteristic vesicular pattern, whereas in partial

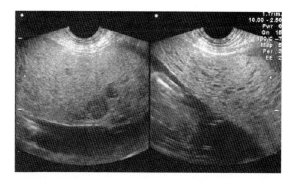

Figure 17.2 Ultrasound image showing a molar placenta in the right panel with part of the normal fetus (nourished by a second placenta). The left panel shows molar cavitations in the placenta. Image courtesy of B. Caspi

mole, only part of the placenta appears normal and the other part exhibits the classic 'snowstorm' pattern. In addition, an aberrant gestational sac and congenital anomalies may also be seen. When a molar-appearing placenta is recognized, high-resolution sonographic equipment is useful to differentiate between a partial mole and a twin pregnancy with a complete mole and a coexisting normal fetus. Doppler velocimetry, where available, may be helpful in confirming the avascular nature of a complete mole.[14] In 50% of the cases, bilateral theca lutein cysts are also present. Interestingly, Steller and colleagues reported that only 68% of patients with hydatidiform mole and coexisting fetus were diagnosed correctly by abdominal ultrasound.[3] This detection rate is even worse in the first trimester before fetal anomalies associated with a partial mole are visualized.

The radiographic appearance of hydatidiform mole is highly variable, depending mainly on the size of the chorionic villi, which range from 1–2 mm up to 3 cm in size. On MR imaging, the cystic mass often yields a high signal on T2-weighted images. Maternal serum α-fetoprotein (MSAFP) helps differentiate between a partial mole and a twin pregnancy with a complete mole and a coexisting normal fetus.[14] MSAFP levels are within the normal range in a twin gestation with a normal fetus and a coexistent complete mole, whereas elevated levels of MSAFP with normal amniotic fluid AFP levels are found in partial molar pregnancy.[15]

A markedly elevated human chorionic gonadotropin (hCG) value may suggest CHM, but this determination is not reliable for the diagnosis, especially in twin pregnancies in which hCG levels can be significantly but normally elevated. It follows that whenever the diagnosis of a molar placenta/coexisting fetus combination is suspected, the diagnosis should be reached by invasive methods.

The histologic appearance of villi as well as standard chromosomal analysis may be inconclusive. Although chromosomal triploidy is diagnostic of a partial mole, a diploid karyotype – typical of a complete mole – has been described in partial moles as well. Thus, the final diagnosis of a complete mole requires elaborate cytogenetic studies to prove the androgenic origin of the chromosomes.[16]

HIGH-ORDER MULTIPLE PREGNANCIES AND COEXISTENT COMPLETE MOLE

The first case of a high-order multiple pregnancy coexistent with hydatidiform mole was reported in 1980 by Sauerbrei and colleagues who described a triplet pregnancy with a complete hydatidiform mole and two fetuses.[17] Since then, more cases have been reported, but unfortunately do not significantly expand the limited information about the natural history of such pregnancies. As usual, high-order multiple gestations carry an increased risk of preterm labor and pre-eclampsia. When accompanied by a mole, however, this risk might be even higher. Chao and associates described six cases of CHM coexisting with either a twin or a triplet pregnancy, with the longest reported gestation being 25 weeks, and no surviving infants.[18]

The management of these rare pregnancies must be individualized utilizing, where possible, available precepts from the treatment of twin gestations.

REFERENCES

1. Fishman DA, Padilla LA, Keh P et al. Management of twin pregnancies consisting of a complete hydatidiform mole and normal fetus. Obstet Gynecol 1998; 91: 546–50.

2. Vejerslev LO. Clinical management and diagnostic possibilities in hydatidiform mole with coexistent fetus. Obstet Gynecol Surv 1991; 46: 577–88.

3. Steller MA, Genest DR, Bernstein MR et al. Clinical features of multiple conception with partial or complete molar pregnancy and coexisting fetuses. J Reprod Med 1994; 39: 147–54.

4. Jones WB, Lauersen NH. Hydatidiform mole with no coexistent fetus. Am J Obstet Gynecol 1975; 122: 267–72.

5. Vassilakos P, Riotton G, Kajii T. Hydatidiform mole: two entities. Am J Obstet Gynecol 1977; 127: 167–70.

6. Bristow RE, Shumway JB, Khouzami AN, Witter FR. Complete hydatidiform mole and surviving coexistent twin. Obstet Gynecol Surv 1996; 51: 705–9.

7. Golubovsky MD. Postzygotic diploidization of triploids as a source of unusual cases of mosaicism, chimerism and twinning. Hum Reprod 2003; 18: 236–42.

8. Vejerslev LO, Sunde L, Hansen BF et al. Hydatidiform mole and fetus with normal karyotype: support of a separate entity. Obstet Gynecol 1991; 77: 868–74.

9. Buckley JD. The epidemiology of molar pregnancy and choriocarcinoma. Clin Obstet Gynecol 1984; 27: 153–9.

10. Sebire NJ, Foskett M, Paradinas FJ et al. Outcome of twin pregnancies with complete hydatidiform mole and healthy co-twin. Lancet 2002; 359: 2165–6.

11. Suzuki M, Matsunobu A, Wakita K et al. Hydatidiform mole with a surviving coexisting fetus. Obstet Gynecol 1980; 56: 384–8.

12. Matsui H, Sekiya S, Hando T et al. Hydatidiform mole coexistent with a twin live fetus: a national collaborative study in Japan. Hum Reprod 2000; 15: 608–11.

13. De George FV. Hydatidiform moles in other pregnancies of mothers of twins. Am J Obstet Gynecol 1970; 108: 369–71.

14. Jauniaux E, de Lannoy E, Moscoso G, Campbell S. Diagnostic prenatal des pathologies molaires associees un fetus: revue de la literature a propos d'uncas. J Gynecol Obstet Biol Reprod 1990; 19: 451.

15. Freeman SB, Priest JH, MacMahon WC, Fernhoff PM, Elsas LJ. Prenatal ascertainment of triploidy by maternal serum alpha-fetoprotein screening. Prenat Diagn 1989; 9: 339–47.

16. Ishii J, Iitsuka Y, Takano H et al. Genetic differentiation of complete hydatidiform moles coexisting with normal fetuses by short tandem repeat-derived deoxyribonucleic acid polymorphism analysis. Am J Obstet Gynecol 1998; 179: 628–34.

17. Sauerbrei EE, Salem S, Fayle B. Coexistent hydatidiform mole and live fetus in the second trimester: an ultrasound study. Radiology 1980; 135: 415–17.

18. Chao AS, Tsai TC, Soong YK. Clinical management of a quadruplet pregnancy combining a triplet pregnancy with a classical hydatidiform mole: case report and review of literature. Prenat Diag 1999; 19: 1073–6.

18

Heterotopic pregnancy

INTRODUCTION

Heterotopic pregnancy is the rare simultaneous coexistence of intrauterine and extrauterine gestational sacs. The fact that practitioners do not regularly see this condition increases its diagnostic and therapeutic challenges. Heterotopic pregnancy is presently thought to result from the implantation of dizygotic twins at widely separated sites. In the modern era of assisted reproductive technologies (ART), heterotopic pregnancy is more common than was the case in the past. As heterotopic pregnancy may present a life-threatening situation, physicians must have a high index of suspicion in order to reach an early diagnosis and institute appropriate treatment.

INCIDENCE

The incidence of spontaneous heterotopic pregnancy is reported variously in the literature. As heterotopic pregnancy is, by definition, a multiple pregnancy with a combination of an intrauterine and an extrauterine pregnancy, its incidence depends on the incidence of each component and both vary with location and time of report. De Voe and Pratt calculated a theoretic figure using the incidence of ectopic pregnancy, 0.37%, multiplied by the rate of dizygotic multiple pregnancies, 0.8%.[1] The result of this calculation was 0.003%. However, they also reported two cases among 13 527 deliveries at the Mayo Clinic in 1947, for an incidence of 0.015%.[1] In 1982, Richards and colleagues[2] performed the identical calculation as De Voe and Pratt and determined an incidence of 0.064%, or 1/15 600 pregnancies, using the incidence of ectopic pregnancies at that time. In 1990, Molloy and colleagues performed 6204 *in vitro* fertilization/gamete intrafallopian transfer (IVF/GIFT) cycles which resulted in 1001 pregnancies, 10 of which were heterotopic, for an incidence of 1%.[3] In the same year, Dimitry and associates reported 1996 IVF cycles from the years 1984–88 which resulted in 315 clinical pregnancies, 9 of which were heterotopic, for an incidence of 2.9%.[4] Shortly thereafter, Dor and co-workers described 4/428 heterotopic pregnancies (0.9%) after 2624 IVF cycles over a period of 9.5 years.[5] In summary, the estimated incidence of heterotopic pregnancy ranges from 1–2/30 000 in the general population to 1/100 with ART.

RISK FACTORS

The precise cause of heterotopic pregnancy is unclear, but it seems to be a non-arithmetic product of factors leading to a multiple pregnancy and to factors related to ectopic pregnancy. Undoubtedly, the most significant factor is the high incidence of multiple pregnancies after fertility treatments. Published rates of 5–10%, 10–30%, and 35% follow clomiphene citrate, human gonadotropins, and IVF therapies, respectively.

Glassner and colleagues described two cases of heterotopic pregnancy in patients treated with clomiphene citrate, and concluded that the incidence of heterotopic pregnancy was 1/900 pregnancies after this treatment.[6] Berger and Taymor previously described two cases of heterotopic pregnancy, the first after treatment with clomiphene citrate, and the second after treatment with gonadotropins.[7] Both patients underwent laparotomy and salpingectomy for a ruptured ectopic pregnancy. Both intrauterine pregnancies continued to term, resulting in the delivery of healthy babies. During the 5-year period in which these two cases had been observed, 204 pregnancies had resulted from the use of clomiphene citrate or gonadotropins, yielding an incidence of 1/100 in this small series.[7]

As IVF treatment is a major risk factor for multiple pregnancy as well as ectopic pregnancy, it is conceivable that IVF results in an increased incidence of heterotopic pregnancies, especially considering that IVF was developed to overcome mechanical infertility, whereby tubal pathology is an independent risk factor for ectopic pregnancy. Goldman and colleagues reviewed 34 heterotopic pregnancies following IVF treatment published between the years 1985 and 1991.[8] Several predisposing factors related to the technique of embryo transfer, the number and quality of transferred embryos, the hormonal milieu, and the chance for superfecundation. These treatments are summarized in Table 18.1 and expanded upon in the following:

(1) Deep insertion of the transfer catheter into the uterine cavity may cause the embryos to migrate from the uterotubal orifice, where they were deposited, into the tubes. Insertion of the transfer catheter into the mid-uterine cavity may help to avoid such migration (Figure 18.1). Embryo migration into the tubes may also be facilitated by gravity because of the use of the head-down tilt position (Trendelenburg's position) after transfer.

(2) A sticky, viscous, and heavy medium (high content of human serum) used in some centers for embryo transfer may contribute to migration of the embryos into the tubes.

(3) A large volume of transfer medium may facilitate the migration of the embryos into the tubes. Limiting the volume of the

Table 18.1 Factors related to increased rate of heterotopic pregnancy in *in vitro* fertilization patients

(1) Transfer of embryos to fundal portion of the uterus
(2) Use of human or animal serum in the medium
(3) Large volume of transfer medium
(4) Large number of embryos transferred to the uterus
(5) High level of estadiol before ovum pick-up
(6) Superfecundation

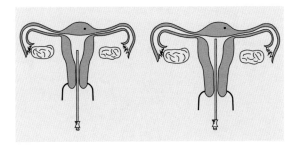

Figure 18.1 Deep insertion of the transfer catheter (right) may increase the risk for heterotopic pregnancy, whereas transferring the embryos to the mid-portion of the uterus (left) may reduce the risk

transfer medium to 10–20 μl may help to avoid ectopic implantation, although heterotopic pregnancy can occur with volumes less than 10 μl.

(4) Heterotopic pregnancy occurs after transfer of 2–6 embryos in a single cycle. The pathogenic role of the number of the embryos is not clear. The transfer of one embryo only eliminates the chance for heterotopic pregnancy. Embryo quality may also be a contributing factor, although a heterotopic pregnancy was described after transferring frozen–thawed embryos, suggesting that even such embryos can implant in the Fallopian tubes.

(5) Some authors suggest a role for the high estrogen levels present just before ovum pick-up in the pathogenesis of ectopic pregnancy. However, reports of heterotopic pregnancies during non-stimulated cycles, when embryos were transferred either after spontaneous ovulation or in synchronized endometrial build-up by controlled estrogen–progesterone replacement therapy, do not support this concept.

(6) Superfecundation can happen if a patient with patent tubes is undergoing IVF treatment. Ectopic/heterotopic gestation may result from the spontaneous fertilization of an unrecovered oocyte, if coitus occurs near the time of ovulation.

DIAGNOSIS AND TREATMENT

The diagnosis of heterotopic pregnancy presents a great clinical challenge. Whereas early diagnosis is undoubtedly difficult, it clearly increases the likelihood of salvaging the intrauterine pregnancy. An awareness of this possibility and high index of suspicion in atypical cases of multiple pregnancy, ectopic pregnancy, and/or abortion is essential for prompt diagnosis. In 1983, Reece and colleagues reviewed 66 cases of heterotopic pregnancy published between 1966 and 1979, including five new cases from their center.[9] The clinical characteristics of these patients was highly variable, and the following unrelated criteria were all helpful in making a diagnosis in the years before ultrasound diagnosis was available:

(1) Uterine fundal height compatible with dates in a patient believed to have an ectopic pregnancy (the absence of a closed cervical os or the presence of vaginal bleeding should not alter the suspicion of heterotopic pregnancy);

(2) Two or more corpora lutea and an enlarged, soft, and globular uterus;

(3) The absence of withdrawal bleeding and the presence of pregnancy symptoms following excision of an ectopic pregnancy;

(4) Hemoperitoneum following the termination of an intrauterine pregnancy;

(5) The combination of abdominal pain, adnexal mass with pain and tenderness, peritoneal irritation, and an enlarged uterus;

(6) Higher serum β-human chorionic gonadotropin (hCG) levels than expected in the presence of an intrauterine singleton pregnancy.

Of the 66 cases reviewed, the most common presenting signs and symptoms were: abdominal pain (81.8%), adnexal mass (43.9%), peritoneal irritation (43.9%), enlarged uterus (42.4%), and vaginal spotting (31.8%).[9] Interestingly, these authors did not relate this group of symptoms to the classic symptoms of ectopic pregnancy, namely amenorrhea, pain, bleeding, etc.

In 1996, Tal and colleagues reviewed 139 cases published from 1971 to 1993.[10] Of these, 111 detailed the clinical course that led to the diagnosis of a heterotopic pregnancy. Diagnosis was made in 59% of cases during emergency laparoscopy or laparotomy. Sonographic detection of an extrauterine gestational sac with or without a fetal pole along with an intrauterine pregnancy was made in another 41% of the patients. Nevertheless, sonographic diagnosis was not always made at the first examination, and was frequently delayed. Approximately 70% of the heterotopic pregnancies were diagnosed between 5 and 8 weeks of gestation, almost 20% between 9 and 10 weeks, and the remaining 10% after the 11th week in this series.

When performing a first-trimester sonographic examination, especially in a patient who has had fertility treatments, it is always advisable to scan both adnexa, to exclude heterotopic pregnancy (Figure 18.2), as the sonographic evidence of an intrauterine multiple pregnancy does not exclude in any manner the diagnosis of a heterotopic pregnancy. Zalel and co-workers described an IVF case in which four embryos were transferred, three of which implanted in the uterus while the fourth

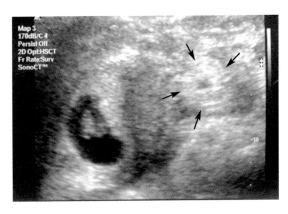

Figure 18.2 Ultrasound scan showing an intrauterine pregnancy together with a tubal ectopic pregnancy (arrows). Image courtesy of Arie Herman, Assaf Harophe Medical Center, Israel

was implanted in the left tube.[11] The diagnosis was established by emergency laparotomy, and salpingectomy was performed. Later, the intrauterine triplets were delivered by cesarean section at 35 weeks. Such a combination has also been described by Muller et al in a 34-year-old nulliparous pregnant woman after ovulation induction with clomiphene, whereby an ectopic pregnancy occurred with a twin intrauterine pregnancy.[12]

Obviously, triplet heterotopic pregnancies are not restricted to intrauterine twins and an ectopic. For example, Hoopmann et al[13] described a case of combined bilateral tubal and intrauterine pregnancy after IVF and embryo transfer. These authors commented that such an occurrence should encourage the transfer of only one embryo. This conclusion may well be true because an intrauterine monochorionic twin pregnancy combined with

an ectopic pregnancy was described after the transfer of two embryos.[14]

The vigilance required regarding the possibility of coexisting ectopic and intrauterine pregnancy following assisted conception, even in entirely asymptomatic cases, was reported by Tan and Ridley.[15] These authors described a case of an asymptomatic woman who conceived after assisted reproduction and was found to have an extrauterine mass on ultrasound and MRI. This complex mass had equivocal imaging features and was eventually found to be a ruptured ovarian heterotopic pregnancy. Cheng and co-workers[16] described a young, multiparous woman, presenting at 6 weeks' gestation, complaining of a dark reddish-brown vaginal discharge and progressive left lower-quadrant discomfort during early pregnancy following a natural conception cycle. A heterotopic pregnancy complicated by hematometra was diagnosed with the help of transvaginal ultrasonography and 3D power Doppler ultrasound angiography.

The most frequent location of the ectopic pregnancy in patients with heterotopic pregnancy is the Fallopian tubes. In Tal's review, 89% implanted mostly in the ampullar portion, and the remaining gestations were found in a tubal stump, isthmus, cornua, and in the fimbria. The authors also reported the extremely rare instances of two gestational sacs implanted in the same tube alongside the intrauterine pregnancy, and a heterotopic quintuplet pregnancy in which there was an intrauterine triplet pregnancy accompanied by two extrauterine gestational sacs, one in each tube.[10] Unusual locations of the ectopic pregnancy were also described as the uterine cervix, the ovary, and the abdominal cavity.[10]

REFERENCES

1. De Voe RW, Pratt JH. Simultaneous intrauterine and extrauterine pregnancy. Am J Obstet Gynecol 1948; 56: 1119–26.

2. Richards SR, Stempel LE, Carlton BD. Heterotopic pregnancy: reappraisal of incidence. Am J Obstet Gynecol 1982; 142: 928–30.

3. Molloy D, Deambrosis W, Keeping D et al. Multiple-sited (heterotopic) pregnancy after in vitro fertilization and gamete intrafallopian transfer. Fertil Steril 1990; 53: 1068–71.

4. Dimitry ES, Subak Sharpe R, Mills M et al. Nine cases of heterotopic pregnancies in 4 years of in vitro fertilization. Fertil Steril 1990; 53: 107–10.

5. Dor J, Seidman DS, Levran D et al. The incidence of combined intrauterine and extrauterine pregnancy after in vitro fertilization and embryo transfer. Fertil Steril 1991; 55: 833–4.

6. Glassner MJ, Aron E, Eskin BA. Ovulation induction with clomiphene and the rise in heterotopic pregnancies. A report of two cases. J Reprod Med 1990; 35: 175–8.

7. Berger MJ, Taymor ML. Simultaneous intrauterine and tubal pregnancies following ovulation induction. Am J Obstet Gynecol 1972; 113: 812–13.

8. Goldman GA, Fisch B, Ovadia J, Tadir Y. Heterotopic pregnancy after assisted reproductive technologies. Obstet Gynecol Surv 1992; 47: 217–21.

9. Reece AE, Roy PH, Sirmans MF et al. Combined intrauterine and extrauterine gestations: a review. Am J Obstet Gynecol 1983; 146: 323–30.

10. Tal J, Haddad S, Gordon N, Timor Tritsch I. Heterotopic pregnancy after ovulation induction and assisted reproductive technologies: a literature review from 1971 to 1993. Fertil Steril 1996; 66: 1–12.

11. Zalel Y, Barash A, Caspi B, Borenstein R. Heterotopic pregnancy – an unusual case report following in vitro fertilization and embryo transfer. J Assist Reprod Genet 1993; 10: 169–71.

12. Muller Vranjes A, Popovic Z, Vlahovic I, Habek D, Kasac Z. Heterotopic trigeminal pregnancy in infertile women after ovulation stimulation and embolisation of a uterine myoma. Fetal Diagn Ther 2006; 21: 81–3.

13. Hoopmann M, Wilhelm L, Possover M, Nawroth F. Heterotopic triplet pregnancy with bilateral tubal and intrauterine pregnancy after IVF. Reprod Biomed Online 2003; 6: 345–8.

14. Nikolaou DS, Lavery S, Bevan R, Margara R, Trew G. Triplet heterotopic pregnancy with an intrauterine monochorionic diamniotic twin pregnancy and an interstitial pregnancy following in vitro fertilisation and transfer of two embryos. J Obstet Gynaecol 2002; 22: 94–5.

15. Tan PL, Ridley LJ. Incidental heterotopic pregnancy demonstrated on magnetic resonance imaging. Australas Radiol 2005; 49: 75–8.

16. Cheng PJ, Chueh HY, Qiu JT. Heterotopic pregnancy in a natural conception cycle presenting as hematometra. Obstet Gynecol 2004; 104: 1195–8.

19

Predicting preterm birth by cervical assessment

INTRODUCTION

The incidence of twin and multiple births has increased in most developed countries by epidemic proportions, with an immediate consequence of an important increase in the numbers of infants born at < 33 weeks (1.7% of singletons, 13.9% of twins, and 41.2% of triplets). Several studies indicate that twin infants originating after *in vitro* fertilization (IVF) have an even greater likelihood of prematurity than naturally conceived twins.[1] Unfortunately, the high rate of perinatal mortality and morbidity associated with twin pregnancy is mainly due to preterm birth. Many strategies have been suggested to remedy this circumstance, but, until now, have failed to prevent spontaneous preterm births (SPB), either in singletons or, more importantly, in multiples. Whereas the infant mortality rate has nearly halved over the past 15 years,[2] the reduction in morbidity related to premature birth has been decidedly less pronounced. Preterm births remain responsible for 70% of neonatal deaths and 50% of neonatal neurological disabilities, including cerebral palsy.[3]

This chapter reviews the issue of cervical assessment to improve early diagnosis of SPB at a stage when it might have an impact on the use of either preventive or therapeutic strategies.

HOW AND WHEN TO ASSESS THE CERVIX

Early diagnosis of twin pregnancy and the membrane status by ultrasound is mandatory and discussed in detail elsewhere in this book (see Chapter 5). This strategy is not only appropriate for planning of antenatal visits, but also to allow the healthcare provider(s) to give information to the parents about potential outcomes. It is important that they not only be told but clearly understand that twin pregnancies represent a risk group for preterm delivery *per se*. This risk is even higher in monochorionic (MC) compared with dichorionic (DC) gestations, and in symptomatic compared with asymptomatic twin pregnancies.

To date, no evidence-based guidelines have been published on how and when to assess the risk of SPB by means of cervical examination. That is not to say that data pertaining to this do not exist. In one study, digital examination was performed in 86 twin gestations at weekly intervals, and a score determined by subtracting the clinical cervical dilatation from the estimated cervical length. Intervals to delivery increased significantly with lower scores, e.g. a short and/or dilated cervix.[4] Regardless, clinical experience suggests that the process of cervical shortening and dilatation of the internal os can be better diagnosed by sonographic than digital cervical examination. Moreover, images from successive examinations and taken by the same or different examiners can be compared to document the progression of change. In addition, three-dimensional multiplanar sonography of the cervix has been proposed to improve the understanding of cervical morphology. The two-dimensional transvaginal approach with probes of 5–8.5 MHz is presently regarded as the most feasible imaging modality for routine detection or exclusion of patients at risk for SPB

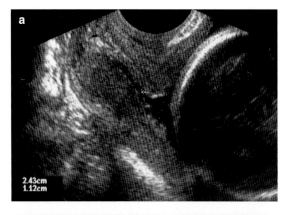

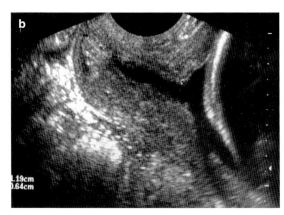

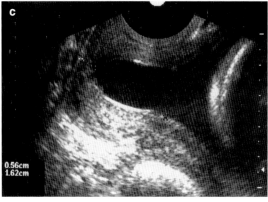

Figure 19.1 Transvaginal sonogram of a cervix of a twin gestation (25 weeks) (a) in the supine position and (b) after 1 min and (c) after 2 min in an upright position, demonstrating increasing opening of the internal os and shortening of the functional endocervical length

based on cervical change, because it provides better resolution than that obtained by the translabial or transabdominal route.

Technique of transvaginal sonography

The urinary bladder should be empty before cervical examination. Recognition of the lowermost edge of the bladder is useful to detect the upper limit of the uterine cervix. When the examiner introduces the vaginal probe into the anterior vaginal fornix, the sonographic image is checked in a sagittal view until the endocervical canal is visualized, after which the examiner retracts the probe to avoid compression of the cervix. The length of the closed portion of the endocervical canal should be visualized in a manner whereby the anterior and posterior cervix appears to be equally thick. The distance between the internal and the external os is not always a straight line, and

in approximately 50% of cases it is visualized as a curve. The ratio of curved/ straight cervix decreases with decreasing length, and therefore the disparity of a curved or a straight cervix does not have essential clinical implications. After serial measurements, the shortest result should be considered.

Cervical length (CL), width and form of the external or internal os, position of the cervix in relation to a horizontal line, and, to some extent, thickness of the endocervical mucus can all be determined from ultrasound images. In patients with dilation of the internal os, the shape (Y- or U-shaped), width, length, and even the area of the internal opening can be described (Figure 19.1). Most healthcare providers perform their examinations with the woman in a supine position, and maternal postural challenge has been advocated by only a few groups in singleton pregnancies. In a pilot study of twin pregnancies, however, the Zwolle

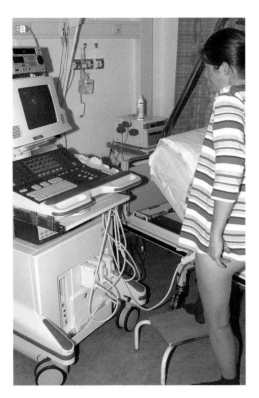 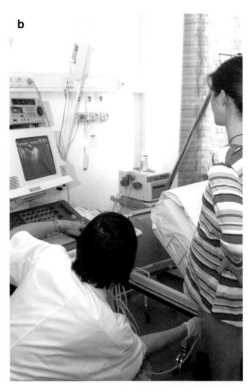

Figure 19.2 A mother pregnant with twins (a) introducing the transvaginal probe and (b) observing the result

(NL) group demonstrated that the closed endocervical length may shorten when the mother assumes the upright position, owing to increasing pressure on the internal os from the uterine contents which lie directly above it (Figure 19.1).[5] Subsequently, these researchers characterized the changes as a risk factor for the occurrence of SPB.[6] More recently, the effect of maternal position on CL measurement was evaluated by a second research group among uncomplicated twin pregnancies.[7] In agreement with the results presented by the Dutch group, these investigators found that the shorter the cervix in the recumbent position, the greater is the difference in CL between the recumbent and upright positions.

To detect early signs of functional cervical incompetence, the Zwolle group currently conducts nearly every examination in both the supine and the upright position, presuming, of course, that the membranes are intact.

At the appropriate time, the patient who previously had been recumbent and now is in the standing position places one foot on a footstool and guides the transvaginal transducer into the lower part of the vagina until it can be directed by the examiner (Figure 19.2). In patients with pre-existing cervical dilatation, not only may the width of the internal os increase in the upright position (Figure 19.1), but the membranes may be shown to progressively bulge or dissociate, indicating the potential for additional risks for membrane activation and preterm premature rupture of the membranes (PROM). These examinations clearly clarify the risk of postural stress for these patients, and may be particularly useful if maternal lifestyle changes are deemed appropriate. Conversely, insignificant changes may motivate the patient to lead a normal life or the physician to avoid unnecessary interventions.

Timing of cervical assessment

In early pregnancy, the space between the cervix and the uterine cavity (the so-called 'virtual internal os') can be identified by high-resolution sonography, visualizing the cervical glands as a hypoechogenic area. If this visualization is impaired, the location of the 'virtual' internal os can be determined using the urinary bladder as a reference point, as it is situated approximately 1.6 cm inwards from the vesico-cervical fold. The entire CL can be assessed as early as 12 weeks' gestation, but it is doubtful that cervical assessment in the first trimester has prognostic value to predict SPB. To date, no data have been collected in twin gestations. Between 12 and 15 weeks, the distance between the gestational sac and the internal os remains nearly unchanged in singleton pregnancies. In high-risk singleton pregnancies, on the other hand, the cervix can begin to shorten as early as 15 weeks of gestation, and the shortening is more rapid in pregnant women who deliver prematurely or who have a history of SPB. Most studies investigating the cervix in twin gestations have used the interval between 20 and 25 gestational weeks

or thereafter for the prediction of SPB, employing either the length of the cervical canal or the width of the internal os as reference (Table 19.1).

Normal values

Gradual cervical changes precede the onset of labor over several weeks. With regard to shortening of the CL and opening of the internal os, differences exist between singleton and twin pregnancies. Data on the CL, width of the internal os, and the anterior angle with a presumed horizontal line, reflecting the degree of curvature, for singleton, twin, and triplet pregnancies in both the supine and upright positions were collected from pregnancies not treated by any interventions to prevent SPB, and which delivered at > 36 weeks. These values were used to determine 'normal' standards for twin pregnancies.[6] It was found that the CL decreased significantly from 15 weeks to term in both (recumbent and upright) positions (Figure 19.3a), and that the values between the two positions were significantly different from 20 weeks onwards. In normal twin pregnancies, a width of the internal os of

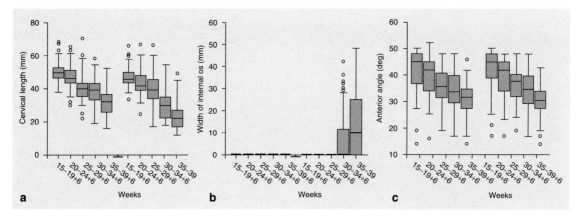

Figure 19.3 Box–whisker plots of (a) cervical length, (b) width of the internal os, and (c) presumed anterior angle with a horizontal line in normal twin pregnancies with delivery ≥ 36 weeks without any intervention to prevent preterm birth (*n* = 71): all boxes on the left side of each diagram signify values in a supine position, all boxes an the right signify values in an upright position. There are five intervals: 15–19 + 6 weeks, 20–24 + 6 weeks, 25–29 + 6 weeks, 30–34 + 6 weeks, and 35–39 + 6 weeks. The 'box' includes 50% of the values between the 25th and 75th centiles and the median; the 'whisker' marks the 1½ time fold of the 25th and 75th centiles

Table 19.1 Comparison of studies dealing with the prediction of spontaneous preterm birth (SPB) in twin pregnancies by detection of cervical length (CL) by transvaginal sonography. 'Variables' include additional investigated parameters

Source	Population (n)	Gestational age at examination (weeks)	Cut-off CL (mm)	Outcome parameter/ threshold of SPB (weeks at birth)	Variables	Study design
Shulman et al, 2002[22]	57	24/27	30	interval to delivery	—	AS–PROS
Vayssiere et al, 2002[10]	251/215	22/27	25	<32/35	FU, FU + TFP	AS–PROS
Soriano et al, 2002[23]	54	18–24	35	>34	WG, BMI, SM, WO	AS–PROS
Skentou et al, 2001[24]	464	18–24	20/25/40/60	<33	—	AS–PROS
Iams et al, 2001[25]	188	24–28	20	<32/35/37	REL	AS–PROS
Shapiro et al, 2000[26]	66	<30	20/25/30	<28/35	—	AS–RET
Venditelli et al, 2001[27]	26	18–36	30	<37	FU	SY–PROS
Persutte et al, 2000[28]	105	20–32	25	<37	—	SY–PROS
Guzman et al, 2000[18]	131	15–20/21–24/25–28	20	<28/30/32/34	FU, CI	AS–PROS
Yang et al, 2000[19]	65	22–24	25/30/35	<35	FU	AS–PROS
Weisz et al, 2000[29]	50	18–22	35	<34	—	AS–PROS
Althusius and Dekker, 1998[30]	101	16–32	30	<34	—	AS–RET
Granovski-Gisaru et al, 1998[31]	43	18–29	30	<34	—	AS–PROS
Souka et al, 1999[32]	215	22–24	15/25/35/45	≤28/30/32/34	—	AS–PROS
Imseis et al, 1997[33]	85	24–26	35	<34 (± intervention)	—	AS–PROS
Crane et al, 1997[34]	26	23–33	30	<34/<37	D, FU	SY–PROS
Wennerholm et al, 1997[35]	121	24–34 (at intervals)	33	<35/37	BV, E, FI	AS–PROS
Goldenberg et al, 1996[17]	147	24–28	25	<32/35/37	BV/FI	AS–PROS

Variables: BMI, body mass index; BV, bacterial vaginosis; CI, cervical index; D, digital examination; E, endotoxin; FI, fibronectin; FU, funneling; REL, relaxin; SM, smoking; TFP, transfundal pressure; WG, weight gain; WO, working during pregnancy
Study design: AS, asymptomatic twin pregnancies; PROS, prospective; RET, retrospective; SY, symptomatic twin pregnancies

more than 5 mm (funneling) was observed in an upright position at > 30 gestational weeks (Figure 19.3b), and differences in funneling between the positions were statistically significant from 25 weeks onwards. The anterior angle decreased in both positions (Figure 19.3c), but differences in the angle between both positions were not significant. Most centers use defined cut-off values to select patients with a risk for SPB. However, not all patients with threatening premature labor are identified at a specific gestational age. Some who have a CL of > 2.5 cm in the supine position still demonstrate a shorter cervix or even funneling in the upright position.

The reference values for different positions in uncomplicated twin pregnancies can be integrated into daily practice. Interventions such as a reduction of physical stress and workload in multiple gestation when values are outside the 50% 'box', e.g. below the 25th centile for CL, may then be recommended. However, the effect of any interventions based on these parameters to date has only been evaluated using historical controls.

Apart from the longitudinal results presented by the Zwolle investigators, others have also described dynamic cervical changes with advancing twin gestation. In the study of Bergelin and Valentin, values of CL decreased from 41 to 31 mm between 24 and 32 gestational weeks.[8] Fujita et al[9] found a correlation between CL measurement and gestational age and that the mean cervical length shortened by approximately 0.8 mm per week, from 47 mm at 13 weeks to 32 mm at 32 weeks, with corresponding lower limits for the 95% prediction intervals of 29 and 15 mm, respectively. A prospective multicenter French study[10] found that for spontaneous delivery before 32 and 35 weeks of gestation, the sensitivity of CL = 30 mm was 46% and 27%, respectively; the specificity was 89% and 90%, respectively. The sensitivity of funneling was 54% and 33%, and its specificity 89% and 91%, respectively. After multivariate analysis, only funneling remained significant for delivery before both 32 and 35 weeks of gestation. For

spontaneous delivery before 32 and 35 weeks of gestation, the sensitivity of CL = 25 mm was 100% and 54%, respectively, and the specificity was 84% and 87%, respectively. The sensitivity of funneling was 86% and 54%, and the specificity 78% and 82%, respectively. After multivariate analysis, both indicators remained significant for delivery before 35 weeks of gestation. These authors concluded that cervical length and funneling both predict the very preterm birth of twins. However, in another French study[11] the accuracies of ultrasound cervical assessment (cervical length and cervical index) and of digital examination (Bishop score and cervical score) in the prediction of spontaneous birth before 34 weeks in twin pregnancies were the same. Transvaginal sonography predicted spontaneous delivery before 34 weeks better than digital examination at the 27-week but not the 22-week examination.

A German study[12] assessed 87 women with twin pregnancies presenting with regular and painful uterine contractions at 24–36 weeks' gestation. Delivery within 7 days of presentation occurred in 22% of these women, and this was inversely related to CL, decreasing from 80% at 1–5 mm, to 46% at 6–10 mm, 29% at 11–15 mm, 21% at 16–20 mm, 7% at 1–25 mm, and 0% at > 25 mm. Logistic regression analysis demonstrated that a significant independent contribution in the prediction of delivery within 7 days was provided by CL.

In agreement with the results shown in Figure 19.3, two studies found that the cervix widened with advancing gestation.[8,13] In patients who had multifetal pregnancy reduction to twins, the CL was compared from 14 to 32 weeks with that in a control group without pregnancy reduction. Despite the likelihood of inflammatory responses and bleeding, the CL across gestation was not significantly affected by multifetal pregnancy reduction.[14] More recently, Fait et al[15] evaluated the application of transvaginal sonography assessment of CL before fetal reduction for predicting spontaneous preterm birth in triplet gestations reduced to twins in a cohort of 25 women. CL at reduction was 4.0 ±

0.85 cm (range: 1.2–5.5). The sensitivity, specificity, positive predictive value, and negative predictive value of CL < 3.5 cm to predict delivery prior to 33 gestational weeks were 67%, 94%, 67%, and 94%, respectively.

PREDICTION OF SPONTANEOUS PRETERM BIRTH BY CERVICAL ASSESSMENT

Most studies using transvaginal sonography to identify women at risk for SPB in singleton and multiple gestations have examined the possibility of using one or two cervical measurements. Wide variations exist among studies with respect to gestational age at testing, definition of abnormality thresholds, and the outcome reference in twin pregnancies (Table 19.1). A recent review identified published studies through different databases and manual searching of bibliographies, and these data were stratified according to singleton or twin pregnancy, gestational age at testing, CL and funneling width thresholds, or reference standards, and pooled to produce summary estimates of likelihood ratios.[16] The given thresholds to predict the likelihood of SPB varied, even if symptomatic and asymptomatic patients were analyzed separately (Table 19.2). Both CL measurement and funneling, whether alone or in combination, appeared to be useful in predicting SPB in twin pregnancies. Another study also demonstrated that CL and funneling both predicted very preterm birth of twins, whereas CL appeared to be the predictor of choice at 27 weeks of gestation; at 22 weeks the diagnostic values of both parameters were comparable.[10]

Table 19.2 Likelihood ratios (LRs, individual and pooled) for predicting spontaneous preterm birth for a range of thresholds for cervical length measurements among asymptomatic and symptomatic twin pregnancies. Adapted from reference 16

Subgroups testing gestational age 'thresholds'	Spontaneous preterm birth before 34–35 weeks	
	+LR (95% CI)	–LR (95% CI)
Asymptomatic		
<20 weeks		
20 mm	59.89 (3.46–103.48)	0.71 (0.52–0.96)
20–24 weeks		
15 mm	7.60 (2.09–27.67)	0.89 (0.81–0.97)
20 mm	4.54 (1.46–14.14)	0.75 (0.64–0.90)
25 mm	5.02 (3.31–7.61)	0.75 (0.54–1.06)
30 mm	2.31 (1.08–4.93)	0.69 (0.91–1.17)
35 mm	1.47 (1.09–1.97)	0.88 (0.69–1.12)
45 mm	1.12 (1.00–1.26)	0.45 (0.15–1.40)
>24 weeks		
20 mm	3.44 (2.05–5.78)	0.41 (0.21–0.80)
25 mm	1.82 (1.26–2.63)	0.83 (0.72–0.95)
30 mm	2.11 (1.43–3.12)	0.61 (0.42–0.87)
35 mm	1.84 (1.48–2.29)	0.29 (0.08–1.09)
Symptomatic		
30 mm	2.33 (1.42–3.82)	0.15 (0.01–2.14)

+LR, positive likelihood ratio; –LR, negative likelihood ratio; CI, confidence interval

Table 19.3 Comparison of the diagnostic values of fibronectin, cervical length, Bishop score, and premature contractions in twin pregnancies at risk for spontaneous preterm birth ($n = 180$ with delivery ≥ 36 weeks, $n = 70$ with delivery < 36 weeks), all parameters detected between 24 and 26 gestational weeks[6]

Parameter	Sensitivity (%)	Specificity (%)	PPV (%)	NPV (%)	+LR	95% CI
Fibronectin	48.5	90.2	64.3	90.2	3.2	2.1–4.2
Cervical length	64.9	81.5	52.1	81.5	2.6	1.5–3.8
Bishop score	65.2	80.0	54.8	80.0	2.5	1.8–3.2
Premature contractions	59.7	83.1	50.0	83.1	2.9	1.7–4.2

PPV, positive predictive value; NPV, negative predictive value; +LR, positive likelihood ratio; CI, confidence interval

Previous studies have shown that once dilatation of the internal os has occurred, the interval to delivery is comparable in patients who subsequently go into either spontaneous term or preterm labor. According to the Zwolle data shown in Figure 19.3, a CL < 25 mm and funneling width ≥ 10 mm between 20 and 28 weeks in both positions predicted a risk for SPB. In addition, disparities of CL and width of the internal os due to the maternal position increased with advanced gestational age and were more pronounced in twin pregnancies at risk for SPB compared with normal controls.[6]

In practice, clinicians should be able to make informed and explicit decisions based on probabilities generated by cervical assessment and other tools with regard to the risk of SPB.

As reported in the first National Institute of Child Health and Human Development Maternal–Fetal Medicine Network preterm prediction study dealing with twin pregnancies, the most widely known risk factors for SPB were not significantly associated with SPB of twins. At 24 weeks, a CL ≤ 25 mm was the best predictor of SPB. Of all other risk factors evaluated at 28 weeks, fetal fibronectin was the only statistically significant predictor of SPB.[17] Others found that a combination of cervical assessment of either CL or funneling in both supine and upright positions and fibronectin were significant predictors of SPB in twin pregnancies between 20 and 28 weeks.[6]

In a more recent study of asymptomatic twin pregnancies, a CL of ≤ 2.0 cm measured between 15 and 28 weeks' gestation appeared to be a reasonable parameter for predicting SPB in twin gestations.[18] The high specificities indicate that CL is better at predicting the absence than the presence of threatening SPB.[18] Both a CL ≤ 30 mm and cervical funneling in twin pregnancies under 26 weeks' gestation were independently and strongly associated with a risk for SPB.[18] Because a long cervix, > 35 mm, is associated with very low risk (4%) for preterm birth, pregnant women with these results can be reassured.[19] After 30 weeks, CL was shown to be not predictive of SPB.

Gibson et al[20] prospectively evaluated CL measurements and fetal fibronectin detection as predictors of spontaneous preterm delivery in an unselected population of twin pregnancies. The spontaneous preterm delivery rate was 16.5% in 91 studied twin pregnancies. A CL = 25 mm at 18 weeks and = 22 mm at 24 weeks were the best predictors of preterm delivery. A shortening of CL = 2.5 mm per week between 18 and 28 weeks' gestation also predicted preterm delivery. There was no relationship between the detection of fetal fibronectin and preterm delivery. Although this study confirms the value of transvaginal ultrasound assessment of CL as a predictor of preterm delivery in twin pregnancies, the poor sensitivity of this test makes it unsuitable as a single predictor of preterm delivery. Moreover, fetal fibronectin testing does not identify twin pregnancies destined to deliver prematurely.

Some authorities use historical and demographic characteristics to predict SPB. Recently, the value of combining maternal characteristics and measurement of CL at 22–24 weeks in the prediction of spontaneous early preterm delivery was examined in 1163 twin pregnancies attending for routine antenatal care.[21] The rate of spontaneous delivery < 32 weeks was 6.5% and the rate of early delivery was inversely related to cervical length. For a false-positive rate of 10%, the detection rate of early delivery was 65.3% compared to the respective 26.4% detection rate for maternal characteristics and obstetric history. Logistic regression analysis demonstrated that the only significant independent predictor of spontaneous early delivery was CL.

In summary, transvaginal sonography can identify impending SPB before advanced cervical dilatation, and may therefore help to indicate maternal (*in utero*) transfer to a level III hospital, tocolytic treatment, or the application of antenatal steroids. It seems that uterine contraction monitoring has a lower sensitivity for detecting women at risk of SPB compared with cervical assessment and fetal fibronectin in the vaginal fluid in twin pregnancies (Table 19.3).[6] The high specificities underline that current use of CL and fetal fibronectin are of importance in situations where negative results can avoid unnecessary interventions. However, obstetricians should be aware that there will always be a group of mothers of twins who deliver preterm unexpectedly. In the future, cervical assessment should be incorporated into the routine care of twin pregnancies by educating patients to recognize first symptoms of spontaneous preterm birth or to reduce physical stress, and by educating physicians to perform transvaginal sonography at regular intervals or even initiate interventions based on sonography results. Specially trained staff and twin clinics are desirable. Cervical assessment allows researchers to target randomization in at-risk patients when evaluating the effectiveness of interventions to prevent spontaneous preterm birth. Collaborative studies are needed with a definition of dynamic thresholds of cervical assessment and defined outcome parameters such as gestational age at delivery, morbidity, mortality, and long-term follow-up separate for mono- and dichorionic twins.

REFERENCES

1. Lambalk CB, van Hooff M. Natural versus induced twinning and pregnancy outcome: a Dutch nationwide survey of primiparous dizygotic twin deliveries. Fertil Steril 2001; 75: 731–6.

2. Guyer B, MacDorman MF, Martin JA et al. Annual summary of vital statistics 1997. Pediatrics 1998; 102: 1333–49.

3. Hack M, Horbar JD, Malloy MH et al. Very low birth weight outcomes of the National Institute of Child Health and Human Development Neonatal Network. Pediatrics 1991; 87: 587–97.

4. Newman RB, Godsey RK, Ellings JM et al. Quantification of cervical change: relationship to preterm delivery in the multifetal gestation. Am J Obstet Gynecol 1991; 165: 264–71.

5. Arabin B, Aardenburg R, van Eyck J. Maternal position and ultrasonic cervical assessment in multiple pregnancy. Preliminary observations. J Reprod Med 1997; 42: 719–24.

6. Arabin B, Hübener M, Halbesma J, van Eyck J. Sonographic diagnosis of cervical incompetence in twin pregnancies. Ultrasound Rev 2001; 1: 340.

7. Bernath T, Brizot ML, Liao AW et al. Effect of maternal position on cervical length measurement in twin pregnancies. Ultrasound Obstet Gynecol 2002; 20: 263–6.

8. Bergelin I, Valentin L. Cervical changes in twin pregnancies observed by transvaginal ultrasound during the latter half of pregnancy: a longitudinal, observational study. Ultrasound Obstet Gynecol 2003; 21: 556–63.

9. Fujita MM, Brizot Mde L, Liao AW et al. Reference range for cervical length in twin pregnancies. Acta Obstet Gynecol Scand 2002; 81: 856–9.

10. Vayssiere C, Favre R, Audibert F et al. Cervical length and funneling at 22 and 27 weeks to predict

spontaneous birth before 32 weeks in twin pregnancies: a French prospective multicenter study. Am J Obstet Gynecol 2002; 187: 1596–604.

11. Vayssiere C, Favre R, Audibert F et al. Research Group in Obstetrics and Gynecology (GROG). Cervical assessment at 22 and 27 weeks for the prediction of spontaneous birth before 34 weeks in twin pregnancies: is transvaginal sonography more accurate than digital examination? Ultrasound Obstet Gynecol 2005; 26: 707–12.

12. Fuchs I, Tsoi E, Henrich W, Dudenhausen JW, Nicolaides KH. Sonographic measurement of cervical length in twin pregnancies in threatened preterm labor. Ultrasound Obstet Gynecol. 2004; 23: 42–5.

13. Eppel W, Schurz B, Frigo P et al. Vaginosonography of the cervix in twin pregnancies. Geburtshilfe Frauenheilkd 1994; 54: 20–6.

14. Rebarber A, Carreno CA, Fipkind H et al. Cervical length after multifetal pregnancy reduction in remaining twin gestations. Am J Obstet Gynecol 2001; 185: 1113–17.

15. Fait G, Har-Toov J, Gull I, Lessing JB, Jaffa A, Wolman I. Cervical length, multifetal pregnancy reduction, and prediction of preterm birth. J Clin Ultrasound 2005; 33: 329–32.

16. Honest H, Bachmann LM, Coomarasamy A et al. Accuracy of cervical transvaginal sonography in predicting preterm birth: a systematic review. Ultrasound Obstet Gynecol 2003; 22: 305–22.

17. Goldenberg RL, Iams JD, Miodovnik M et al. The preterm prediction study: risk factors in twin gestations. National Institute of Child Health and Human Development Maternal–Fetal Medicine Units Network. Am J Obstet Gynecol 1996; 175: 1047–53.

18. Guzman ER, Walters C, O'Reilly-Green C et al. Use of cervical ultrasonography in prediction of spontaneous preterm birth in twin gestations. Am J Obstet Gynecol 2000; 183: 1103–7.

19. Yang JH, Kuhlman K, Daly S, Berghella V. Prediction of preterm birth by second trimester cervical sonography in twin pregnancies. Ultrasound Obstet Gynecol 2000; 15: 288–91.

20. Gibson JL, Macara LM, Owen P, Young D, Macauley J, Mackenzie F. Prediction of preterm delivery in twin pregnancy: a prospective, observational study of cervical length and fetal fibronectin testing. Ultrasound Obstet Gynecol 2004; 23: 561–6.

21. To MS, Fonseca EB, Molina FS, Cacho AM, Nicolaides KH. Maternal characteristics and cervical length in the prediction of spontaneous early preterm delivery in twins. Am J Obstet Gynecol 2006; 194: 1360–5.

22. Shulman A, Jauniaux E, Holmes A et al. Vaginal sonography of the cervix for the prediction of 'time to delivery' in ART twin gestations. Twin Res 2002; 5: 255–9.

23. Soriano D, Weisz B, Seidman DS et al. The role of sonographic assessment of cervical length in the prediction of preterm birth in primigravidae with twin gestation conceived after infertility treatment. Acta Obstet Gynecol Scand 2002; 81: 39–43.

24. Skentou C, Soulea AP, To MS et al. Prediction of preterm delivery in twins by cervical assessment at 23 weeks. Ultrasound Obstet Gynecol 2001; 17: 7–10.

25. Iams JD, Goldenberg RL, Mercer BM et al. The preterm prediction study: can low-risk women destined for spotaneous preterm birth be identified? Am J Obstet Gynecol 2001; 184: 652–5.

26. Shapiro JL, Kung R, Barrett JF. Cervical length as a predictor of pre-term birth in twin gestations. Twin Res 2000; 3: 213–16.

27. Vendittelli F, Mamelle N, Munoz F, Janky E. Transvaginal ultrasonography of the uterine cervix in hospitalized women with preterm labor. Int J Gynecol Obstet 2001; 72: 117–25.

28. Persutte W et al. Cervical length in twins. Am J Obstet Gynecol 2000; 182: 118.

29. Weisz B et al. Risk factors for premature birth in primigravidae with twin gestation and the role of transvaginal ultrasonographic assessment of the cervix. Am J Obstet Gynecol 2000; 182: 115.

30. Althusius S, Dekker G. Short cervical length predicts preterm delivery in twin gestations. Am J Obstet Gynecol 1998; 178: 194.

31. Granovski-Gisaru S et al. Is a single ultrasound measurement of cervical length a predictor of the risk of preterm delivery in multifetal pregnancy? Am J Obstet Gynecol 1998; 178: 191.

32. Souka AP, Heath V, Flint S et al. Cervical length at 23 weeks in twins in predicting spontaneous preterm delivery. Obstet Gynecol 1999; 94: 450–4.

33. Imseis HM, Albert TA, Iams JD. Identifying twin gestations at low risk for preterm birth with a transvaginal ultrasonographic cervical measurement at 24 to 26 weeks' gestation. Am J Obstet Gynecol 1997; 177: 1149–55.

34. Crane JM, Van den Hof M, Armson BA, Liston R. Transvaginal ultrasound in the prediction of preterm delivery: singleton and twin gestations. Obstet Gynecol 1997; 90: 357–63.

35. Wennerholm UB, Holm B, Mattsby-Baltzer I et al. Fetal fibronectin, endotoxin, bacterial vaginosis and cervical length as predictors of preterm birth and neonatal morbidity in twin pregnancies. Br J Obstet Gynaecol 1997; 104: 1398–404.

Biophysical assessment

20

INTRODUCTION

Many biophysical techniques are used to assess fetal well-being in multiple pregnancy, including ultrasonography, Doppler velocimetry, and cardiotocography. Considering the specific characteristics of multiple pregnancies in terms of higher rate of preterm delivery, higher incidence of fetal growth restriction, and higher rates of obstetric complications as compared with singleton gestation, as well as specific problems related to chorionicity and to the number of fetuses, it is difficult to generally summarize the usefulness and role of each specific technique, or to provide a general standard of management. Rather, it is advisable to assess and manage each case individually on the basis of the presence of recognized risk factors, making use of each technique or of a combination of different techniques according to the specific information desired. These complexities also demand that the information obtained should be interpreted on the basis of a thorough understanding of the pathophysiology involved. In twin pregnancy, the development of chronic and acute hypoxemia is a major contributor to morbidity and mortality. The criteria for diagnosis and management of specific conditions of twin pregnancy linked to alterations in fetal oxygen supply, such as discordant fetal growth, twin-to-twin transfusion syndrome, and alterations in placentation, are addressed in other chapters of this book.

The aim of this chapter is to summarize the current evidence related to the role of the fetal biophysical profile and cardiotocographic evaluation in the diagnosis of fetal oxygen deficiency.

THE BIOPHYSICAL PROFILE IN MULTIPLE PREGNANCY

Reports on the usefulness of the fetal biophysical profile in multiple pregnancy are few. One of the first regarding twin gestation was published in 1986 by Lodeiro and associates.[1] These authors used the Vintzileos scoring system in 49 twin gestations as a means of follow-up of a non-reactive non-stress test (NST). Sixty-four fetuses had a reactive NST, and in all of them the biophysical profile score was 8. Of these, only two died of prematurity. Of the 34 fetuses with a non-reactive NST, about 82% had a biophysical profile score of 8 and all had a favorable outcome. In contrast, 18% had a biophysical profile score of < 8, and all were compromised at birth. In a prospective study of the biophysical profile in twins, Medina and associates[2] demonstrated that the use of Manning's sonographic criteria to predict stillbirth had a sensitivity of 66.7%, a specificity of 98.8%, a positive predictive value of 50%, and a negative predictive value of 99.4%. The biophysical profile has been recommended in high-order multiple gestations when cardiotocography is technically difficult to perform. However, the biophysical profile can be difficult too, because of problems arising in the assessment of the amniotic fluid volume.

The presence of synchronous patterns of fetal activity might also interfere in interpretation because, independent of chorionicity, gross body movements, breathing movements, and accelerations of the fetal heart rate, may be synchronous in 25, 50, and 50–60%, respectively.[3] Elliot and Finberg[4] reported on the use of the biophysical profile in 18 sets of triplets and 6 sets of quadruplets. The biophysical profile was used as the primary method of fetal surveillance and was performed twice weekly starting from 28 weeks' gestation. Scoring was based on Manning's recommendations. Six pregnancies (25%, 9 fetuses of five triplet sets and 2 fetuses of one quadruplet set) with 2/8 scores were delivered because of the low biophysical scores and clinical situation, with good outcome. There was no morbidity or mortality in the 19 babies delivered because of an abnormal biophysical profile. Four pregnancies had poor outcome despite a normal (8/8) biophysical score. Despite these conflicting findings, these authors concluded that the biophysical profile appeared to be a reliable antepartum test of fetal well-being in triplets and quadruplets.

One of the more difficult variables to assess in multiple pregnancies is the amniotic fluid volume, because abnormalities occur more frequently than in singletons secondary to placental insufficiency, placental vascular anastomoses, and maternal hemodynamic alterations. No agreement exists on the optimal sonographic method of evaluating amniotic fluid volume in multiple pregnancies, and no method has been validated for predicting perinatal outcome in multiple gestation. Chau and colleagues found that the amniotic fluid index (AFI), the vertical depths, and the two diameter pockets measured at 2-week intervals were not significantly different between dichorionic and monochorionic pregnancies.[5]

Gerson et al[6] described a methodology for a two-pocket AFI for each fetus of a twin gestation. Data included 216 pairs of measurements that were analyzed to yield regressions (curves) for all observations, as well as for the larger and smaller AFI of each observation on a particular set of twins. The twin AFI increased non-linearly until week 27. From week 27 to week 36, however, decreasing linear trends were found. Intra-observer variation in evaluating the amniotic fluid volume in diamniotic twin pregnancy was about 2–3%, approximately the figure cited for singleton pregnancies.

In a study to determine the accuracy of amniotic fluid volume estimation, Magann and co-workers[7] compared the estimates of the volume of each sac in 23 sets of diamniotic twin pregnancies made by a second-year obstetric resident, nurse sonographer, maternal–fetal medicine fellow, and maternal–fetal medicine staff members, respectively. The actual volume was confirmed by amniocentesis and a dye-dilution technique. The authors found no difference in the total number of correct estimates of volume by level of operator experience, ultrasonography technique, or combined subjective versus objective correct estimates. Identification of low volume was not different among the four evaluators, but the percentage of correct estimates was generally poor and ranged from 7 to 29%.

The accuracy of the 2×2 cm pocket as a cut-off value for low amniotic fluid volume in twin pregnancies was also studied by Magann and associates.[8] Among amniotic sacs of the 60 twin pairs, oligohydramnios was found in 33 amniotic sacs, normal volume in 80 sacs, and high volume in 7. An amniotic fluid pocket smaller than 2×2 cm was identified in only 2 of the 120 twin amniotic sacs. These results led to the conclusion that judging amniotic fluid volume on the basis of a 2×2 cm pocket misses more than 90% of cases of oligohydramnios in twins.

INTRAPARTUM FETAL SURVEILLANCE

It is outside the aim of this chapter to discuss in detail the interpretation of cardiotocographic patterns. Nonetheless, it is important to underline some of the problems linked with the clinical use of this technique. Most of these are common for both singleton and multiple pregnancy, whereas some are more specifically related to the latter.

Continuous fetal heart rate and uterine contraction recording (cardiotocography or CTG) is widely used to assess fetal well-being during labor. This method has, however, certain limitations. A normal CTG trace reflects optimal fetal oxygenation and is of reassurance regarding fetal condition. In contrast, the significance of fetal heart rate changes is often unclear and therefore difficult to interpret. In the clinical setting, this can potentially result in unnecessary interventions for suspected fetal hypoxia or in inappropriate delays in action, with potentially disastrous consequences for the fetus. Some of these difficulties can be overcome by better training of the medical and nursing staff. Evidence also suggests that the use of expert systems for decision-making would provide a valuable contribution toward improving the detection and clinical management of cases with abnormal CTG patterns. However, it is also evident that there are situations in which the CTG changes are not specific enough for the presence of fetal hypoxia, and additional information is necessary for appropriate decision-making. Thus, the limitations of cardiotocography in the term fetus are mainly linked to the difficulty of interpretation of abnormal fetal heart rate (FHR) patterns and to the poor specificity of the technique in identifying threatening hypoxia.

Significant interobserver differences in interpretation of FHR of twins may not be a real problem for dedicated personnel. For example, a Portuguese study of interobserver agreement in antepartum estimation of FHR baselines in twins evaluated the assessments of two residents and one specialist in obstetrics and gynecology. All participants had special interest in FHR monitoring and independently estimated baselines in 162 consecutive antepartum FHR tracings recorded in 24 twins.[9] Tracings were obtained with a dual-channel fetal monitor for the simultaneous recording of both twins' heart rates. Baselines were estimated, as single values corresponding to the mean of the lowest stable FHR segment, in the absence of fetal movements and uterine contractions, within physiologic limits (110–150 beats per minute). Interobserver agreement in antepartum estimation of fetal heart rate

baselines in twins was excellent with the baseline concept used in this study.[9]

Twin pregnancy is often complicated by the threat of preterm delivery. Assessment of fetal well-being in the preterm fetus by analysis of the fetal heart rate presents, in addition to the limitations described, further and specific difficulties. The antepartum non-stress test, of recognized value in term fetuses, has less clinical value in the preterm fetus, owing to greater uncertainty in the relationship between baseline heart rate, reactivity, and fetal conditions. During preterm labor, the incidence of abnormal findings from intrapartum monitoring is higher, compared with term labor, when the same set of criteria for interpretation is used for both groups. The fetal heart rate is regulated through changes in the autonomic nervous system. Due to the immaturity of the fetal autonomic nervous system, the usual diagnostic and interpretative criteria for fetal heart rate analysis used for term fetuses are not entirely appropriate. In particular, in the preterm fetus, the maturational process in the patterns of fetal heart rate results in a progressive decrease in baseline fetal heart rate, in a progressive increase in the amplitude of fetal heart rate accelerations, and in a progressive increase in long-term fetal heart rate variability with advancing gestation.

The interpretation of fetal heart rate patterns in the preterm fetus is also complicated by the impact of specific drugs more frequently used in women with threatened or actual preterm labor. It is well known, for example, that the administration of steroids or magnesium sulfate exerts a negative effect on fetal heart rate variability, and that administration of β-receptor agonists affects both fetal heart rate variability and baseline heart rate. A Dutch group recently performed a prospective study to determine whether betamethasone had similar effects on FHR and behavior in preterm twin pregnancy as in singletons and whether the effects occur similarly in both twin members.[10] Eighteen women who were carrying twins received optimal corticosteroid treatment. Simultaneous recordings were made on twins

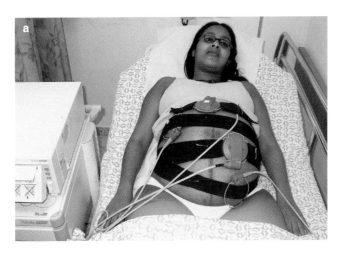
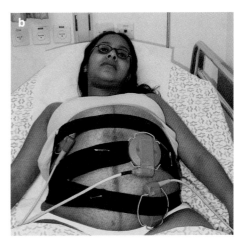

Figure 20.1 (a) Dual cardiotocography (CTG) in a twin pregnancy using two monitors. Note the two transducers for fetal heart rate and two transducers to record contractions. The output comprises two different strips, one for each fetus. (b) Dual CTG in a twin pregnancy using one monitor. Modern CTG monitors have the ability to differentiate between signals of twins. Note the two transducers for fetal heart rate and one transducer to record contractions. The output comprises one strip, with both fetal heart tracings. Images courtesy of I. Blickstein

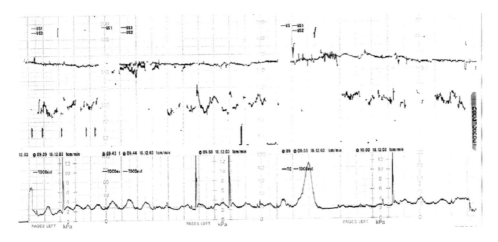

Figure 20.2 Difficult antepartum tracing may be encountered in some cases. In this tracing, one twin was surrounded by polyhydramnios and was constantly moving, and hence its fetal heart rate tracing (lower part) is not interpretable. The other twin shows a 'silent' pattern, with reduced long-term variability. Image courtesy of I. Blickstein

before (day 0), during (days 1–2), and after (days 3–4) corticosteroid therapy using separate cardiotocography and ultrasound machines. Betamethasone administration was associated with significant transient decreases in basal FHR (day 1), FHR variability (days 2 and 3), and body and breathing movements (day 2).

The overall changes in twins were similar to those previously found in singleton pregnancies. There was a high degree of association of response to betamethasone among individual members of twin pairs. The betamethasone-induced effects were unrelated to fetal sex, positioning, chorionicity, and discordance in

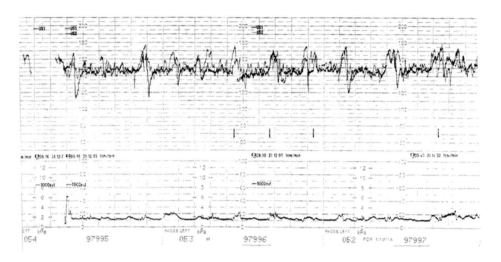

Figure 20.3   Reassuring antepartum tracing of both twins. Image courtesy of I. Blickstein

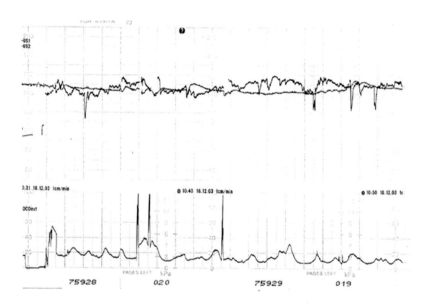

Figure 20.4   Non-reassuring antepartum tracing in monoamniotic twins. There is loss of variability in one twin, whereas the other twin shows short variable decelerations. This case was complicated by cord entanglement. Image courtesy of I. Blickstein

size, but there was an effect of gestation on FHR. It is reasonable to conclude that the current regimen of antenatal corticosteroids used in preterm twin pregnancies results in observable physiologic and behavioral changes in twin pairs irrespective of their composition. It also follows that the assessment of fetal well-being in the preterm fetus by electronic fetal monitoring requires further study to develop interpretative criteria considering the specific physiologic aspects of the maturing fetus.

Maeda and co-workers studied the synchronization of phases of diurnal rhythms in FHR baseline between twin fetuses and the

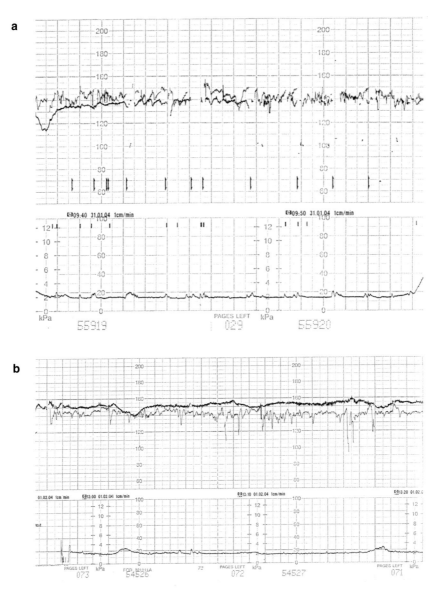

Figure 20.5 (a) Dual antepartum tracing at 28 weeks in a case of twin–twin transfusion. The tracings are reassuring. (b) Dual antepartum tracing at 30 weeks of the same twins as in (a). Cardiotocography of one twin shows almost absent variability. Images courtesy of I. Blickstein

occurrence of sustained fetal tachycardia.[11] The FHR was simultaneously recorded in twins for 24 h in 7 monochorionic–diamniotic and 8 dichorionic–diamniotic twin pregnancies at 35 to 38 weeks' gestation. The results of this study revealed that the diurnal rhythms in the FHR baseline correlated well between twins, and that the occurrences of sustained fetal tachycardia were completely independent.

Another problem related to cardiotocographic fetal monitoring in twin pregnancy is

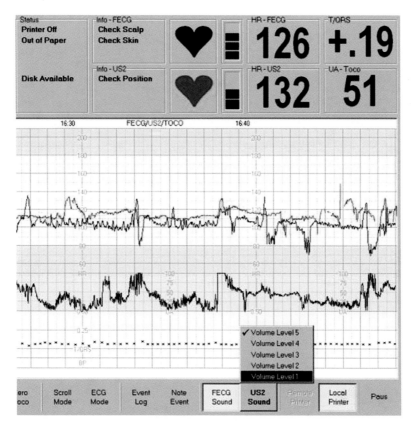

Figure 20.6 Example of intrapartum cardiotocography (CTG) tracing in a twin pregnancy in labor. Twin 1 CTG fetal heart rate is recorded by a scalp clip (black trace) while the fetal heart rate of twin 2 is recorded externally (pink trace)

that associated with the difficulty of obtaining a reliable dual tracing (Figure 20.1a and b). This difficulty can give rise to errors linked to double recording of the same heart rate, or inadvertent recording of the maternal heart rate that can be erroneously interpreted as fetal. Some examples of normal and abnormal antepartum tracings are shown in Figures 20.3–20.5.

During labor and after membrane rupture, it is advisable to record the heart rate of the first twin by means of a scalp clip (Figure 20.6). Intrapartum FHR recordings in twins were compared for fetal signal loss during stages of labor to assess the quality of these recordings

by the method that had been used: external ultrasound or directly via a scalp electrode.[12] Recordings obtained via ultrasound demonstrated significantly more fetal signal loss than those obtained via the direct mode, particularly in the second stage. Approximately 26–33% of first-stage and 41–63% of second-stage ultrasound intrapartum FHR recordings in twins exceeded the International Federation of Gynecology and Obstetrics (FIGO) criteria for fetal signal loss. These authors concluded that intrapartum FHR monitoring via ultrasound provides far poorer quality FHR signals than the direct mode (via scalp electrode).

REFERENCES

1. Lodeiro JG, Vintzileos AM, Feinstein SJ et al. Fetal biophysical profile in twin gestations. Obstet Gynecol 1986; 67: 824–7.

2. Medina D, Vargas N, Bustos JC et al. Biophysical profile in twin pregnancy: prospective study. Rev Chil Obstet Ginecol 1994; 59: 343–8.

3. Zimmer EZ, Goldstein I, Alglay S. Simultaneous recording of fetal breathing movements and body movements in twin pregnancy. J Perinat Med 1988; 16: 109–12.

4. Elliot JP, Finberg HJ. Biophysical profile testing as an indicator of fetal well-being in high-order multiple gestations. Am J Obstet Gynecol 1995; 172: 508–12.

5. Chau AC, Kjos SL, Kovacs BW. Ultrasonographic measurement of amniotic fluid volume in normal diamniotic twin pregnancies. Am J Obstet Gynecol 1996; 174: 1003–7.

6. Gerson A, Free SM Jr, Russino J et al. Amniotic fluid index in twin gestation. Ultrasound Obstet Gynecol. 1997; 10: 98–102.

7. Magann EF, Chauhan SP, Whitworth NS, Anfanger P, Rinehart BK, Morrison JC. Determination of amniotic fluid volume in twin pregnancies: ultrasonographic evaluation versus operator estimation. Am J Obstet Gynecol 2000; 182: 1606–9.

8. Magann EF, Nevils BG, Chauhan SP et al. Low amniotic fluid volume is poorly identified in singleton and twin pregnancies using the 2×2 cm pocket technique of the biophysical profile. South Med J 1999; 92: 802–5.

9. Bernardes J, Costa-Pereira A, Calejo L et al. Fetal heart rate baselines in twins. Interobserver agreement in antepartum estimation. J Reprod Med 2000; 45: 105–8.

10. Mulder EJ, Derks JB, Visser GH. Effects of antenatal betamethasone administration on fetal heart rate and behavior in twin pregnancy. Pediatr Res 2004; 56: 35–9.

11. Maeda Y, Muro M, Shono M, Shono H, Iwasaka T. Diurnal rhythms in fetal heart rate baseline and sustained fetal tachycardia in twin pregnancy. Early Hum Dev 2006; 82: 637–44.

12. Bakker PC, Colenbrander GJ, Verstraeten AA, Van Geijn HP. Quality of intrapartum cardiotocography in twin deliveries. Am J Obstet Gynecol 2004; 191: 2114–19.

21

Zygosity testing

INTRODUCTION

Twins are currently classified into two main types, monozygotic (MZ) and dizygotic (DZ). A more complex classification was proposed some years ago by Keith and Oleszczuk to recognize some of the problems that may attach to the simplistic MZ–DZ paradigm (see below for details). DZ twins occur when two oocytes are fertilized by two spermatozoa. MZ twins occur when one oocyte is fertilized by one spermatozoon and at some later time divides to form two embryos. The causes of this split are uncertain. Familial MZ twinning is rare, but does occur. Similarly, many families appear to be 'twin' prone, but controversy exists on the exact cause of this phenomenon. MZ twins occur at approximately two to three times the normal rate in pregnancies resulting from assisted reproductive technologies (ART),[1,2] be they *in vitro* fertilization (IVF) or ovulation induction.

WHY ZYGOSITY TESTING?

In the antenatal period, the issue of zygosity is usually not considered and is less important than chorionicity (although chorionicity may provide some clues to zygosity) (see Chapter 5). This is because chorionicity and external genital sex are the only means by which zygosity can be assessed at this early stage of pregnancy. Unfortunately both methods (chorionicity and confirmation of external genital sex) are imperfect means of assessing zygosity.

When unlike-sex twins are born, no question exists regarding their zygosity. They are,

by definition, DZ. On the other hand, when like-sexed twins are born, the issue of zygosity becomes paramount. Unless chorionicity has been demonstrated accurately and correctly interpreted in the delivery room (and/or by the pathology department) (see Chapter 5), parents are at risk for the most common mistake in zygosity assignment based on placentation and membranes – that is, the assumption that their (like-sexed) twins are DZ because they are determined to be dichorionic (DC) at birth. The genesis of this error is the widespread lack of recognition that like-sexed DC twins (with fused or separate placental disks) may be DZ or MZ (approximately 25% are MZ). The perpetuation of this error is assured when parents report this misinformation to their children. Indeed, twins often proceed through life wondering why, having been told that they are DZ, they look so much alike but are not perfectly 'identical'.

The term 'identical' is commonly used as a short-cut for MZ, but as shown below, in this chapter and Chapter 3 of this monograph this too is a serious misnomer. Rarely if ever are MZ twins 'identical' in their phenotypic appearance, even if they carry the same genetic patrimony at the time of the original zygotic split. Having provided this disclaimer, important medical and social reasons underlie the need for twins to know their zygosity. From a medical point of view, the allegedly identical genes of an MZ twin pair will usually (but not always) exhibit concordance in many major and chronic disorders, such as diabetes, asthma, Alzheimer's disease, depression, cancer, etc. Similarly, matched genetic complement is of paramount importance when one member of a twin pair requires organ transplantation. In suitable circumstances, the co-twin is an ideal donor, with no need for anti-rejection therapy.[3] Moreover, should one MZ twin develop cancer, the other could be considered at similar risk, and careful assessment on an ongoing, preventive basis is necessary. Finally, from a social point of view, one could argue that the twins themselves have a unique right to this information and that to withhold it is to deny their birthright. Just as it is unethical forcibly to separate twins (or other multiples) for adoption, it is unethical to deny twins knowledge of a fundamental biologic fact because of its supposed frivolity or presumed cost.

WHEN TO TEST?

The optimal time to determine zygosity is at delivery. This assessment is most easily and efficiently achieved by the obstetrician, alone or in consultation with the pathologist (see Chapter 3). The benefits of such assessments include: first, the ability to state to the parents with certainty, and in writing, that their monochorionic (MC) twins are MZ, and second, institution of formal zygosity testing, using placental tissue, in all like-sexed DC twins, recognizing that about 25% of these twins are MZ and the remainder, DZ. If these opportunities are lost, twins' families may draw false conclusions and/or will of necessity be forced to resort to other methods of zygosity testing later in life.

AVAILABLE METHODS

Historical background (Weinberg methodology)

In 1874, the French mathematician Bertillon assumed that the sex of each zygote of a pair of DZ twins would be determined independently. He then postulated that the number of DZ pairs was equal to twice the number of unlike-sexed pairs, with the remainder of the like-sexed pairs presumably MZ. This concept was restated in 1902 by Weinberg, and subsequently became entrenched in the literature as 'Weinberg's rule'. It was criticized, however, almost from its inception, and is still subject to intense negative interpretation. Its usefulness is purely confined to statistical samples, and it cannot be applied to the zygosity determination of a given pair of multiples.

Assessment of physical characteristics

Any comprehensive review of the use of physical characteristics for zygosity determination must recognize the extraordinary contribution of the late Luigi Gedda, then Director of the Gregor Mendal Institute, Rome, in his monumental volume, *Twins in History and Science*.[4] Among the characteristics studied and reviewed by Gedda were biometric parameters, skeletal structures, skin, hair and dermatoglyphics, ocular and orbital anatomy, nasal and dental characteristics, and specularity (mirrored or reversed asymmetry). Unfortunately, many such physical structures or characteristics, are poorly developed in newborns, if present at all. Moreover, later in life, comparisons of various physical characteristics are often not sufficiently robust to determine a definitive diagnosis of zygosity. Among the characteristics used in such analyses, albeit with varying degrees of efficacy, are: ear forms, patterns of ridging on the tongue and dental eruption patterns, as well as tooth morphology.[4] Fingerprints obtained from MZ twins, which one might intuitively suppose would be identical or nearly so, are never completely identical. Moreover, the fingerprint system first proposed by Bertillon was for exact identification of criminals rather than diagnosis of zygosity. The same may be said for the use of iris identification, the most recent advance in commercial and governmental security applications. The probability of two different irises agreeing by chance in more than 70% of their phase sequence is about one in 7 billion.[5]

According to the older literature (see Gedda), the ideal test for zygosity was concomitant intertwin acceptance of skin grafts. Not only is this intervention invasive in nature, costly, and fraught with potential for morbid consequences, it is currently considered unethical in view of the many other methods that exist. Indeed, it is the use of more precise methods of zygosity determination that has furthered the ability of MZ twins to undergo organ transplantation without rejection.

CURRENTLY APPLICABLE METHODS OF ZYGOSITY DETERMINATION

Blood groups

A commonly used and relatively inexpensive method of zygosity determination is the use of blood groups and human leukocyte antigens (HLA). A complete discussion is provided by Bryan.[6] Zygosity can be determined from blood by studying common population variants known as polymorphisms. These include the common blood groups, HLA types, serum proteins, enzyme polymorphisms, and, most recently, DNA polymorphisms. In the case of ABO blood groups, for example, if the father of twins is blood group AB and the mother is group O, the offspring may be either group A or group B. If one twin is group A and the other is group B, the pair is clearly DZ. If both are A or B, however, zygosity is unproven. There is a one in two chance that these same parents will produce a group A zygote that goes on to produce MZ twins. The chance of producing two DZ group A zygotes is a half of one in two, or one in four. In clinical calculations this number is usually shown as the relative chance (or odds) of DZ:MZ, which in this case would be 1/4:1/2, or 0.25:0.5. This process can be repeated for many other sets of polymorphisms, with the intent of establishing differences (diagnostic of DZ) or, alternatively, a high statistical probability of MZ on the basis of failing to detect any differences. It is important to note that the higher is the statistical probability desired, the more difficult it is to achieve (see Table 21.1).

Table 21.2 clearly shows that the more complex, multiple allele systems are not necessarily more efficient for determining zygosity, at least in this data set. For example, the rhesus (Rh) system is less efficient than several simple blood group systems. Also, nothing is gained by differentiating between the A_1 and A_2 antigens in the ABO system.

DNA

The most sophisticated form of zygosity detection from blood is commonly characterized as 'DNA fingerprinting'.[9–11] Whereas many writers describe this analysis as being most accurate, it is not always the case, for reasons stated below. DNA testing analyzes the genes directly rather than their protein products. In this type of analysis, several genetic loci are tested at the same time, and a pattern unique to each individual is quickly assembled. Using this technology, MZ twins share identical genomic patterns in some studies, whereas the probability that a DZ pair would also exhibit superimposable patterns may be as low as 3×10^{-14}. At first glance, calculations such as these suggest that technology is the most accurate available for zygosity testing. However, like many emerging technologies, DNA fingerprinting is not perfect, and is associated with disadvantages as well as advantages. Advantages include that only small amounts of DNA (from blood, placenta, etc.) need to be obtained. Additionally, dried biologic specimens such as semen and hair can be used. Indeed, because of the stability of DNA, the zygosity of stillborn fetuses can be established in cases where proteins have already disaggregated; in other instances, archival histologic tissue blocks can be treated to yield high-quality DNA from any pair of twins. The major disadvantages of DNA testing include its alleged high cost and its relative unavailability in comparison with more standard laboratory methods. In reality, however, DNA fingerprinting is not more expensive compared with extensive and full blood group analysis. Moreover, batched sampling and analysis can further reduce cost per

Table 21.1 An example of the determination of chances of dizygosity in a pair of twins alike for all blood group and biochemical markers and of the most common phenotype of all loci. From reference 6

Marker system*	Phenotype	Relative chance of dizygosity for a particular system	Relative chance of monozygosity for a particular system
Initial odds		0.7000	0.3
Sex	Female	0.5000	1.0
ABO	A	0.6945	1.0
MNSs	MS	0.5161	1.0
Rh	$R_1 r$	0.5400	1.0
Kell	K-	0.9548	1.0
Secretor	Sec	0.8681	1.0
Duffy	Fy(a+)	0.8099	1.0
Kldd	Jk(a+)	0.8616	1.0
Dombrock	Do(a+)	0.8094	1.0
Xg	Xg(a+)	0.9573	1.0
Pl	I	0.7006	1.0
PGM_3	I	0.7569	1.0
ACP_1	I	0.6320	1.0
ADA	I	0.9409	1.0
ES-D	I	0.9054	1.0
GPT	2–1	0.6250	1.0
Gc	I	0.7569	1.0
Pi	I	0.9555	1.0
Combined test after testing		0.00056	0.3
Chance of dizygosity = 0.00560/0.3056 = 0.0183			

*P, YI and Hp have not been used as they are not fully developed in the newborn, and Lu, PGM_1 and AK because they are linked to Sec, Rh and ABO, respectively

Table 21.2 Efficiencies of eight common blood group systems. Adapted from references 7 and 8 by permission of the authors and WB Saunders Co Ltd

	Secretor (Le)	Kell (K)	Duffy (Fy)	ABO	A_1A_2BO	MNSs	Rh
Number of alleles	2	2	2	3	4	4	8
Minimum p (concordance|DZ)	0.5937	0.5937	0.5937	0.4630	0.4023	0.4023	0.3198
p (concordance|DZ)	0.5947	0.9050	0.5938	0.5933	0.5651	0.4351	0.4647
Efficiency	0.9977	0.2337	0.9997	0.7572	0.7277	0.9451	0.7870

test. Commercial kits that look for severely limited numbers of specific DNA polymorphisms are now available. Whereas these are convenient because DNA can be extracted in sufficient quantity from mouthwashes or buccal brushings, for example, the risk of insufficient statistical power to exclude dizygosity is high (see below). With further refinements and a standardization of loci, DNA kits might possibly become more robust, thus making them fully acceptable and avoiding the need to obtain blood samples. This would be particularly attractive to the parents of young children if archival placental tissue is not available. Whether and how soon this might happen is unknown.

The major problem in DNA analysis for the determination of zygosity relates to the existence of small-scale mutations, the process by which DNA is mutated in specific zones, e.g. point mutations, deletions and insertions, trinucleotide repeat sequences (such as are found in X-linked mental retardation and Huntington's disease) and tandem repeat sequences. When Derom and colleagues[9] reported their initial DNA finding in 1985, they examined six different polymorphic sites using four restriction enzymes and six DNA probes in a sample of 22 pairs with known zygosity determined by placentation. Their sample was placental DNA. Within the 12 MZ pairs, concordance was complete, and only one of the ten DZ pairs was not demonstrably different. In the same year, Hill and Jeffreys[10] reported the use of similar technology on umbilical cord blood samples collected at delivery, or peripheral blood samples (0.5–1.0 ml) obtained from each baby the day after birth. Their sample consisted of five twin pairs and two sets of triplets. Their conclusion was, 'mini satellite DNA probes provide a single genetic test that should allow positive determination of zygosity in all cases of multiple pregnancy'. The discussion on the appropriateness of using this technology continues, however, and standardization of the number of microsatellite probes, also called variable number of tandem repeat markers (VNTR), or their specific

nature for the purpose of zygosity determination has yet to be accomplished.

In an effort to avoid the complexities and costs of DNA evaluation of blood or placental tissues, some laboratories turn their attention to 'mouthwash' kits because of their ease of use. Such kits, often popularized in the lay media or advertised to the public, may be used at home or in field studies and then analyzed later at a remote location. Although we have not performed a survey and/or analysis of existing kits of this type, Dr Geoffrey Machin (personal communication, 2002) suggests that their general application should be viewed with caution for at least two reasons: first, the lay press reports of such kits fail to state the number of genetic probes used, and second, the accuracy of these tests, which clearly is related to the number of probes, is often unknown to the public. According to Machin, who used the best available mouthwash polymerase chain reaction (PCR) kit in Edmonton, Canada to test 50 pairs of twins who were known to be DZ by VNTR Southern blot, the kit failed to find genetic differences between one of these DZ pairs, thus yielding a false MZ result.

INCREASING POSTNATAL DISCORDANCE

This specific phenomenon underlies the fact that MZ twins are not truly 'identical'. It is currently unclear how many mutations occur, under what circumstances they occur and to what degree they continue to occur. The senior author (LK) has observed more than 20 000 sets of twins over the years at the Twins Day Festival in Ohio, most of whom exhibited variations in body phenotype under close scrutiny. Only one pair stands out as being indistinguishable on an individual basis. These elderly gentlemen invariably puzzled the most sophisticated and experienced judges of the twin contest. It is not possible to say whether the phenomenon of post-zygotic mutational change affecting phenotype was not operational in this pair. It is also not known whether DNA tests were ever obtained from these individuals. Figure 21.1 is a

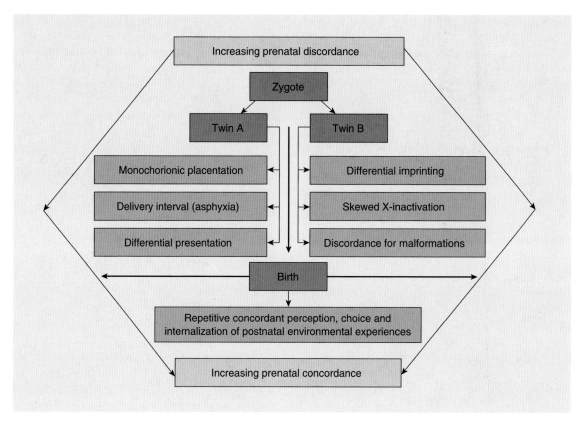

Figure 21.1 Acquisition of discordance in twins from conception to mature extrauterine existence. Adapted from reference 12

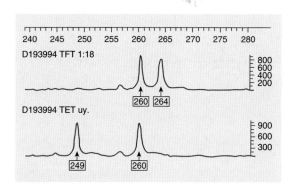

Figure 21.2 Absorption spectra of genetic material from Louis Keith and his twin brother, Donald, showing a difference in one area (all others identical). Courtesy of Dr Andreas Busjahn, Max Delbruck Center for Molecular Medicine and the Franz Volhard Clinic of Humboldt University, Berlin

composite describing various phenomena affecting post-zygotic discordancy.

Keeping this in mind, Figure 21.2 is the absorption spectrum obtained from a mouth-wash sample of one of the authors (LK) and his co-twin, Donald Keith. A difference was found in one DNA zone where multiple repeat sequences were present, whereas the other zones gave identical results. Despite this, the Keith twins were later confirmed to be MZ using restriction fragment length polymorphism (RFLP) technology in two different reference laboratories (Figure 21.3). The clinical paradox occasioned by the different interpretation derived from Figures 21.2 and 21.3 is explained by the fact that RFLP methodology examines segments of DNA at 'lesser magnification', as it were. It therefore

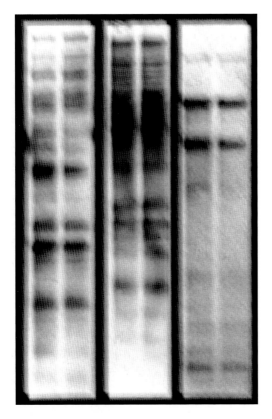

Figure 21.3 DNA fingerprints of the Keith twins, courtesy of Dr Fiona Bamforth, University of Alberta, Edmonton, Alberta, Canada

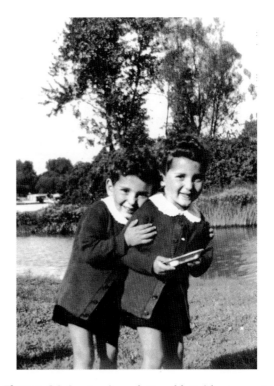

Figure 21.4 Louis and Donald Keith at age 4. Photo by Myron Keith

provides a 'broad brush-stroke' diagnosis of monozygosity by failing to pick up the inevitable, smaller, post-zygotic mutational differences that are now thought to be present in most, if not all, MZ twin pairs. RFLP technology is the type that is generally used for forensic purposes, paternity testing, etc. In contrast, the tandem repeat sequences could be considered too sensitive for use in zygosity testing, although the fact that they can be obtained from a mouthwash sample versus blood is an advantage. Figures 21.4–21.7 show Louis and Donald Keith at ages 4, 7, 32, and 67. Close inspection of these figures shows subtle changes in facial phenotypic features that increase with age. Whether these relate to post-zygotic changes or the effects of the environment, lifestyle, and diet is not known. Possibly

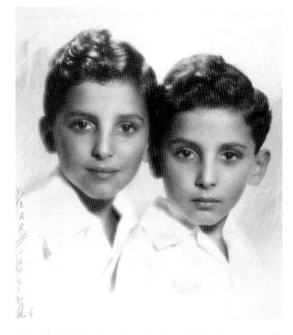

Figure 21.5 Louis and Donald Keith at age 7. Photo by Harry Johnson

223

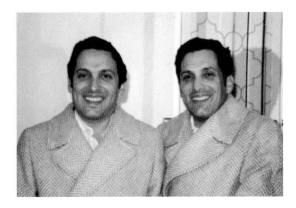

Figure 21.6 Louis and Donald Keith at age 32. Photo by Myron Keith

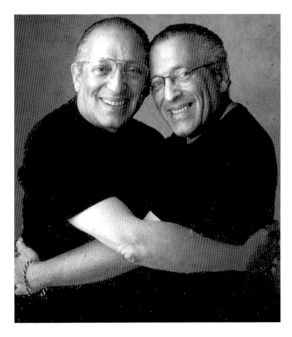

Figure 21.7 Louis and Donald Keith at age 67. Close inspection of Figures 21.4–21.7 shows subtle changes in facial phenotypic features that increase with age. Photo courtesy of Marc Hauser, Chicago. © 2003

some changes relate to the phenomenon of post-zygotic changes, with the exception of the nasal difference, as Donald incurred a broken nose in childhood. At present, neither Louis nor Donald is able to identify himself in the pictures obtained at age 4 and 7. It is precisely

the difference in technology and the lack of standardization of the number and types of markers that stands in the way of DNA fingerprinting becoming a more useful tool for clinical zygosity determination. In summary, no DNA gold standard currently exists and it is not clear when one will be developed.

Because of the uncertainties just described, the use of combinations of tests has been proposed. One author[13] recorded global impressions of zygosity obtained by two objective (based upon physical resemblance questionnaire; dermatoglyphic analysis) and two subjective procedures (parental impressions and physician's impressions), which were then compared with blood typing of 53 twin pairs. The judgments of the investigator furnished the most accurate indication of zygosity (94–96% accuracy). Laboratory tests were repeated for five pairs when the results proved incompatible with the investigator's ratings. In all five instances, the investigator's judgments were confirmed, indicating that a laboratory error had occurred. It appears that the opinion of a skilled observer of twins can provide a convenient and highly effective alternative to blood typing or even DNA analysis.

The repeated observations that zygosity tests are not error-free has prompted some investigators to develop self- or parental-administered questionnaires to assess zygosity, most often with results that are considered more than 90% reliable. In one of the most recent studies, Ooki and Asaka[14] examined zygosity in 224 childhood age twin pairs identified by genetic markers including DNA samples, by a simple questionnaire administered to the twins' mothers and to the twins themselves. The questionnaire items included twin similarity of physical features, degree of similarity, and frequency of being mistaken (confusion of identity) when twins were about 1 year of age. The twins themselves responded to three questionnaire items dealing with only confusion of identity items. The results were calculated with logistic regression analysis, which showed that the total accuracy of mothers' questionnaires was 91.5% when using only the items dealing with confusion of identity. This accuracy was slightly lower than that obtained by twins' self-reports answered by both twins separately, with 93.3% accuracy. The total accuracy of mothers' questionnaire responses rose to 95.1% when the authors used all 19 items. This study concluded, 'twin zygosity can be estimated by the use of the mother's simple questionnaire with sufficient accuracy even in young twins about 1 year of age'.

IMPLICATIONS FOR CLINICAL PRACTICE

The following implications for practice derive from recognition of the complex nature of zygosity testing, its long and continuing evolution and recent advances in ultrasound and molecular genetics:

(1) All MC twins are MZ, but they may be discordant for genetic disease, malformations, etc., and also some DNA tests of zygosity if sufficiently detailed and exhaustive tests are used.

(2) Unlike-sexed twins are DZ.

(3) Not all like-sexed DC twins are DZ. In fact, about 25% in the Caucasian twin population resident in the United States and Europe are MZ.

(4) Not all like-sexed twins conceived using ART are DZ.

(5) Not all twins who are discordant for genetic disease, chromosome constitution or a major malformation are DZ. If a major malformation is present in MZ twins, it may affect only one of the pair or may be phenotypically less severe in the other member of the pair.

(6) Selective termination in discordant twins and higher-order multiples must be approached with caution and only after great efforts to establish chorionicity definitively. Because the presence of fetal vascular anastomoses may lead to the death of both twins if traditional means are used, selective termination can be achieved only by umbilical vessel occlusion in MC–MZ twins discordant for lethal malformations or chromosomal abnormalities.

(7) All like-sexed DZ twins have the right to know their zygosity, and this should become the standard practice in perinatal medicine. Likewise, all parents of MC twins should be informed in writing that their twins are MZ. The ultimate responsibility for this endeavor might be assumed by the department of obstetrics, pathology, or neonatology so that parents of all surviving MC twins would receive a letter declaring the twins to be MZ rather than identical. A copy of this letter would be retained in both the maternal and pediatric hospital records.

(8) Correct terminology, monozygotic/dizygotic, should always be used rather than misleading and inaccurate lay-terms such as identical/fraternal. Parents are able to understand and accept these terms. For parents of MZ twins, it is a relief to understand that MZ twins are seldom, if ever, absolutely identical. This settles the issue of zygosity for them.

A LOOK TOWARDS THE FUTURE

In the context of zygosity, future nomenclature should include qualifying descriptions of those characteristics which are phenotypically and or genetically discordant, in order to provide a more precise diagnosis of zygosity. Whereas it may be sufficiently accurate to characterize a pair of twins as DZ, it may be imprecise to characterize a pair as MZ with no further qualification, especially when such qualifications would clearly explain phenotypic or other types of discordance. For example, a pair of twins might be more accurately characterized as MZ-discordant for schizophrenia, MZ-discordant for breast cancer or MZ-discordant for Duchenne muscular dystrophy. In this regard, based upon analysis of childhood sleep patterns, it has already been postulated that there are three clinical types of MZ twins: those who are identical in every sense of the word, those who are opposite in every sense of the word and the remainder who share some, but not all similarities and dissimilarities.[15]

SPECIAL CONSIDERATIONS

Josef Mengele, also known as Auschwitz's 'Angel of Death', held a fascination with twins. As Auschwitz's senior 'physician', he conducted so-called and never-published 'genetic experiments' on nearly 1500 sets of twins between 1943 and 1944. For this purpose, he selected twin sets from the lines of prisoners coming off the cattle cars. With the blessing and support of his senior mentor, Baron Otmar Von Verscher at the Kaiser Wilhelm Institute in Berlin, Mengele tested various genetic theories with the aim of illuminating Hitler's racial dogmas. Twins were considered particularly useful, because so-called identical twins were thought to be an identical gene pool and their responses to mutual treatments could be monitored with this in mind.

REFERENCES

1. Derom C, Vlietinck R, Derom R et al. Increased monozygotic twinning rate after ovulation induction. Lancet 1987; 1: 1236–8.
2. Edwards RG, Mettler L, Walters DE. Identical twins and in vitro-fertilization. J In Vitro Fert Embryo Transf 1986; 3: 114–17.
3. Tilney NL. Renal transplantation between identical twins: a review. World J Surg 1986; 10: 381–8.
4. Gedda L. Twins in History and Science. Springfield, IL: Charles C Thomas, 1961.
5. Daugman J, Downing C. Epigenetic randomness, complexity and singularity of human iris patterns. Proc R Soc Lond B 2001; 268: 1737–40.
6. Bryan EM. Twins and Higher Order Multiple Births: A Guide To Their Nature and Nurture. London: Edward Arnold, 1992.
7. Selvin S. Efficiency of genetic systems for diagnosis of twin zygosity. Acta Genet Med Gemellol Roma 1977; 26: 81–2.
8. Corney G, Robson EB. Types of twinnings and determination of zygosity. In: MacGillivray I, Nylander PPS, Corney G, eds. Human Multiple Reproduction. London: WB Saunders, 1975.
9. Derom C, Bakker E, Vlietinck R et al. Zygosity determination in newborn twins using DNA variants. J Med Genet 1985; 22: 279–82.
10. Hill AVS, Jeffreys AJ. Use of minisatellite DNA probes for determination of twin zygosity at birth. Lancet 1985; 2: 1394–5.
11. Erdmann J, Nothen MM, Stratmann M et al. The use of microsatellites in zygosity diagnosis of twins. Acta Genet Med Gemellol Roma 1993; 42: 45–51.
12. Keith L, Machin G. Zygosity testing. Current status and evolving issues. J Reprod Med 1997; 42: 699–707.
13. Segal NL. Zygosity testing: laboratory and the investigator's judgment. Acta Genet Med Gemellol Roma 1984; 33: 515–21.
14. Ooki S, Asaka A. Zygosity diagnosis in young twins by questionnaire for twins' mothers and twins' self-reports. Twin Res 2004; 7: 5–12.
15. Golbin A, Golbin I, Keith L et al. Mirror imaging in twins: biological polarization – an evolving hypothesis. Acta Genet Med Gemellol Roma 1993; 42: 237–43.

Index